Ontogeny of hematopoiesis
Aplastic anemia

Ontogénie de l'hématopoïèse
Aplasie médullaire

British Library Cataloguing in Publication Data

A catalogue record for this book
is available from the British Library

ISBN 2-7420-0103-4
ISSN 0768-3154

First published in 1995 by

Editions John Libbey Eurotext
127, avenue de la République, 92120 Montrouge, France.
(33) (1) 46 73 06 60
ISBN 2-7420-0103-4

John Libbey and Company Ltd
13 Smiths Yard, Summerley Street, London SW18 4HR,
England.
(44) (81) 947 27 77

Institut National de la Santé et de la Recherche Médicale
101, rue de Tolbiac, 75654 Paris Cedex 13, France.
(33) (1) 44 23 60 00
ISBN 2-85598-626-5

ISSN 0768-3154

© 1995 Colloques INSERM/John Libbey Eurotext Ltd,
All rights reserved
Unauthorized publication contravenes applicable laws

Ontogeny of hematopoiesis
Aplastic anemia

Ontogénie de l'hématopoïèse
Aplasie médullaire

Proceedings of the joint international workshop on
"Foetal and neonatal hematopoiesis and mechanisms
of bone marrow failure", Paris (France), April 3-6, 1995

Edited by
Eliane Gluckman Pr, MD
Laure Coulombel, MD

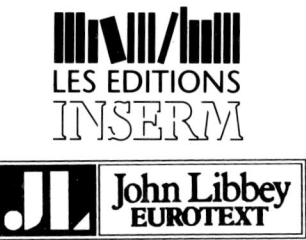

Editorial

The origin of blood, symbol of life, has not yet revealed all its secrets. At the beginning is the mythical totipotent stem cell with its potential to differentiate into more specialized cells. What are the signals, the regulatory mechanisms and the cellular interactions which govern the formation of the first clusters of primitive haematopoietic stem cells, make them travel along the body's newly formed blood vessels and circulate when the heart first begins to beat? Are these stem cells identical to those of the adult or do they possess specific potentialities which could be restored in the fully developed individual thanks to therapeutic intervention? These novel questions were addressed during the first symposium on foetal and neonatal haematopoiesis in a multidisciplinary setting where geneticists, haematologists, immunologists, embryologists and clinicians exchanged their views.

The second part of this meeting was devoted to the study of the mechanisms of aplastic anaemia. It was a valuable chance to address epidemiologic, molecular and genetic aspects of the subject and to exchange recent data arising from the therapeutic use of allogeneic transplantation, immunosuppressive agents, haematopoietic growth factors and gene therapy.

Unfortunately, this book cannot reflect the lively, friendly, informative and interactive atmosphere which contributed so strongly to the character of the meeting. It is however a true reflection of current knowledge in the fields of foetal and neonatal haematopoiesis and mechanisms of bone marrow failure.

Professor Eliane GLUCKMAN

Editorial

L'origine du sang, symbole de la vie, n'a pas encore livré tous ses secrets. Au début, c'est une cellule souche mythique qui possède en elle toutes les potentialités pour se différencier vers des cellules plus spécialisées. Quels sont les signaux, les mécanismes régulateurs, les interactions intercellulaires qui permettront de former les premiers nids de cellules souches hématopoïétiques, de les faire cheminer le long des vaisseaux nouvellement formés et circuler au premier battement du cœur ? Ces cellules souches sont-elles identiques à celles de l'adulte, ou ont-elles des possibilités différentes, perdues à l'âge adulte, mais qu'il sera possible de restituer chez l'homme dans un but thérapeutique ? C'est au cours du premier symposium sur l'hématopoïèse fœtale et néonatale que ces questions ont été posées par une approche multidisciplinaire où des généticiens, des hématologistes, des embryologistes, des immunologistes, des transplanteurs et des cliniciens ont échangé leurs vues sur ces problèmes.

La deuxième partie de cette réunion a été consacrée à l'étude du mécanisme des insuffisances médullaires. Cette approche, plus clinique, a permis d'aborder des aspects épidémiologiques, moléculaires et génétiques des insuffisances médullaires. Le point a été fait sur les différentes méthodes thérapeutiques incluant la transplantation, l'utilisation de facteurs de croissance hématopoïétiques, les traitements immunosuppresseurs et la thérapie génique.

Ce livre résume les connaissances actuelles sur ce sujet, mais, malheureusement, il ne reflète qu'en partie l'ambiance du meeting, vivante, dense, amicale et très instructive.

Professeur Eliane GLUCKMAN

Acknowledgments

We would like to extend our gratitude to:
   Mr Philippe Lazar, General Director of INSERM.

We wish to thank the following Institutions for their support:
   The "Institut National de la Santé et de la Recherche Médicale" (INSERM), particularly the "Département Information et Communication, Bureau des Colloques et des Conférences",
   The "Ministère de l'Enseignement et de la Recherche",
   The National Institutes of Health, National Heart, Lung and Blood Institute (USA),
   The European Haematology Association,
   The European School of Haematology,
   The "Association pour la Recherche sur les Transplantations Médullaires" (ARTM),
   The AFMF (Association for Fanconi Anemia).

We wish to thank the following industries for their contribution:
   Amgen, Baxter, Cell Pro, Glaxo, Merrel Dow, Roche, Roger Bellon, Sandoz, Upjohn, Zimogenetics.

We are very grateful to Yvette Coadou, Sandrine Laudrel, Ghyslaine Lebougault, Karen Harris and Didi Jobin for their marvellous help.

Sincere thanks are also due to the chairpersons and the members of the scientific committee who have played a major role for the preparation of the sessions and during general discussion:
A.E. Auerbach, M. Boiron, H.E. Broxmeyer, E. Buchwald, B. Camitta, D. Charron, M.D. Cooper, L. Coulombel, J. Deeg, C. Eaves, A. Gratwohl, M. Horowitz, L. Luzzatto, N. Young, E. Zanjani.

We are very grateful to the contributors who have provided their expertise, shared their experience, created new collaborations and drawn the lessons for future clinical trials and new research.

Remerciements

Nous remercions les institutions suivantes pour leur aide et leur contribution à l'organisation du Symposium :
> L'Institut National de la Santé et de la Recherche Médicale (INSERM), particulièrement le Département Information et Communication, Bureau des Colloques et des Conférences,
> Le Ministère de l'Enseignement Supérieur et de la Recherche (MESR),
> «The National Institutes of Health, National Heart, Lung and Blood Institutes» (USA),
> L'Association Européenne d'Hématologie (EHA),
> l'Ecole Européenne d'Hématologie (ESH),
> L'Association pour la Recherche sur les Transplantations Médullaires (ARTM),
> L'AFMF, Association Loi 1901 relative à la maladie de Fanconi.

Nous remercions les laboratoires pharmaceutiques suivants :
> Amgen, Baxter, Cell Pro, Glaxo, Merrel Dow, Roche, Roger Bellon, Sandoz, Upjohn, Zimogenetics.

Nous remercions Yvette Coadou, Sandrine Laudrel, Ghyslaine Lebougault, Karen Harris et Didi Jobin pour leur aide très efficace.

Nous remercions les présidents de session et les membres du comité scientifique qui ont joué un rôle essentiel dans l'organisation des sessions et pour les discussions générales, vivantes et stimulantes :
A.E. Auerbach, M. Boiron, H.E. Broxmeyer, E. Buchwald, B. Camitta, D. Charron, M.D. Cooper, L. Coulombel, J. Deeg, C. Eaves, A. Gratwohl, M. Horowitz, L. Luzzatto, N. Young, E. Zanjani.

Nous sommes très reconnaissants aux participants qui ont apporté leur expérience, partagé leur savoir-faire, créé de nouvelles collaborations et tiré les leçons pour de nouveaux essais cliniques et de nouvelles recherches.

Contents
Sommaire

VII Preface
VIII Préface
IX Acknowledgments
XI Remerciements
XIX List and address of speakers
Liste et adresse des orateurs

I. ONTOGENY OF HEMATOPOIESIS / *ONTOGÉNIE DE L'HÉMATOPOÏÈSE*

1) EMBRYONIC DEVELOPMENT OF HEMATOPOIESIS / *DÉVELOPPEMENT EMBRYONNAIRE DE L'HÉMATOPOÏÈSE*

5 F. Dieterlen-Lièvre, I. Godin, L. Pardanaud, A. Cumano, M.-L. Gaspar, M. Marcos, J. Garcia-Porrero
Sites of hemopoietic stem cell production in early embryogenesis
Sites de la production de cellules souches hématopoïétiques au cours de l'embryogenèse précoce

13 E. Dzierzak, A. Müller, A. Sinclair, C. Miles, N. Gillett, B. Daly, M.-J. Sanchez, A. Medvinsky
Development of hematopoietic stem cell activity in the mouse embryo
Développement de l'hématopoïèse chez l'embryon de souris

17 L.I. Zon, M. Kieran, B. Paw, M. Thompson, D. Ransom, A. Brownlie, F. Y. Chan, L. Barone, H. McClennan, S. Ziegler, S. Pratt, H. W. Detrich III
The zebrafish: a new model for studying embryonic hematopoiesis
Le poisson zèbre : un nouveau modèle pour l'étude de l'hématopoïèse

23 M.-T. Mitjavila, M.-D. Filippi, F. Le Pesteur, W. Vainchenker, F. Sainteny
Models of developmental hematopoiesis: embryonic stem cells - hematopoietic development
Modèles de développement de l'hématopoïèse : cellules souches embryonnaires - développement hématopoïétique

27 D. Vittet, M.-H. Prandini, R. Berthier, A. Schweitzer, H. Martin-Sisteron, G. Uzan, E. Dejana
Endothelial differentiation of embryonic stem cells *in vitro*: a model of early vasculogenesis
Différenciation endothéliale in vitro *des cellules souches embryonnaires : un modèle d'angiogenèse précoce*

33 L.S. Lu, S.J. Wang, R. Auerbarch
Primitive hematopoietic stem cells and endothelial cells in the mouse yolk sac
Cellules souches hématopoïétiques primitives et cellules endothéliales dans la vésicule vitelline de souris

37 M. Tavian, P. Charbord, L. Humeau, L. Coulombel, D. Luton, F. Dieterlen-Lièvre, B. Péault
Embryonic and early fetal development of the human hematopoietic system in the yolk sac, dorsal aorta, liver and bone marrow
Développement embryonnaire et fœtal précoce du système hématopoïétique humain dans le sac vitellin, l'aorte dorsale, le foie et la moelle osseuse

43 L. Coulombel, A. Huyhn, M. Dommergues, B. Izac, A. Katz, W. Vainchenker
Characterization of hematopoietic progenitor cells in the human extraembryonic yolk sac and in the human embryo
Caractérisation des progéniteurs clonogéniques dans la vésicule vitelline et l'embryon humain

49 P.M. Lansdorp, V.I. Rebel, W. Dragowska, M.T.E. Little, T.E. Thomas, R.K. Humphries, C.J. Eaves, H. Mayani
Proliferative and differentiation potential of neonatal and fetal hematopoietic stem cells
Capacité de prolifération et de différenciation des cellules souches hématopoïétiques fœtales et néonatales

55 C.L. Miller, V.I. Rebel, C.D. Helgason, M.E. Lemieux, R.K. Humphries, P.M. Lansdorp, C. J. Eaves
Differential role of Steel factor on hematopoietic stem cells during ontogeny, in adults and after bone marrow transplantation
Rôle différentiel du Steel facteur au cours de l'ontogénie, chez l'adulte et après greffe de moelle

2) ONTOGENY OF THE IMMUNE SYSTEM / *ONTOGÉNIE DU SYSTÈME IMMUNITAIRE*

63 J.P. Di Santo
Cytokine/receptor control points in murine T cell development
Contrôle des rapports cytokine/récepteur au cours du développement T chez la souris

71 G. Chaouat
Materno foetal relationship
Relations materno-fœtales

81 A. Cumano, F. Dieterlen-Lièvre, C.J. Paige, I. Godin
Hematopoietic cell commitment during embryonic development
Rôle des cellules souches hématopoïétiques au cours du développement embryonnaire

3) ANIMAL MODELS / *MODÈLES ANIMAUX*

89 G. Almeida-Porada, A.W. Flake, C. Porada, J. Ruthven, J. Ruthven, E. D. Zanjani
Human stem cell engraftment in sheep
Greffe de cellules souches humaines chez le mouton

97 J.E. Dick, T. Lapidot, J. Vormoor, A. Larochelle, D. Bonnet, J. Wang
Human hematopoiesis in SCID mice
Développement de l'hématopoïèse humaine dans un modèle de souris SCID

103 F. Pflumio, B. Izac, A. Katz, W. Vainchenker, L. Coulombel
Characteristics of human clonogenic and primitive cells engrafted into SCID mice
Caractérisation des progéniteurs hématopoïétiques humains greffés dans la souris SCID

4) GENE TRANSFER IN CORD BLOOD HEMATOPOIETIC STEM CELLS / *TRANSFERT DE GÈNES DANS LES CELLULES SOUCHES DU SANG DE CORDON*

109 H.E. Broxmeyer, S. Cooper, M. Etienne-Julan, S. Braun, L. Lu, S.D. Lyman, A. Srivastava
Cord blood hematopoietic stem/progenitor cell growth and gene transduction using adeno-associated and retroviral vectors
Prolifération des progéniteurs hématopoïétiques du sang de cordon et transfert de gènes dans les cellules par l'intermédiaire d'adéno-associated virus (AAV) et de rétrovirus

115 L. Lu, Z.H. Li, Y. Ge, H.E. Broxmeyer
Retroviral-mediated cell transfer into hematopoietic stem/progenitor cells from fresh and cryopreserved umbilical cord blood
Transfert de gènes dans les progéniteurs de sang de cordon frais ou après congélation

5) IMMUNOLOGICAL DEVELOPMENT / *DÉVELOPPEMENT IMMUNOLOGIQUE*

123 F. Garban, J.-P. Truman, C. Roucard, C. Choqueux-Séébold, D. Charron, N. Mooney
Conformation and function of MHC class II molecules on foetal B lymphocytes
Structure et fonction des molécules du complexe majeur d'histocompatibilité de classe II à la surface des lymphocytes B fœtaux

131 P. Le Bouteiller, A.-M. Rodriguez
Classical and non classical HLA class I genes in the human trophoblast cells: expression, regulation and possible function(s)
Etude des gènes de classe I classiques et non classiques dans les cellules de trophoblaste humain : expression, régulation et fonction(s) potentielle(s)

143 M. Kirszenbaum, E. Carosella
HLA-G expression in fetal and neonatal hematopoietic cells
Expression de HLA-G sur les cellules hématopoïétiques fœtales et néonatales

149 V. Schiavon, E. Carosella, I.-G. Mansur, E. Gluckman, S. El Marsafy, L. Boumsell, A. Bensussan
BY55 mAb delineates within human adult peripheral blood, newborn cord blood and adult bone marrow lymphocytes distinct cell subsets mediating cytotoxic activity
L'anticorps monoclonal BY reconnaît des sous-populations cytotoxiques différentes dans le sang, la moelle adulte et le sang placentaire

6) CLINICAL RESULTS OF CORD BLOOD TRANSPLANT / *RÉSULTATS CLINIQUES DES GREFFES DE SANG DE CORDON*

163 O. Ringdén, M. Westgren, S. Eik-Nes, S. Ek, A.M. Brubakk, T.H. Bui, A. Giambona, C. Jakil, T. Kiserud, A. Kjaeldgaard, A. Maggio, L. Markling, O. Olerup, B.M. Svahn, F. Orlandi
Intrauterine transplantations of foetal hematopoietic stem cells to four foetuses with haemoglobinopathies
Transplantations intra-utérines de cellules souches hématopoïétiques fœtales chez quatre fœtus atteints d'hémoglobinopathie

169 J.-L. Touraine
In utero transplantation of fetal liver stem cells into human fetuses for immunodeficiency and thalassemia treatment
Transplantation in utero *de cellules de foie fœtal, chez des fœtus humains, pour le traitement des déficits immunitaires et des thalassémies*

177 J.E. Wagner
Allogeneic umbilical cord blood transplantation: report of the international cord blood transplant registry
Greffe allogénique de sang de cordon ombilical : résultats du registre international des greffes de sang de cordon

183 E. Gluckman
Advantages of using foetal and neonatal cells for treatment of hematological diseases in human
Avantages de l'utilisation des cellules fœtales et néonatales pour le traitement des maladies hématologiques chez l'homme.

II. APLASTIC ANEMIA / *APLASIES MÉDULLAIRES*

1) MECHANISMS OF APLASTIC ANEMIA / *MÉCANISMES DES APLASIES MÉDULLAIRES*

191 N.S. Young, J.P. Maciejewski, C. Serelli, T. Sato, A. Nisticò, K.E. Brown, S.W. Green, S. Wong, S. Anderson
The pathophysiology of acquired aplastic anemia
Physiopathologie des aplasies médullaires acquises

203 A. Bacigalupo, G. Piaggio, M. Podesta, M. Valbonesi, G. Lercari, O. Figari, G. Sogno, E. Tedone, M.R. Raffo, L. Grassia, M.T. Van Lint, A.M. Marmont
Mobilization of peripheral blood hemopoietic progenitors (PBHP) from patients with severe aplastic anemia (SAA) after prolonged administration of G-CSF
Mobilisation des cellules souches périphériques chez des patients atteints d'aplasie médullaire sévère après administration prolongée de G-CSF

209 R. Huss, C.A. Hoy, H.J. Deeg
Stroma derived hemopoietic progenitors: cell cycle dependent proliferation and differentiation
Progéniteurs hématopoïétiques dérivés du stroma : prolifération et différenciation dépendantes du cycle

2) CLONALITY / *CLONALITE*

217 G. Socié
Is aplastic anemia a preleukemic disorder ? Facts and hypotheses
L'aplasie médullaire est-elle une pathologie pré-leucémique ? Faits et hypothèses

223 A. Wodnar-Filipowicz, C.Y. Manz, E. Schklovskaya, M.S. Krieger, A. Gratwohl, A. Tichelli, B. Speck, C. Nissen
Tyrosine kinase receptors and their ligands in aplastic anemia
Récepteurs à tyrosine kinase et leurs ligands dans les aplasies médullaires

233 A. Raghavachar, H. Schrezenmeier
The aplastic anemia - paroxysmal nocturnal hemoglobinuria syndrome
Aplasie médullaire - syndrome d'hémoglobinurie paroxystique nocturne

3) FANCONI ANEMIA / *ANÉMIE DE FANCONI*

241 B.P. Alter
Fanconi's anemia : clinical aspects and diagnosis
Anémie de Fanconi : aspects cliniques et diagnostic

249 M. Buchwald, M. Chen, F. Krasnoshtein, R. Cumming, J. Lightfoot, L. Parker, A. Savoia
Isolation and characterization of the Fanconi anemia genes
Isolement et caractérisation des gènes de la maladie de Fanconi

257 A.D. Auerbach, P.C. Verlander
Mutation analysis of the Fanconi anemia gene *FAC*
Analyse et mutations du gène FAC de la maladie de Fanconi

265 H. Joenje
Classification of Fanconi anemia patients by complementation analysis
Classification des malades atteints d'anémie de Fanconi par étude des groupes de complémentation

271 D. Papadopoulo, A. Laquerbe, E. Moustacchi
Mechanisms of mutagenesis in Fanconi anemia. Possible relation with predisposition to AML
Mécanismes de la mutagenèse dans la maladie de Fanconi. Relation possible avec la prédisposition à la leucémie aiguë myéloblastique

4) EPIDEMIOLOGY / *ÉPIDÉMIOLOGIE*

281 S. Issaragrisil
Preliminary results on epidemiology of aplastic anemia in Thailand
Etude épidémiologique des aplasies médullaires en Thaïlande : résultats préliminaires

291 J.Y. Mary, M. Guiguet, E. Baumelou
Epidemiology of aplastic anemia: the French experience
Epidémiologie des aplasies médullaires : l'expérience française

5) TREATMENT OF APLASTIC ANEMIA / *TRAITEMENT DES APLASIES MÉDULLAIRES*

307 H.J. Deeg, K. Doney, C. Anasetti, R. Storb
Transplant and nontransplant therapy for patients with severe aplastic anemia: an update of the Seattle experience
Traitement des aplasies médullaires par transplantation ou nontransplantation : actualisation des résultats de Seattle

313 M.M. Horowitz, J. R. Passweg, K.A. Sobocinski, M. Nugent, J.P. Klein
Bone marrow transplantation for severe aplastic anemia - a report from the International Bone Marrow Transplant Registry
Rapport du Registre International des Greffes de Moelle Osseuse - Résultats dans les aplasies médullaires graves

319 E. Gluckman
Allogeneic bone marrow transplantation in Fanconi anemia
Greffe de moelle osseuse allogénique dans la maladie de Fanconi

325 **B. Camitta, H.J. Deeg, H. Castro-Malaspina, N.K.C. Ramsay**
Unrelated or mismatched bone marrow transplants for aplastic anemia: experience at four major centers
Greffe de moelle non apparentée ou HLA incompatible pour aplasie médullaire : expérience de quatre grands centres

331 **J. Hows, A. Bacigalupo, T. Downie, R. Brand**
Alternative donor bone marrow transplantation for severe aplastic anaemia: the European experience
Expérience européenne de greffe de moelle pour aplasie médullaire à partir de donneurs non apparentés.

335 **N. Frickhofen, H. Schrezenmeier, A. Bacigalupo**
Results of European trials of immunosuppression for treatment of aplastic anemia
Résultats d'essais européens de traitements immunosuppresseurs dans les aplasies médullaires

345 **A. Gratwohl**
Hematopoietic growth factors in the treatment of aplastic anemia. Emphasis on European studies
Facteurs de croissance hématopoïétiques dans le traitement des aplasies médullaires : études européennes

353 **S.D. Nimer**
The role of cytokines in the pathogenesis and treatment of aplastic anemia and myelodysplastic syndromes
Rôle des cytokines dans la pathogénie et le traitement des aplasies médullaires et des syndromes myélodysplasiques

361 **J.M. Liu**
Molecular approaches to the treatment of Fanconi anemia
Approches moléculaires du traitement de la maladie de Fanconi

371 **Author index**
Index des auteurs

List and address of speakers
Liste et adresse des orateurs

ALTER Blanche
Children's Hospital, C3-42 Pediatric Hematology-Oncology Division, University of Texas - Medical branch, Galveston TX 77555, USA;
tel. : (409) 772-2341, fax : (409) 772-4599

AUERBACH Arleen
Investigative Dermatology, The Rockefeller University, Room W-218, Hospital Building, 1230 York Avenue, New York, NY 10021-6399, USA;
tel. : (212) 327 7533, fax : (212) 327 8232

AUERBACH Robert
Center for Developmental Biology, 1117 West Johnson street, WI 53706 Madison, USA;
tel. : (212) 327 7533, fax : (212) 327 8232

BACIGALUPO Andrea
Ospedal San Martino, Centro Trapianti di Midollo Osseo, Divisione Ematologia 2, Viale Benedetto XV, 16148 Genova, Italy;
tel. : (39 10) 35 54 69, fax : (39 10) 35 55 83

BENSUSSAN Armand
Unité INSERM 93, Centre Hayem, Hôpital Saint-Louis, 1, avenue Claude Vellefaux, 75475 Paris Cedex 10, France;
tel. : (33 1) 42 39 17 63, fax : (33 1) 42 06 84 54

BROXMEYER Hal. E.
Walther Oncology Center, Indiana University School of Medicine, 975 West Walnut Street, IB-501, Indianapolis IN 46202-5121, USA;
tel. : (317) 274 7510, fax : (317) 274 7592

BUCHWALD Manuel
Research Institute, The Hospital for Sick Children, Department of Genetics, 555 University Avenue, Toronto, Ontario M5G 1X8, Canada;
tel. : (416) 813 63 50, fax : (416) 813 49 31

CAMITTA Bruce
Medical College of Wise, Department of Pediatrics, 8701 Watertown Plank Road, WI 53226 Milwaukee, USA;
tel. : (414) 266 41 70, fax : (414) 266 46 23

CHAOUAT Gérard
INSERM CJF 92-09, Hôpital Antoine Béclère, Biologie Cellulaire et Moléculaire, de la Relation Materno-Foetale, Bâtiment de Gynécologie-Obstétrique, Avenue de la Porte de Trivaux, 92140 Clamart, France;
tel. and fax : 45 37 44 50

CHARRON Dominique
INSERM U 396, Institut Biomédical des Cordeliers, 75006 Paris, France;
tel. : (33 1) 42 49 90 81, fax : (33 1) 42 49 44 49

COULOMBEL Laure
INSERM U 362, Institut Gustave Roussy, 39, avenue Camille Desmoulins, 94805 Villejuif Cedex, France;
tel. : (33 1) 45 59 42 33, fax : (33 1) 46 77 84 37

CUMANO Ana
Unité INSERM 277, Biologie cellulaire du gène, Institut Pasteur, 2, rue du Dr Rouoc, 75015 Paris, France;
tel. : (33 1) 45 68 85 45, fax : (33 1) 45 68 85 48

DEEG Joachim
Fred Hutchinson Cancer Research Center, 1124 Columbia Street, Seattle WA 98104, USA;
tel. : (206) 667 5985, fax : (206) 667 6124

DI SANTO James
Institut Fédératif de Recherche, INSERM U 429, Hôpital Necker-Enfants Malades, 149, rue de Sèvres, 75015 Paris, France;
fax : (33 1) 46 77 84 37

DICK John
The Hospital for Sick Children, Department of Genetics, 555 University Avenue, Toronto, Ontario M5G 1X8, Canada;
tel. : (416) 813 6354, fax : (416) 813 4931

DIETERLEN-LIEVRE Françoise
Institut d'Embryologie Cellulaire, 49 bis, rue de la Belle Gabrielle, 94736 Nogent-sur-Marne Cedex, France;
tel. : (33 1) 48 73 60 90, fax : (33 1) 48 73 43 77

DZIERZAK Elaine
Medical Research Council, National Institute for Medical Research, The Ridgeway - Mill-Hill, London NW7 1AA, UK;
tel. : (81) 959 3666, fax : (91) 906 4477

FRICKHOFEN Norbert
Hematology-Oncology Department, University of Ulm, Robert Koch Street 8, D-89081 Ulm, Germany;
tel. : (49 73) 15 02 43 99, fax : (49 73) 15 02 43 93

GLUCKMAN Eliane
Service de greffe de moelle osseuse, Hôpital Saint-Louis, 1, avenue Claude Vellefaux, 75475 Paris Cedex 10, France;
tel. : (33 1) 42 49 96 44, fax : (33 1) 42 49 96 34

GRATWOHL Alois
Hematology - Internal Medicine, Kantonsspital Basel, CH-4031 Basel, Switzerland;
tel. : (4161) 26 54 254, fax : (4161) 26 54 450

HOROWITZ Mary M.
Statistical Center, Medical College of Wisconsin, 8701 Watertown Plank Road, P.O. Box 26509, Milwaukee WI 53226, USA;
tel. : (414) 456 8325, fax : (414) 266 8471

HOWS Jill M.
Department of Haematology, Bristol University, Southmead Hospital, Westbury-on-Trym, Bristol BS10 5NB, U. K.
tel. : (44) 272 50 50 50, fax : (44) 272 59 31 54

HUSS Ralf
Virchowstr. 171, Institut für Immunologie, Universitätsklinikum, D-45122 Essen, Germany;
tel. : (49) 201 723 4200, fax : (49) 201 723 5936

ISSARAGRISIL Surapol
Division of Hematology, Department of Medicine, Faculty of Medicine, Siriraj Hospital, Mahidol University, 10700 Bangkok, Thailand;
tel. : (662) 411 2012, fax : (662) 412 9783

JOENJE Hans
Free University, Department of Human Genetics, Van der Boechorststraat 7, NL 1081 BT Amsterdam, The Netherlands;
tel. : (31 20) 548 27 64, fax : (31 20) 548 33 29

KIRSZENBAUM Marek
Unité de Recherche sur la Biologie des Cellules Souches Hématopoïetiques, Hôpital Saint-Louis, Centre Hayem, 1, avenue Claude Vellefaux, 75475 Paris Cedex 10, France;
tel. : (33 1) 42 49 98 24, fax : (33 1) 48 03 19 60

LANSDORP Peter
Plesmanlaan 125, University of Amsterdam, C.L.B. dpt. of I.H., 1066 CX Amsterdam, The Netherlands;
tel. : (604) 877 6070, fax : (607) 877 0712

LE BOUTEILLER Philippe
INSERM U 395, CHU Purpan, BP 3028, 31024 Toulouse Cedex, France;
tel. : (33) 61 49 36 33, fax : (33) 61 49 97 52

LIU Johnson M.
N.I.H, Building 10 Acrf, Room 7C103, MD 20205 Bethesda, USA;
tel. : (301) 496 5093, fax : (301) 496 8396

LU Li
Walther Oncology Center, Medical Research and Library Bldg, Room 501, 975 W. Walnut Street, Indianapolis IN 46202-5121, USA;
tel. : 317 274 7501, fax : 317 274 7592

MARY Jean-Yves
Université Paris VII D-Diderot, INSERM U 263 - Case 7113, 2, place Jussieu, 75251 Paris Cedex 05, France;
tel. : (33 1) 44 27 78 86, fax : (33 1) 44 27 69 12

MILLER Cindy
The Terry Fox Laboratory, 601, West 10th Avenue, British Columbia, Vancouver V5Z 1L3, Canada;
tel. : (604) 877 6070, fax : (604) 877 0712

MOUSTACCHI Ethel
Laboratoire de Génotoxicologie, URA 1292 CNRS, Section de Biologie, Institut Curie, 26, rue d'Ulm, 75005 Paris, France;
tel. : (33 1) 40 51 67 10, fax : (33 1) 46 33 30 16

NIMER Stephen
Hematology Service, Memorial Sloan Kettering Cancer Center, 1275 York Avenue, Box 575, New York, NY 10021, USA;
tel. : (212) 639 7871, fax : (212) 794 5849

PEAULT Bruno
Institut d'Embryologie Cellulaire, 49 bis, rue de la Belle Gabrielle, 94736 Nogent-sur-Marne Cedex, France;
tel. : (33 1) 48 73 60 00, fax : (33 1) 48 73 43 77

PFLUMIO Françoise
INSERM U 362, Institut Gustave Roussy, 39, avenue Camille Desmoulins, 94805 Villejuif, France;
tel. : (33 1) 45 59 42 33, fax : (33 1) 45 26 92 74

RAGHAVACHAR Aruna
University of Ulm, Department of Internal Medicine III, Robert-Koch Street 8, D-89081 Ulm, Germany;
tel. : (49 731) 502 44 02, fax : (49 731) 502 43 93

RINGDEN Olle
Department of Clinical Immunology, Huddinge Hospital, F-79, S-141 86 Huddinge, Sweden;
tel. : (46 8) 746 57 23, fax : (46 8) 746 68 69

SAINTENY Françoise
INSERM U 362, Institut Gustave Roussy, 39, avenue Camille Desmoulins, 94805 Villejuif Cedex, France;
tel. : (33 1) 45 59 42 33, fax : (33 1) 47 26 92 74

SOCIE Gérard
Unité de Recherche sur la Biologie des Cellules Souches Hématopoïétiques, Hôpital Saint-Louis, Centre Hayem, 1, avenue Claude Vellefaux, 75475 Paris Cedex 10, France;
tel. : (33 1) 42 49 98 24, fax : (33 1) 48 03 19 60

TOURAINE Jean-Louis
Hôpital Edouard Herriot, Pavillon P / Médecine de Transplantation, Immunologie Clinique, Place d'Arsonval, 69437 Lyon Cedex 03, France;
tel. : (33) 72 11 01 51, fax : (33) 72 11 02 71

VITTET Daniel
INSERM U 217, DBMS-CENG, 17, rue des Martyrs, 38054 Grenoble Cedex 09, France;
tel. : (33) 76 88 40 35, fax : (33) 76 88 51 23

WAGNER John E.
University of Minnesota, Pediatrics, Box 366 UMHC, 420 Delaware Street, S.E Minneapolis MN55455, USA;
tel. : (612) 626 2778, fax : (612) 626 2815

WODNAR - FILIPOWICZ Alexandra
Kantonsspital Basel, Department Research, Hebel Street 20, 4031 Basel, Switzerland;
tel. : (41 61) 265 42 54, fax : (41 61) 265 44 50

YOUNG Neal S.
N.I.H, Room 7C103, Building 10 Acrf, Bethesda MD 20205, USA;
tel. : (301) 496 5093, fax : (301) 496 8396

ZANJANI Esmail
VA Medical Center, 1000 Locust Street, Reno NV 89520, USA;
tel. : (702) 786 7200, fax : (702) 328 1745

ZON Leonard
Howard Hughes Medical Institute, Research Laboratories, Children's Hospital, 300 Longwood Avenue, Boston MA 02115, USA;
tel. : (617) 735 7781, fax : (617) 730 0506

I. ONTOGENY OF HEMATOPOIESIS
I. ONTOGÉNIE DE L'HÉMATOPOÏÈSE

1) Embryonic development of hematopoiesis

1) *Développement embryonnaire de l'hématopoïèse*

Sites of hemopoietic stem cell production in early embryogenesis

Françoise Dieterlen-Lièvre[1], Isabelle Godin[1], Luc Pardanaud[1],
Ana Cumano[2], Maria-Luisa Gaspar[3], Miguel Marcos[3]
and Juan Garcia-Porrero[4]

[1] Institut d'Embryologie cellulaire et moléculaire du CNRS et du Collège de France, 49bis, avenue de la Belle Gabrielle, 94736 Nogent-sur-Marne Cedex, France, tel.: (33 1) 48 73 60 90, fax: (33 1) 48 73 43 77;
[2] Unité de Biologie Moléculaire du Gène, Institut Pasteur, 25, rue du Docteur-Roux, 75015 Paris;
[3] Universidad autonoma de Madrid, Centro de Biologia Molecular, 28049 Madrid, España;
[4] Universidad de Cantabria, Departamento de Anatomia y Biologia Cellular, Avenida Cardenal Herrera Oria, s/n, 39011 Santander, España

Abstract

The yolk sac is the only embryonic organ that produces hemopoietic stem cells (HSC) in situ. All other rudiments are colonized by extrinsic HSC. Analysis of chimeras constructed between a quail embryo and a chick yolk sac have yielded proof that, in birds, yolk sac HSC become extinct without giving rise to a self renewing pool and that a new population of HSC of intraembryonic origin seed the rudiments of the definitive hemopoietic organs. The site where these cells emerge was identified through interspecific transplantations and in vitro clonal assays as the aortic ventral endothelium and the surrounding mesenchymal layers of the 3-4 day embryo. A homologous region from the mouse embryo, the "paraaortic splanchnopleura" (P-Sp), retrieved at stages between 10 and 25 pairs of somites (8.5 to 9.5 dpc), harbours growing numbers of HSC, capable of differentiating into several lineages when tested by in vivo *or* in vitro *methods. In parallel the yolk sac (YS) also produces a wave of HSC. These HSC appear in P-Sp and YS prior to liver rudiment colonization, at a time when primary erythropoiesis is full blown in the yolk sac. A cytological study reveals hemopoietic cell aggregates in postumbilical arteries at the period involved. The antigenic phenotype and gene expression profile of cells in the P-Sp is under study. The role of these HSC in the ontogeny of the hemopoietic system is discussed.*

Hemopoietic stem cells (HSC), endowed with self-renewal capacity and pluripotency, are present in the bone marrow of vertebrates from the time it develops. Like all other hemopoietic organ rudiments except the yolk sac, the bone marrow is colonized by extrinsic HSC, distinct in their embryonic lignage from the stromal cells of the organ. This fundamental rule has been repeatedly verified by embryonic transplantation experiments, in amphibians, birds and mammals. Provided that a rudiment is obtained from the donor embryo at an early stage, prior to the beginning of HSC entry, it becomes colonized by HSC from the host where it is engrafted. In these experiments donor and host are selected so as to differ by appropriate cell markers [1, 2]. The only exception to this rule is the yolk sac, which produces its own HSC at the initiation of the hemopoietic activity, but later receives fresh ones from an extrinsic origin [3].

The circumstances through which HSC emerge during ontogeny are obviously central to the function of the hemopoietic system. For many years the whole contingent of HSC was supposed to form in the yolk sac during a unique commitment event and to colonize sequentially the rudiments according to their developmental schedule [4]. An experimental model was then devised in birds, in which an embryo was grafted onto a foreign yolk sac through micromanipulation [5]. Upon analysis of blood and host/donor makeup of organs in these "yolk sac chimeras", blood progenitors of yolk sac origin were found to function transiently and become extinct while the self-renewable HSC pool originated from the embryo proper [6, 7].

The production of intraembryonic HSC could be ascribed to the mesodermal region surrounding and comprising the aorta [8-10]. In the present report, we shall review recent evidence about the emergence of HSC in a homologous region of the mouse embryo, that we designate as the paraaortic splanchnopleura (P-Sp). The tissue distribution, phenotype, potentialities and gene expressions displayed by these HSC will be summarized and considered in the context of blood-forming potency mapping in avian embryos.

Mapping mesodermal commitment to the hemangioblastic lineage in birds

A common ontogenic origin has been postulated for the endothelial and hemopoietic lineages, from a presumed " hemangioblastic" lineage. Indeed early endothelia and hemopoietic progenitors display intimate connexions in young embryos, both in the extraembryonic area (future yolk sac) and in the intraembryonic area (region of the aorta). Furthermore early hemopoietic progenitors share an assortment of surface antigens with endothelial cells (EC). One of these shared antigens is QH1, a glycosylated protein antigen present in the quail species on the surface of EC and hemopoietic progenitors. The monoclonal antibody that recognizes this molecule has no affinity for any chick cells thus QH1 labeling is an excellent marker for quail EC and hemopoietic cells in avian interspecific combinations [11]. To map the hemangioblastic capacities of the mesoderm, structures into which the mesoderm subdivides (*Figure 1*) were dissected from quail embryos and grafted into heterotopic or orthotopic sites of chicken host embryos. The two layers of lateral plate mesoderm from 2-day old embryos (E2) were thus shown to differ completely in their capacities to yield derivatives from the blood forming system. The splanchnic mesoderm, grafted either in the limb bud or in the vicinity of the dorsal mesentery, gave rise to both EC and hemopoietic cells, while the somatic mesoderm did not [12-14]. The somatic mesoderm or framework of the body wall and limbs built its endothelial network from immigrating endothelial precursors. These emerge from the axial mesoderm, namely the somites [15].

Like the splanchnic mesoderm from E2 embryos, the dorsal aorta and surrounding mesoderm from slightly older embryos (E3-4) gave rise to abundant hemopoietic progenitors, when transplanted from the quail into the dorsal mesentery of the chick embryo. The hemopoietic and endothelial potencies of these different structures were monitored *in situ* by the expression of two nuclear protooncogenes, c-*myb* and c-*ets*1. In the adult, c-*myb* is known to be specifically expressed during amplification of hemopoietic progenitors, while c-*ets*1 is expressed during multiplication of lymphoid cells. In the course of a recent study, the c-*ets*1 message was found, by *in situ* hybridization, to co-localize in the embryo with EC and their forerunners and probably with their common hemangioblastic precursor [16]. In the mesodermal substructures described above, c-*ets*1 expression is intense in the splanchnic layer of mesoderm and patchy in the somatic layer [17], a pattern in good agreement with the transplantation results, according to which only the splanchnic layer has the hemangioblastic potentiality.

In E3-4 embryos, c-*myb* expression is restricted to the ventrolateral aspects of the aortic endothelium, all along the trunk, a region where the aortic endothelium buds aggregates of cells into

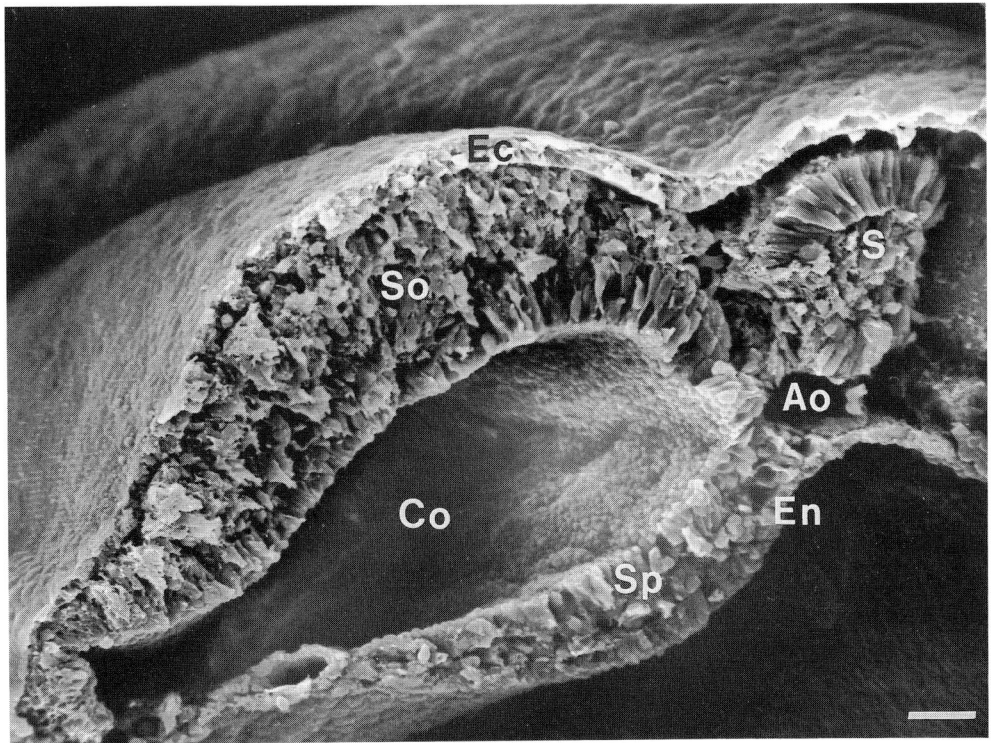

Figure 1. Scanning electron micrograph of the germ layers in a 2 day chick embryo; transverse break at trunk level. The neural tube and notochord to the right of the picture are not visible in this view which depicts the germ layers on one side of the embryo. Ao = aorta; Co = coelom; Ec = ectoderm; En = endoderm; S = Somite; So = Somatic mesoderm; Sp = Splanchnic mesoderm; Bar = 20 mm.

the lumen of the vessel. c-*ets*1 messages, probably coexpressed with c-*myb* in the ventrolateral cells, are widely distributed in the endothelial network.

To summarize, in the avian embryo, transplantation experiments and some gene expressions point to the splanchnic mesoderm first in the extraembryonic area and secondly in the aorta of the embryo as capable of giving rise to both EC and hemopoietic cells. The avian background provides the guidelines that prompted mouse experiments.

The P-Sp of the 10-25 somite mouse embryo, a candidate region for the production of a secondary HSC population; experimental and cytological arguments

A sequence of hemopoietic sites is recognized during mouse embryogenesis *(Figure 2)*. The main organs involved are the yolk sac, the fetal liver, the thymus, the omentum, the spleen and the bone marrow. Our aim is to find out whether one or several new inputs of HSC may seed

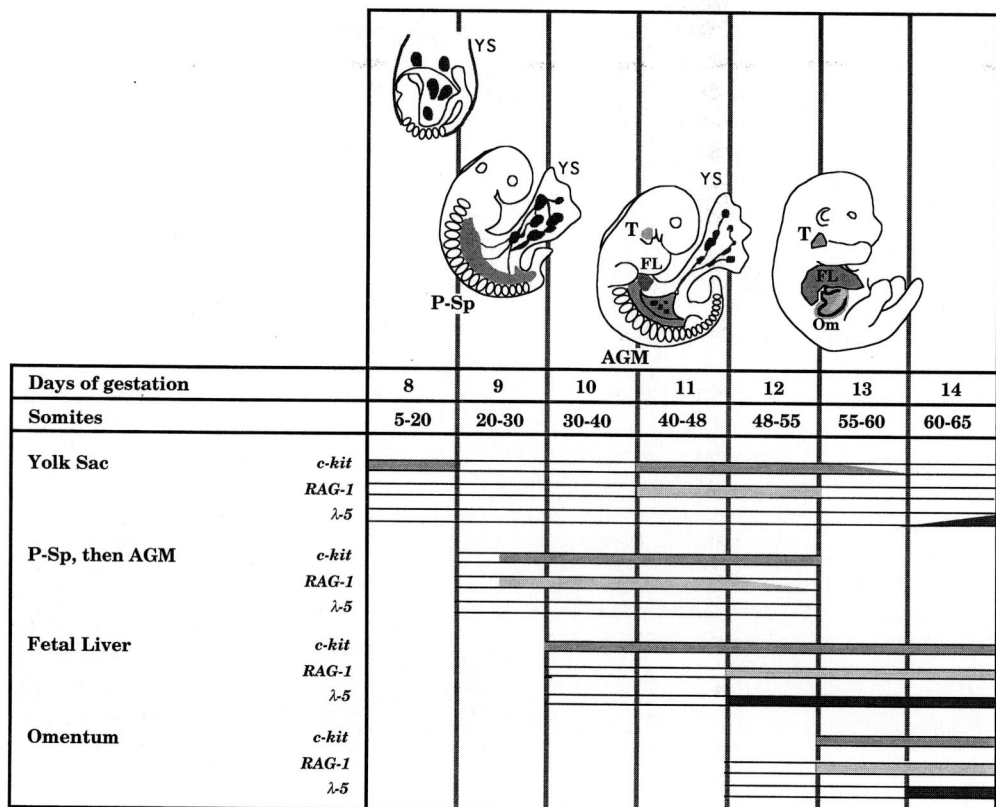

Figure 2. Diagramme of the sequential sites of hemopoiesis in a mouse embryo with developmental schedule and gene expressions analyzed in [22].

the system after the initial pool has emerged from the yolk sac. The omentum has been considered as a candidate; its possible role will not be discussed here. We have been looking for an earlier source of HSC, which might be active before the time when fetal liver seeding is initiated at the 28-32 somite stages, *i.e.* early 10 dpc (days post coitum).

The region we selected for testing is homologous but not identical to the paraaortic region of avian embryos, since this is too small to dissect in the mouse. This region comprises the splanchnopleure derivatives neighbouring the aorta, namely the digestive tube endoderm surrounded by the splanchnic mesoderm in which are embedded the two dorsal aortae (later to fuse into a single vessel) and the omphalomesenteric artery [18]. The dissection proceeded from the level of the liver rudiment caudalwards, because in a previous study progenitors were detected in the caudal but not the cephalic half of the embryonic body [19]. Retaining only the caudal half of the P-Sp insured that the structures obtained were devoid of liver rudiment. The tissues were tested by *in vivo* and *in vitro* approaches. For *in vivo* testing, the whole structure was grafted under the kidney capsule of adult SCID (Severe Combined Immuno-Deficiency) mice and the extent of host immune system reconstitution was investigated. In these specific experimental conditions, the Bla subset of the B lymphoid system became reconstituted [19], as well as the

T cell compartment (unpublished results). The biased reconstitution of the B cell compartment was probably circumstancial. Indeed by means of *in vitro* amplification and differentiation of the progenitors present in the P-Sp, the following points could be established or precised:

1) progenitors with a B lymphoid potential may be present at least as early as the 10-somite stage in the P-Sp, their presence became regular from the stage of 15 somites onwards; their number increased progressively and reached a means of 15 per embryo at the stage of 25 somites. Single micromanipulated cells from the P-Sp, enriched in AA4.1$^+$ progenitors by panning, yielded clones that differentiated into the myeloid, B or T lymphoid pathways according to the culture conditions they were subdivided into [20; details in 21];

2) progenitors with a similar potential appeared in parallel in the yolk sac; their total number followed the same chronological evolution as described in the P-Sp; however as the yolk sac is a much larger structure than the P-Sp, the concentration of progenitors is 10 fold higher in the latter;

3) the meanwhile, no progenitors were found in the remainder of the embryo, from which P-Sp and yolk sac had been dissected away.

Cytological correlates were looked for on sections from 9 to 11.5 dpc embryos. Two types of cell arrangements answered the criteria, *i.e.* they displayed hemopoiesis features and were not enclosed in discrete hemopoietic organs. The earliest of these cell arrangements are cell aggregates, several layer thick, that sit inside the lumen of arteries in close association with the endothelium. Differently from the avian situation, truncal aorta cell aggregates are very small. Very large aggregates are present in the other main arteries in the postumbilical part of the embryo, namely, the omphalomesenteric artery, the umbilical arteries, and the recurved distal parts of the aorta. Typically these aggregates are polarized onto one aspect of the artery, proximal to the coelomic cavity. The second type of cell arrangement consists in blood island-like structures that are located in the mesentery around the gut epithelium. Abundant towards the somite stage, they evolve from clusters of homogeneous dense cells to endothelium-wrapped hemocytoblast-filled structures that finally acquire a lumen and transform into capillaries.

Antigenic phenotype of the candidate intraembryonic progenitors and expression profiles of relevant genes [22]

This recent study aims at defining *ex vivo* the cell progenitors that can be amplified and orientated *in vitro* into various hemopoietic pathways. The antigen display was analyzed by fluorescence activated sorting and the gene expression by RT-PCR. At the 25-somite stage these cells are characterized by the expression of the AA4.1 antigen and, surprisingly, by the absence of the Sca-1 antigen, which is the hallmark of hemopoietic progenitors in murine fetal liver and bone marrow. Of the genes studied, c-*kit* and CD34 were not restricted to the P-Sp, an expected finding since the c-*kit* receptor is expressed not only in hemopoietic progenitors but also in melanoblasts and primordial germ cells, and since CD34 is expressed on endothelial cells.

The expression of B lymphoid specific genes was revealing *(Figure 2)*. Rag-l, first expressed at 9.5 dpc in the P-Sp, became down regulated at 11 dpc. In the yolk sac, Rag-l was lower and detectable only from 10 dpc onwards. Expression of two other B lineage specific genes really set apart the P-Sp from the more conventional sites. The surrogate light chain l5 transcripts were never detected there nor in the YS or embryo remainder at the early stages of our study. This gene started to be expressed only in 12 dpc liver, despite the fact that B genes are being rearranged, since Rag-1 is expressed. Finally IgH DJ rearrangements were biased in P-Sp cells towards J4 usage, while the four J segments became equally used in post 13 dpc liver cells.

Conclusion

We review recent functional and cytological evidence, indicating that a secondary wave of HSC emerges in the mouse embryo proper, at least 24 hours after the primary generation that gives rise to the nucleated red cells of the yolk sac. These HSC clearly represent a secondary set because of their kinetics of appearance. They display a specific antigenic phenotype and express specific sets of genes. Secondary HSC emerge simultaneously in the yolk sac. We think that this is a programmed event that occurs in all regions of the conceptus from about the stage of l0 somites. A similar programme unfolds in the avian embryo, where the secondary wave of HSC gives rise to erythrocytes characterized by a specific assortment of hemoglobins (hbs), distinct by reference to hbs present in the primary erythroid lineage. In the avian chimeras, these secondary stem cells were respectively chick (from the YS) and quail (from the embryos) and thus were definitely known not to belong to a common circulating pool. Such a formal proof is not available yet in the murine model. We hope that the comparison of genes expressed by the progeny of these HSC during the differentiation process with these expressed by homologous populations active at other times of ontogeny may lead us to solve this issue and determine whether several distinct generations of HSC might be successively involved in the ontogeny of the blood system.

Finally it is important to emphasize that a region, identified in 11 dpc embryos as AMG (Aorta-Mesonephros-Gonads), has been shown to contain long-term repopulating HSC [23, 24]. The AMG contains tissues (or organs) derived from the P-Sp; P-Sp and AMG must be considered as a continuum, which clearly has a specific role in the ontogeny of the hemopoietic system.

References

1. Metcalf D, Moore, MAS. Embryonic aspects of haemopoiesis, In *Haemopoietic cells*, A Neuberger & EL Tatum, ed, North Holland Publ, Amderdan, p. 127, 1971.
2. Le Douarin NM, Dieterlen-Lièvre F, Oliver, PD. Ontogeny of primary lymphoid organs and lymphoid stem cells, *Am J Anat* 1984; 170: 261-299.
3. Beaupain D, Martin C, Dieterlen-Lièvre F. Are developmental hemoglobin changes related to the origin of stem cells and site of erythropoiesis ? *Blood* 1979; 2: 212-225.
4. Moore MAS, Owen JJT. Experimental studies on the development of the thymus, *J Exp Med* 1967; 126: 715-725.
5. Martin C. Technique d'explantation *in ovo* de blastodermes d'embryons d'oiseaux. *C R Soc. Biol* 1972; 116: 283-285.
6. Dieterlen-Lièvre, F. On the origin of haemopoietic stem cells in the avian embryo: an experimental approach. *J Embryol Exp Morphol* 1975; 33: 607-619.
7. Dieterlen-Lièvre F. Hemopoiesis during avian ontogeny. *Poultry Science Reviews* 1994; 5: 273-305.
8. Dieterlen-Lièvre F. Emergence of intraembryonic blood stem cells in avian chimeras by means of monoclonal antibodies. *Dev Comp Immunol* 1984; supplt 3: 75-80.
9. Cormier F, de Paz P, Dieterlen-Lièvre F. *In vitro* detection of cells with monocytic potentiality in the wall of the chick embryo aorta. *Dev Biol* 1986; 118: 167-175.
10. Cormier F, Dieterlen-Lièvre F. The wall of the chick embryo aorta harbours M-CFC, G-CFC, GM-CFC and BFU-E. *Development* 1988; 102: 279-285.
11. Pardanaud L, Altmann C, Kitos P, Dieterlen-Lièvre F, Buck C. Vasculogenesis in the early quail blastodisc as studied with a monoclonal antibody recognizing endothelial cells. *Development* 1987; 100: 339-349.
12. Pardanaud L; Yassine F, Dieterlen-Lièvre F. Relationship between vasculogenesis, angiogenesis and haemopoiesis during avian ontogeny. *Development* 1989; 105: 473-485.
13. Pardanaud L, Dieterlen-Lièvre F. Emergence of endothelial and hemopoietic cells in the avian embryo. *Anat and Embryol* 1993; 187: 107-114.

14. Pardanaud L, Dieterlen-Lièvre F. Does the paraxial mesoderm of the avian embryo have hemangioblastic capacities ? *Anat & Embryol* 1995; In press.
15. Pardanaud L, Luton D, Bourcheix LM, Catala M, Dieterlen-Lièvre F. Mapping body wall colonization by angioblasts from the somites in the avian embryo. Submitted.
16. Vandenbunder B, Pardanaud L, Jaffredo T, Mirabel MA, Stéhelin D. Complementary patterns of expression of c-*ets*1, c-*myb* and c-*myc* in the blood-forming system of the chick embryo. *Development* 1989; 106: 265-274.
17. Pardanaud L, Dieterlen-Lièvre F. Expression of c-ets1 in early chick embryo mesoderm: relationship to the hemangioblastic lineage. *Cell Adh & Comm* 1993; 1: 119-132.
18. Godin I, Garcia-Porrero J, Coutinho A, Dieterlen-Lièvre F, Marcos MAR, Paraaortic splanchnopleura from early mouse embryo contains B1a-cell progenitors. *Nature* 1993; 364: 67-70.
19. Cumano A, Paige CJ, Iscove NN, Brady G. Bipotential precursors of B cells and macrophages in murine fetal liver. *Nature* 1992; 356: 612-615.
20. Godin I, Dieterlen-Lièvre F, Cumano A. Emergence of multipotent hematopoietic cells in the yolk sac and paraaortic splanchnopleura of 8.5 dpc mouse embryos. *Proc Natl Acad Sci* 1995; 92: 773-777.
21. Cumano A, Dieterlen-Lièvre F, Paige CJ, Godin I. Hematopoietic cell commitment during embryonic development. This volume.
22. Gaspar ML, Morales S, Godin I, Dieterlen-Lièvre F, Copin SG, Marcos M. Two phases of lymphohemopoiesis in the early mouse embryo. Submitted.
23. Medvinsky AL, Somoylina NL, Müller AM, Dzierzak EA. An early pre-liver intra-embryonic source of CFU-S in the developing mouse. *Nature* 1993; 364: 64-66.
24. Müller AM, Medvinsky A, Strouboulis J, Grosveld F, Dzierzak EA. Development of hematopoietic stem cell activity in the mouse embryo. *Immunity* 1994; 1: 291-301.

Résumé

Le sac vitellin est le seul organe embryonnaire qui produit des cellules souches hématopoïétiques (CSH) *in situ*. Les ébauches des autres organes hématopoïétiques sont toutes colonisées par des CSH extrinsèques. Des chimères créées par micromanipulation entre un embryon de caille et un sac vitellin de poulet ont fourni la preuve que, chez l'oiseau, les CSH du sac vitellin ont une durée de vie éphémère et sont remplacées par des CSH autorenouvelables d'origine intraembryonnaire, responsables de la colonisation des organes hématopoïétiques définitifs. Le mésoderme périaortique a été identifié comme le site d'émergence de ces CSH chez l'embryon d'oiseau de 3-4 jours.

La « splanchnopleure paraaortique » (Sp-P), région homologue chez l'embryon de souris, disséquée aux stades de 10 à 25 paires de somites (soit 8,5 à 9,5 jours postcoïtum) avant le développement de l'ébauche hépatique, donne des CSH capables de se différencier selon différentes lignées, qui ont été détectées soit *in vivo*, soit *in vitro*. L'étude cytologique révèle à ces stades des bourgeonnements de cellules intraartériels postombilicaux, ainsi que des îlots sanguins dans le mésentère, qui sont équivalents aux agrégats de cellules hématopoïétiques intra- et para-aortiques aviaires. Le phénotype antigénique et les profils d'expression de certains gènes dans les cellules de la Sp-P ont été analysés et comparés à ceux du sac vitellin, du foie fœtal et du sang périphérique.

Development of hematopoietic stem cell activity in the mouse embryo

E. Dzierzak, A. Müller, A. Sinclair, C. Miles, N. Gillett, B. Daly, M.-J. Sanchez and A. Medvinsky

National Institute for Medical Research, The Ridgeway, Mill Hill, London, NW7 1AA, England, tel.: (81) 959 3666, fax: (91) 906 4477

Summary

Mammalian hematopoietic stem cell development has been studied in an in vivo *transplantation model with donor cells from various mouse embryonic tissues. While it has been previously shown that differentiated hematopoietic cells and committed progenitors begin to appear at day 7 in mouse embryogenesis, transplantable stem cell activity does not appear until much later. We have found long term, pluripotential hematopoietic stem cell activity in the intra-embryonic AGM region of the mouse on day 10. This site is analogous with the site of definitive hematopoietic activity in other vertebrates. At day 11, stem cell activity is found in the AGM region as well as two other sites; the yolk sac and liver. Such information on the appearance of the earliest transplantable hematopoietic stem cells in mammalian embryonic development may lead to a better understanding of stem cell maintenance, expansion and lineage potential.*

The stem cells for the hematopoietic system of adult mammals reside in the bone marrow and are responsible for the continuous supply of mature blood cells through-out life. The origin of the hematopoietic system is known to be within the mesodermal germ layer of the developing embryo. However, the precise embryonic location of definitive hematopoietic stem cell (HSC) production is uncertain. Previously, *in vitro* hematopoietic colony formation and *in vivo* transplantation assays with embryonic yolk sac have led to the general acceptance of the yolk sac origin of mammalian HSCs [1]. However, only recently have other regions of the developing mammalian embryo been examined for hematopoietic activity [2-5]. We review here our results demonstrating the presence of potent CFU-S progenitor [2] and HSC [3] activity in the intra-embryonic AGM (aorta, genital ridge, mesonephros) region of the developing mouse embryo. Analogies with the developing hematopoietic system of other vertebrates suggest that the AGM region is very important for the development of the adult mammalian hematopoietic system.

Hematopoietic progenitors appear early in mouse embryogenesis

Previously, the yolk sac has been the tissue most extensively analyzed for CFU-C and CFU-S progenitor activity in the developing mouse embryo [1, 6]. Precursors for granulocyte and macrophages have been found as early as day 7 in the mouse yolk sac by CFU-C assays. CFU-S activity has been found beginning day 9 in the yolk sac. We examined the intra-embryonic AGM region of day 8, 9, 10 and 11 mouse embryos and compared the number and frequency of $CFU-S_8$ and $CFU-S_{11}$ progenitors in this tissue with those found in the yolk sac [2]. Statistically significant numbers of CFU-S were found beginning at day 9 in both the yolk sac and AGM region. However, the number and frequency of the progenitors in the AGM region surpassed those in the yolk sac up until day 11. At this time there was a rapid decrease in CFU-S activity in the AGM and this coincided with an increase in activity in the liver. During the peak of activity in the AGM region, the frequency CFU-S progenitors was equivalent to that found in adult bone marrow.

Hematopoietic stem cell activity in the AGM region appears at 10-11 dpc

The ability of various embryonic tissues to long term repopulate the hematopoietic system was examined in mouse radiation chimeras [3]. Genetically marked cells from the yolk sac, AGM region or the liver of day 8, 9, 10 and 11 embryos were transplanted into mouse recipients and analyzed for multi-lineage and serial repopulation at 8 months post-transplantation. While cells from day 11 yolk sac, AGM and liver were able to repopulate all hematopoietic lineages in transplant recipients, only AGM cells from late day 10 embryos were found to have this activity. This activity was found to be transplantable into secondary and tertiary recipients, thus demonstrating the presence of genuine HSCs. At day 10 HSCs are probably present in the AGM region in limited numbers since the success of repopulation was only 3 out of 100 adult recipients when each recipient received cells from one AGM tissue equivalent. Although we cannot rule out the presence of low level HSC activity in the yolk sac and liver of day 10 embryos, it appears that the AGM region is probably the region where HSCs first appear.

The two sites of hematopoietic activity in non-mammalian vertebrates

Generally in avian [7] and amphibian [8] embryos, hematopoiesis takes place in two mesodermally derived regions; the ventral mesoderm yielding the yolk sac/ ventral blood island analogue and the dorsal mesoderm yielding the intra-embryonic region containing the dorsal aorta and pro/mesonephros. It has been shown by embryo grafting experiments in birds that the cells contributing to the adult hematopoietic system are derived from the intra-embryonic region while the embryonic hematopoietic system is yolk sac derived and only transient. Similarly, the yolk sac analogue of amphibians contributes to transient embryonic hematopoiesis while the intra-embryonic region contributes stable adult hematopoiesis (although there is some additional contribution by the yolk sac analogue). The generation of intra-embryonic hematopoietic activity in amphibians has been localized to the pronephros and the activity in birds has been thought to be produced in the region of the dorsal aorta. Recent studies by in situ hybridization in fish have demonstrated a dorsal mesodermal location (pronephros) of definitive hematopoietic activity [9, 10]. Thus, the adult hematopoietic activity of non-mammalian vertebrates is derived predominantly from the intra-embryonic mesoderm with some contribution from the yolk sac.

Is the intra-embryonic AGM region of the mouse the site of origin/development/expansion of the HSC?

The demonstration of intra-embryonic HSC and progenitor activity in the developing mouse has opened the way for comparisons of mammalian hematopoietic development with other vertebrate models [6, 7, 11]. Although grafting of mouse embryos is not yet possible, functional transplantation experiments *in vivo* and *in vitro* colony forming assays for hematopoietic progenitors have suggested that there are two waves of hematopoietic activity (yolk sac and AGM) entering the fetal liver in the developing mouse embryo [3, 5, 6, 11]. The development of the activities contained in these two waves of colonization appears to parallel the generation of hematopoietic activities in non-mammalian vertebrates and strongly suggests that mammals are not the exception but probably follow general vertebrate rules for embryonic and definitive hematopoiesis. Further support for this hypothesis is the demonstration that the germ layer fate mate of the mouse gastrula is very similar to the fate maps of fish, amphibians and birds [12] and that mesodermal inducing factors [8] are conserved between the mouse and other vertebrates. Thus, the mouse AGM region may generate *de novo* definitive adult HSCs. Alternatively, the AGM region may provide the microenvironment necessary for the progression of pre-stem cells to full adult HSCs and/or expand a single HSC (through novel competency and/or expansion factors) to the numbers found in the adult bone marrow. Future isolation and functional analysis of individual cells in the AGM region should help in understanding definitive HSC development, expansion and maintenance.

References

1. Moore MAS, Metcalf D. Ontogeny of the haemopoietic system: yolk sac origin of *in vivo* and *in vitro* colony forming cells in the developing mouse embryo. *Br J Haematol* 1970 18: 279-296.
2. Medvinsky AL, Samoylina NL, Müller AM, Dzierzak EA. An early pre-liver intraembryonic source of CFU-S in the developing mouse. *Nature* 1993 364: 64-67.
3. Müller AM, Medvinsky A, Strouboulis J, Grosveld F, Dzierzak, E. Development of hematopoietic stem cell activity in the mouse embryo. *Immunity* 1994 1: 291-301.
4. Godin IE, Garcia-Porrero JA, Coutinho A, Dieterlen-Lievre F, Marcos MAR. Para-aortic splanchnopleura from early mouse embryos contains B1a cell progenitors. *Nature* 1993 364: 67-70.
5. Godin I, Dieterlen-Lievre F, Cumano A. Emergence of multipotent hemopoietic cells in the yolk sac and paraaortic splanchnopleura in mouse embryos, beginning at 8.5 dpc. *Proc Natl Acad Sci* 1995 92: 773-777.
6. Medvinsky AL. Ontogeny of the mouse hematopoietic system. *Seminars Devel Biol* 1993 4: 333-340.
7. Dieterlen-Lievre F, Le Douarin NM. Developmental rules in the hematopoietic and immune systems of birds: how general are they? *Seminars Devel Biol* 1993 4: 325-332.
8. mith JC, Albano RM. Mesoderm induction and erythroid differentiation in early vertebrate development. *Seminars Devel Biol* 1993 4: 315-324.
9. Neave B, Rodaway A, Wilson SW, Patient R, Holder N. Evidence that gta (GATA 3) is involved in specification of cell fate during gastrulation, neurulation and haematopoiesis in zebrafish. *Mech Dev* 1994 (in press).

10. Detrich HW, Kieran MW, Chan FY, Barone LM, Yee K, Rundstadler JA, Zon LI. Intra-embryonic hematopoietic cell migration during vertebrate development. *Proc Natl Acad Sci* 1995 (in press).
11. Dzierzak E, Medvinsky A. Mouse embryonic hematopoeisis. *Trends Gen* 1995 (in press).
12. Lawson KA, Meneses JJ, Pedersen RA. Clonal analysis of epiblast fate during germ layer formation in the mouse embryo. *Devel* 1991 113: 891-911.

Acknowledgements

We thank F Grosveld for his continuous support and encouragement. This work is supported by the MRC (UK), the Wellcome Foundation and the Leukemia Society of America.

Résumé

Le développement des cellules souches hématopoïétiques de mammifères a été étudié dans un modèle de transplantation *in vivo* de cellules de donneur issues de différents tissus embryonnaires murins. Comme il a été montré que les cellules souches hématopoïétiques différenciées ainsi que les cellules progénitrices d'une lignée spécifique commencent à apparaître au jour 7 au cours de l'embryogenèse chez la souris, la capacité reconstitutrice des cellules souches doit apparaître beaucoup plus tard. Nous avons déterminé une activité pluripotente à long terme des cellules souches hématopoïétiques dans la région AGM intra-embryonnaire chez la souris au jour 10. Cette région est analogue au site d'activité hématopoïétique définitive chez les autres vertébrés. Au jour 11, l'activité des cellules souches est détectée dans la région AGM ainsi que dans 2 autres sites : le sac vitellin et le foie. Cette information concernant l'apparition, au cours du développement embryonnaire chez les mammifères, des cellules souches hématopoïétiques les plus précoces et capables de reconstitution, devrait conduire à une meilleure compréhension du maintien des cellules souches, de leur prolifération et de leur pluripotence.

The zebrafish: a new model for studying embryonic hematopoiesis

Leonard I. Zon[1,2], Mark Kieran[1], Barry Paw[1], Margaret Tompson[1], David Ransom[1,2], Alison Brownlie[1], Fung Yee Chan[2], Lauren Barone[2], Heather McClennan[1], Sandra Ziegler[1], Stephen Pratt[1] and H. William Detrich III[1,3]

[1] Division of Hematology/Oncology, Children's Hospital and Dana-Farber Cancer Institute, Department of Pediatrics, Harvard Medical School, Children's Hospital, Boston, MA 02115, USA, tel.: (617) 735 7781, fax: (617) 730 0506; [2] Howard Hughes Medical Institute, USA; [3] Department of Biology, Northeastern University, USA

Abstract

The zebrafish is a powerful molecular and developmental system for studying early events during embryogenesis. We have recently utilized the system to study embryonic hematopoiesis. We isolated cDNA clones, encoding zebrafish GATA-1 and GATA-2, and demonstrated their expression in an inter-embryonic location known as the intermediate cell mass of Oellacher. GATA-1 is initially expressed at the onset of gastrulation in the paraxial mesoderm that lines the embryo and then in the intermediate cell mass. GATA-2 is expressed in a similar distribution, but also is expressed in a very posterior population that resembles hematopoietic stem cells and neural cells. Using GATA-1 and GATA-2 as probes, we studied their expression pattern in three mutations effecting blood formation. In the bloodless *mutation and* spadetail *mutation, GATA-1 and GATA-2 expression are absent in the anterior ICM, but GATA-2 is expressed in the very posterior region where the stem cells are located. Thus, it appears that these two mutations have defects in their ability to differentiate hematopoietic stem cells. In the* cloche *mutation, all GATA-1 and GATA-2 staining in the tail region is deficient, indicating that* cloche *affects the genesis of the stem cell population. Interestingly,* cloche *also has a defect in endothelial and endocardial cell formation, thus supporting the concept that a hemangioblast may exist. Thus, the hematopoietic program appears to be conserved throughout vertebrate evolution and the zebrafish has provided us with interesting mutations affecting blood formation.*

Most vertebrate embryonic hematopoiesis initially occurs on the yolk sac [1]. In mammals, the hematopoietic mesoderm is derived from the epiblast, which in vaginates and enters an extra-embryonic position. This extra-embryonic mesoderm then migrates further onto the yolk sac and forms the blood island. The blood island consists of mesoderm, including erythrocytes and endothelial cells, as well as an endodermal base. The endodermal base is thought to support and induce the hematopoietic program.

The zebrafish is a new molecular developmental system for studying early pattern formation [2-4]. The embryo is perfectly clear during early development, allowing a direct visualization of various organigenesis processes. In addition, it is diploid and can be made haploid through fertilization of eggs with inactivated sperm. The availability of haploid organisms is a benefit to study recessive mutations. In addition, screens have been done for hematopoietic mutants, and the mutants are currently available. Finally, a genetic map [5] has been constructed that will ultimately allow positioning of genes and mutations for their ultimate isolation and characterization.

We initiated our studies of zebrafish hematopoiesis by examining the expression of globin in the early embryo. At about 24 hours after fertilization, benzedine-expressing cells [6, 7] are found in the tail of the embryo in a dorsal location above the yolk tube. This mass of erythroid cells has been called the intermediate cell mass of Oellacher, which was described in 1872 [8]. The mass is capable of producing hematopoietic cells, as well as vascular endothelial cells [6, 9, 10]. For many years, it has been thought that most teleosts form blood in this location and that this is a contradiction to the rule of yolk sac hematopoiesis of most vertebrate species. We examined the derivation of the intermediate cell mass of Oellacher by studying GATA-1 RNA expression during early embryogenesis by whole embryo *in situ* analysis [11] *(Figures 1 and 2)*. Antisense digoxigenin-labelled GATA-1 RNA was used to probe embryos staged from zero somites to 29 hours after fertilization. We demonstrated that GATA-1 was initially expressed at the two-somite stage in two lines of paraxial mesoderm that exist adjacent to the yolk syncytial layer. Later, these two lines converge medially and meet first anteriorly, then posteriorly, to form the intermediate cell mass. Thus, it appears that during gastrolation, the zebrafish utilizes a similar program as other vertebrates with extra-embryonic mesoderm becoming hematopoietic. However, the yolk sac does not play as prominent a role during this early time period as it does in higher vertebrates.

The zebrafish is also incredibly visible with respect to whole embryo *in situ* patterns. We studied the expression of GATA-1 and GATA-2 and demonstrated a relatively similar pattern of expression with respect to the intermediate cell mass [11]. However, GATA-2 is also expressed in a slightly posterior postulation of cells in the tail *(Figure 3)*. Sections through embryos in this region demonstrate cells with a blast-like morphology, potentially indicating a stem cell pool in the early embryo that is GATA-2 positive, but GATA-1 negative. Thus, the visualization of *in*

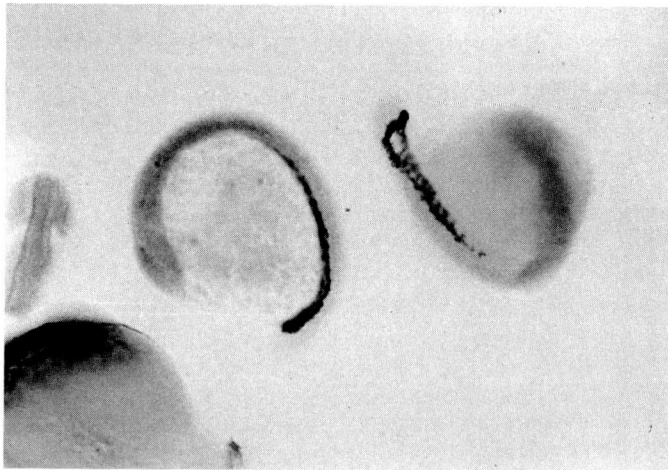

Figure 1. GATA-1 mRNA expression at 22 hours as detected by whole embryo *in situ* analysis. GATA-1 is present in a dorsal location in the tail known as the intermediate cell mass of Oellacher (arrow).

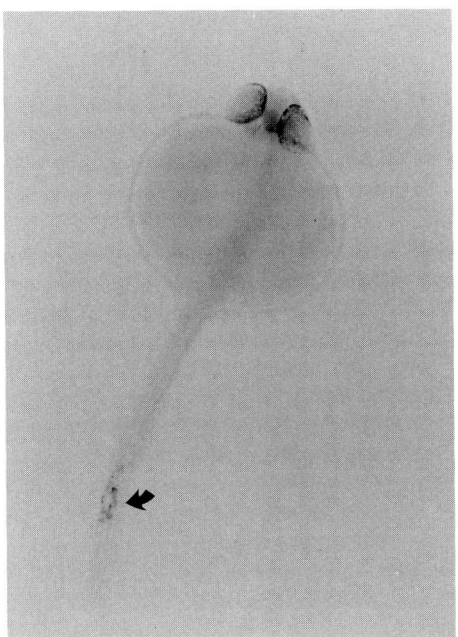

Figure 2. GATA-1 mRNA expression at 29 hours.

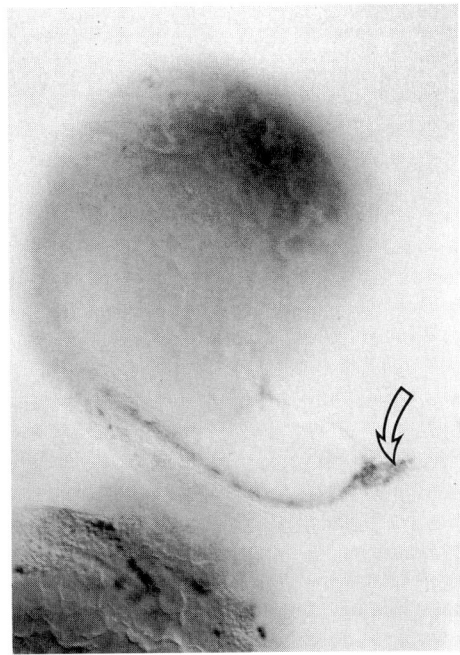

Figure 3. GATA-2 mRNA expression at 20 hours as detected by whole embryo *in situ* analysis. GATA-2 is detected in the intermediate cell mass. There is a posterior population of cells that are GATA-2$^+$, but GATA-1$^-$. These cells are likely to be early progenitors and/or hematopoietic stem cells. GATA-2 mRNA is also detected in some neural cells.

situ analysis may allow you to determine subpopulations of cells, such as the stem cells, from the more committed erythroid progenitors.

We followed the expression of GATA-1 from 24 hours to 29 hours and demonstrated a migration of hematopoietic cells, from the intermediate cell mass anteriorly over the yolk tube to the yolk sac [11]. The cells remain on the yolk sac for a brief period of time and appear to differentiate. Later these cells are channeled into the ducts of Cuvier and finally into the heart, at which time they are pumped through circulation. This migration patterning is very reminiscent of dorsal hematopoiesis in higher vertebrates, as has been described in frogs, chickens, and mice [12-15]. In these organisms, hematopoietic cells are present in the dorsal mesentery near the ducts of Cuvier and will ultimately will form the definitive hematopoiesis in higher vertebrates. Thus, the zebrafish has apparently deleted its ventral hematopoietic program and has a dorsal population that follows a migration pattern similar to that of higher vertebrates.

There are several mutant zebrafish that have been characterized. The *bloodless* and *spadetail* mutations [16] do not express GATA-1, but have posterior expression of GATA-2 consistent with the stem cell population. Therefore, these mutations appear to be defects in which the hematopoietic stem cells cannot differentiate. *Cloche* is a mutation of both the endocardial, endothelial, and hematopoietic cells [17]. In its mutation, the endocardium is missing, and the GATA-1 and GATA-2 staining in the tail is also absent. This would indicate that this mutation affects the genesis of the stem cell population. The concept of a mutant in vertebrates that affects both endothelial and hematopoietic lineages has been lacking, and this may be the first indication genetically that a "hemangioblast" [18] may exist.

We next studied normal hematopoiesis in the zebrafish. The intermediate cell mass forms embryonic blood cells. This is later taken over by the pronephros, and then later, the mesonephros [6]. In the adult, the kidney is the hematopoietic organ. We stained peripheral blood smears to demonstrate that the early cells from the intermediate cell mass appear to be a typical embryonic blood formation with a "normoblast" type of morphology. These cells differentiate over a five day period to a more characteristic embryonic erythrocyte. Later, definitive populations are present in the circulation. All major forms of erythroid progenitors, as well as myeloid progenitors, can be identified in the kidney. Thus, it appears to be the homolog of the bone marrow.

We recently attempted to do methylcellulose cultures of hematopoietic progenitors using the kidney as a source. Hematopoietic progenitors were plated in the presence of anemic carp serum (as a source of erythropoietin) or in cultured supernatant from a cell line, ZF-4. Erythroid and myeloid colonies were derived with characteristic morphology. Thus, hematopoietic cultures could be obtained and are, thus, useful for the analysis of the mutations.

In an effort to obtain homozygote mutant embryos that can be raised to adulthood, we have utilized a transplantation technique. Cells from the kidney were obtained and labeled with the dye PKH-26. These cells were then layered on to a 2-day old embryo within the ducts of Cuvier. These cells quickly entered the circulation over half an hour and then migrated to the tail region where they became hematopoietic. Cells remained in circulation for many days after analysis. Thus, it appears that the transplantation protocol will work. We are in the process of formally demonstrating hematopoietic reconstitution using progenitors that carry a transgene.

In summary, the zebrafish offers a potent system for genetic analysis of embryonic hematopoiesis. Most of the studies of normal hematopoiesis are comparable now to that of mice, and what remains is to isolate novel genes that are involved in these processes.

Acknowledgments

We would like to acknowledge the help of Jim Turpin. This work was supported by NIH grant P50 DK49216-01. L.I.Z. is an Assistant Investigator of the HHMI.

References

1. Tavassoli M (1991). Embryonic and fetal hemopoiesis: an overview. *Blood Cells* **1,** 269-281.
2. Mullins MC and Nusslein-Volhard C (1994). Mutational approaches to studying embryonic pattern formation in the zebrafish. *Current Opinion in Genetics and Development* **3,** 648-54.
3. Rossant J and Hopkins N (1992). Of fin and fur: mutational analysis of vertebrate development. *Genes and Development* **6,** 1-13.
4. Solonica-Krezel L, Schier AF and Driever W (1994). Efficient recovery of ENU-induced mutations from the zebrafish germline. *Genetics* **136,** 1401-1420.
5. Postlethwait JH, Johnson SL, Midson CN, Talbot WS, Gates M, Ballinger EW, Africa D, Andrews R, Carl T, Eisen JS and al, e (1994). A genetic linkage map for the zebrafish. *Science* **264,** 699-703.
6. Al-Adhami MA and Kunz YW (1977). Ontogenesis of haematopoietic sites in brachydanio rerio. *Develop. Growth And Differ* **19,** 171-9.
7. Iuchi I and Yamamoto M (1983). Erythropoiesis in the developing rainbow trout, salmo gairdneri deus: histochemical and immunological detection of erythropoietic organs. *J Exp Zool* **226,** 409-417.
8. Oellacher J (1872). Beitrage zur Entwicklungsgeschichte der Knochenfische nach Beobachtungen am Bachforelleneie. *Zeitschrift f wiss Zool* **23,** 373-421.
9. Al-Adhami MA and Kunz YW (1976). Hematopoietic centres in the developing angelfish, Pterophyllum scalere (Cuvier and Valenciennes). *Wilh Roux Archives* **179,** 393-401.
10. Reib J (1973). La Circulation Sanguine Chez L'Embryon De Brachydanio Rerio (Teleosteens, Cyprinidae). *Annales D'Embryologie Et De Morphogenese* **6,** 43-54.
11. Detrich HW, Kieran MW, Chan FY, Barone LM, Yee K, Rundstadler JA and Zon LI (1995). Intra-embryonic hematopoietic cell migration during vertebrate development. *Proc Nat Acad Sci USA,* in press.
12. Dieterlen LF and Martin C (1981). Diffuse intraembryonic hemopoiesis in normal and chimeric avian development. *Dev Biol* **88,** 180-191.
13. Godin IE, Garcia-Porrere JA, Coutinho A, Dieterlen-Lievre F and Marcos MAR (1993). Para-aortic splanchnopleura from early mouse embryos contains B1a cell progenitors. *Nature* **364,** 67-70.
14. Medvinsky AL, Samoylina NL, Muller AM and Dzierzak EA (1993). An early pre-liver intraembryonic source of CFU-S in the developing mouse. *Nature* **364,** 64-7.
15. Turpen JB, Knudson CM and Hoefen PS (1981). The early ontogeny of hematopoietic cells studied by grafting cytogenetically labeled tissue anlagen: localization of a prospective stem cell compartment. *Dev Biol* **85,** 99-112.
16. Kimmel CB, Kane DA, Walker C, Warga RM and Rothman MB (1989). A mutation that changes cell movement and cell fate in the zebrafish embryo. *Nature* **337,** 358-362.
17. Stanier DYR, Weinstein BM, Detrich HW, Zon LI and Fishman MC (1995). Cloche, a zebrafish gene required for normal vasculogenesis and hematopoiesis, provides evidence for a common progenitor. *Development* , submitted.
18. His W (1900). Lecithoblast und Angioblast der Wirbelthiere. *Abhandl KS Ges Wiss Math-Phys* **22,** 171-328.

Résumé

Le poisson zèbre est un modèle expérimental très performant pour l'analyse des événements survenant très précocement au cours du développement. Nous avons récemment cloné les ADNc des gènes *Gata-1* et *Gata-2* chez le poisson zèbre et nous avons analysé leur expression par hybridation *in situ*. L'ARN codant pour *Gata-1* est exprimé initialement dans le mésoderme paraaxial. Ces régions vont ensuite converger pour former la masse intermédiaire. L'ARN de *Gata-2* a la même distribution mais en plus est exprimé dans des cellules de type hématopoïétique primitif situées dans une région très caudale qui n'exprime pas *Gata-1*. L'analyse de l'expression de *Gata-1* et *Gata-2* a également été faite dans des poissons porteurs de plusieurs mutations : les mutations *bloodless* et *spadetail* sont caractérisées par une absence d'expression des ARN *Gata-1* et *Gata-2* dans la masse intermédiaire, mais l'expression de *Gata-2* dans la région caudale est conservée, suggérant que la mutation affecte la différenciation hématopoïétique des cellules souches. Dans la mutation *cloche,* il n'y a pas d'expression de *Gata-1* et *Gata-2* dans la région caudale, suggérant que la mutation affecte la genèse des cellules souches. Il est intéressant de noter qu'à ce phénotype s'associent des anomalies des cellules endothéliales, suggérant l'existence d'un progéniteur commun endothélial-hématopoïétique. Une analyse plus détaillée de ces mutations devrait donner des informations utiles à la compréhension du développement hématopoïétique.

Models of developmental hematopoiesis: embryonic stem cells – hematopoietic development
Improvement of the hematopoietic potential of ES cells by a stromal cell line

M.-T. Mitjavila, M.-D. Filippi, F. Le Pesteur, W. Vainchenker and F. Sainteny

INSERM U 362, Hématopoïèse et Cellules Souches, Institut Gustave-Roussy, Pavillon de Recherche 1, 39, rue Camille-Desmoulins, 94805 Villejuif Cedex, France, tel.: (33 1) 45 59 42 33, fax: (33 1) 47 26 92

Embryonic stem (ES) cells are continuously growing cell lines derived from the inner mass of mouse blastocyst [1, 2]. They are unique in that they can be maintained *in vitro* as totipotent cell lines for a number of generations in the presence of leukemia inhibitory factor (LIF). When introduced back into a mouse blastocyst, ES cells will contribute to all tissue types of the embryo [3]. In addition, LIF removal from the culture medium results in the differentiation of ES cells to various tissues including hematopoietic cells [4, 5]. The ES *in vitro* model of differentiation to hematological lineages is potentially of interest to investigate the molecular events involved in the first steps of lineage determination.

The work we report here was aimed at (i) improving the commitment of ES cells towards hematopoiesis *in vitro*. For that, we have developped a system of coculture of ES cells with a stromal cell line, MS-5. The choice of this cell line was based on previous data demonstrating that MS-5 cells, derived from adherent layer of LTBMC [6], have a potent hematopoietic promoting activity since they promote the maintenance of murine pre-CFU-S and the expansion of d12 and d8 CFU-S and myeloid progenitors in long-term culture [7]; (ii) to develop a sequential study of the long-term repopulating potential of ES cell-derived hematopoietic cells.

The system of ES cell differentiation towards hematopoietic cell lines we used is the two step system in methylcellulose. ES cells are cultured in methylcellulose and give rise to embryoid bodies (EBs) which spontaneously differentiate to hemoglobinized cells even in the absence of exogenous stimulators, except for the components of fetal calf serum. Replating EBs disrupted at different times of differentiation (from 6 to 14 days) in conventional progenitor assays results in the development of all types of myeloid progenitors in a well-defined temporal order [4, 5]. MS-5 cells were added to the cutures either during the first step of differentiation, from ES to EBs, or during the second step, from EB to progenitors, or during both. On one hand the progenitor output was determined. On the other hand, in order to detect the presence of cells with long-term repopulating ability, EBs were collected at different times of differentiation and were injected into irradiated mice for long-term survival observation.

The effect of MS-5 cells on the hematopoietic potential of ES cells *in vitro* was first investigated

When MS-5 cells were added during the ES-EB step, a positive dose effect of MS-5 on the formation of EBs was observed. The cloning efficiency of ES cells was about 10% in the absence of MS-5. It was increased almost 3 folds in the presence of 40,000 MS-5 cells when ES cells were plated at low concentration. The effect of MS-5 was less potent when ES cells were plated at higher concentrations. Interestingly, no effect of MS-5 on the expansion of ES cells was observed since we found no changes in EB cellularity whatever the time of EB differentiation, day 6 or day 10. The addition of MS-5 during the ES-EB step resulted in a clear positive dose effect on the progeny of pooled day 6 or day 10 EBs. In fact, the number of progenitors generated per 10^5 cells from day 6 EBs increased seven folds in the presence of 40,000 MS-5 cells. The curve obtained with day 10 EBs was below because the progenitor content of control (day 10 EBs grown without MS-5) was lower than day 6 EBs. This suggests an early commitment of ES cells to primitive stem cells within the EBs. We found two reasons for this increase in the concentration of progenitors. First of all, an increase in the incidence of positive EBs: when day 6 EBs were individually replated and assayed for their progenitor content, there was a positive dose effect of MS-5 cells on the proportion of EB-containing progenitors. Secondly, MS-5 induced an increase in the number of progenitors per EB: never more than 7 colonies per EB was observed in control EB grown without MS-5, whereas with MS-5, as much as 27 colonies per EB could be detected.

Whether the addition of MS-5 cells during the ES-EB step has an effect on the distribution of the progenitors generated by EBs have also been examined. Increasing numbers of MS-5 cells did not result in significant changes in the repartition of day 6 EB-derived progenitors. However, trends can be observed such as increase in G + M + GM+MK-CFU, decrease in BFU-E, increase in Mix colony numbers. No changes at all in the repartition of the types of progenitors generated day 10 EBs were observed.

Since MS-5 cells increase the hematopoietic potential of ES cells, we decided to investigate whether the presence of MS-5 cells would result in an increase in the expression of hematopoietic specific cell-surface markers. This would allow an easier phenotypical charaterisation of the steps of hematological differentiation within the EBs. In fact it is very difficult to do flow cytometry on EB cells. First of all, technically, because of the strong adhesion of embryoid body cells, secondly, because of the low concentration of hematopoietic cells in EBs and last we are concerned by the fact that the markers of adult bone marrow stem cells might not be expressed on EBs cells. AA4.1 has originally been described as being specific for murine fetal liver stem cells [9]. However a recent paper argue against this specificity [10]. The expression of this antigen increases during EB differentiation. This phenomenon was increased in the presence of MS-5. The same profile was obtained with the CD 45 antigen which might suggest that AA 4-1 does not reveal only primitive cells. These preliminary data must be confirmed.

The addition of MS-5 during the step of progenitor generation by embryoid bodies was then examined. A positive effect of MS-5 on the cloning efficiency of progenitors contained in EBs was observed. This effect was higher on day 6 than on day 10 EBs, again suggesting a stronger hematopoietic potential of early EBs.

Lastly, MS-5 cells were added both during the ES-EB and during the EB-progenitor steps. The presence of MS-5 during the growth of progenitors was able to further amplify the effect of MS-5 on the first step of differentiation since a cumulative effect of MS-5 cells on the production of progenitors was found. This represents the optimal conditions for the production of progenitors from ES cells with a progenitor output of one progenitor for five ES cells initially plated.

The effect of MS-5 cells on the hematopoietic potential of ES cells *in vivo* was then examined

EBs grown either in the presence or in the absence of MS-5 cells were injected together with 10^5 syngeneic bone marrow cells to irradiated mice. Since ES cells are male, EB cells were injected to female recipients to allow the determination of the origin of reconstitution. Preliminary data show that 90% of mice grafted with 6 day EBs grown in the absence or in the presence of MS-5 cells, 60% of mice grafted only with syngeneic bone marrow were dead 70 days post-grafting, whereas 60% of mice grafted with EBs plus syngeneic bone marrow cells and 100% of mice grafted with EBs grown on the MS-5 cell line plus syngeneic bone marrow cells were alive. Similar survival curves were observed when cells from 10 day EBs were used. Evaluations of the proportions of ES-derived donor cells in bone marrow, spleen, thymus of the recipient mice are currently under study. We have also experiments in progress where cells from EBs were injected directly into the spleen of irradiated mice or I.V. into newborn mice.

In summary, these preliminary data show that, (1) MS-5 cells enhances the potential of ES cells to differenciate towards hematopoiesis *in vitro* as demonstrated by the increase in the cloning efficiency of ES cells, in the frequency of EB-containing hematopoietic progenitors, in the progenitor EB contents when MS-5 cells were added to the step of EB formation. The presence of MS-5 cells during the development of progenitors from EB cells further increases the progenitor output; (2) the highest percentage of survival (100%) two months after grafting differentiating ES cells wasobtained when mice received, in addition to syngeneic bone marrow, cells from EBs grown in the presence of MS-5.

References

1. Evans MJ, Kaufmann MH. Establishment in culture of pluripotential cells from mouse embryos. *Nature* 1981; 292: 154-156.
2. Martin GR. Isolation of a pluripotent cell line from early mouse embryos cultured in medium conditioned by teratocarcinoma stem cells. *Proc Natln Acad Sci USA* 1981; 78: 7634-7638.
3. Bradley A, Evans M, Kaufman MH, Robertson E. Formation of germ-line chimeras from embryo-derived teratocarcinoma cell lines.*Nature* 1984; 309: 255-256.
4. Doetschmann TC, Eistetter H, Katz M, Schmidt W, Kemler R. The *in vitro* development of blastocyst-derived embryonic stem cell lines: formation of visceral yolk sac, blood islands and myocardium. *J Embryol Exp Morphol* 1985; 87: 27-45.
5. Burket U, Von Rüden T, Wagner EF. Early fetal hematopoïetic development from *in vitro* differential embryonic stem cells. *The New Biologist* 1991; 3: 698-708.
6. Itoh K, Tezuka H, Sakoda H, Konno H, Nagata K, Uchiyama T, Uchino H, Mori KJ. Reproducible establishment of hemopoïetic supportive stromal cell lines from murine bone marrow. *Exp Hematol* 1989; 17: 145-153.
7. Kohari L, Dubart A, Le Pesteur F, Vainchenker W, Sainteny F. Hematopoïetic-promoting activity of the murine stromal cell line MS-5 is not related to the expression of the major hematopoïetic cytokines. *J. Cell Physiol* 1995; 163: 295-304.
8. Keller G, Kennedy M, Papayannopoulou T, Wiles M. Hematopoïetic commitment during embryonic stem cell differentiation in culture. *Mol Cell Biol* 1993; 13, 473-486.
9. Jordan CT, Mc Kearn JP, Lemischka IR. Cellular and developmental properties of fetal hematopoïetic stem cells. *Cell* 1990; 61: 953-963.
10. Trevisan M, Iscove NN. Phenotypic analysis of murine long-term hemopoïetic reconstituting cells quantitated competitively *in vivo* and comparison with more advanced colony-forming progeny. *J Exp Med* 1995; 181: 93-103.

Résumé

MS-5 augmente le potentiel des cellules ES à se différencier vers l'hématopoïèse ; cela a été démontré par l'augmentation de l'efficacité de clonage, de la fréquence des corps embryonnaires, du contenu des corps embryonnaires quand des cellules MS-5 ont été ajoutées à l'étape de formation des corps embryonnaires. La présence des cellules MS-5 pendant le développement des progéniteurs à partir des corps embryoïdes augmente la production des progéniteurs. Par ailleurs, le plus grand pourcentage de survie deux mois après le greffe de corps embryoïdes en voie de différenciation a été obtenu quand les souris ont reçu en plus de la moelle syngénique des cellules de corps embryonnaire cultivées en présence de MS-5.

Ontogeny of hematopoiesis. Aplastic anemia. Eds E. Gluckman, L. Coulombel.
Colloque INSERM/John Libbey Eurotext Ltd. © 1995, Vol. 235, pp. 27-32.

Endothelial differentiation of embryonic stem cells *in vitro:* a model of early vasculogenesis

Daniel Vittet, Marie-Hélène Prandini, Rolande Berthier, Annie Schweitzer, Hervé Martin-Sisteron, Georges Uzan and Elisabetta Dejana

CEA, Laboratoire d'Hématologie, INSERM U 217, DBMS CENG, 17, rue des Martyrs, 38054 Grenoble Cedex 9, France, tel.: (33) 76 88 40 35, fax: (33) 76 88 51 23

Abstract

Mechanisms involved in the regulation of vasculogenesis, the process during which angioblasts differentiate to form blood vessels, remain unclear in mammals. Several studies have outlined that embryonic stem (ES) cells may represent a suitable in vitro *model to study molecular events involved in vascular development. Indeed, blood islands formation and the development of vascular channels have been reported in ES-derived embryoid bodies (EBs). Although their definitive identification as blood vessels was difficult, by the lack of a specific endothelial marker, it was suggested that both primary endothelial differentiation and further vascular maturation were intrinsic to the ES cell culture system.*

Cloning of several specific endothelial markers and generation of related antibodies reacting with presumptive murine endothelial precursors allowed us to study the kinetics of ES cell differentiation to endothelial cells.

Results of both RT-PCR and/or immunofluorescence analysis allow the distinction of successive endothelial maturation stages during spontaneous ES cell differentiation. Expression of PECAM, Flk-1, and tie-2 can be observed in day 4- EBs. Double staining experiments showed that the same cell clusters were expressing both PECAM and Flk-1. Moreover, the development of elongated processes which look like vascular structures can thereafter be observed in day-6 EBs, concomitantly with the appearance of tie-1, MECA-32 antigen and VE-cadherin expression. The presence of vascular structures expressing all these markers was evident in day-11 EBs.

In conclusion, a spontaneous endothelial differentiation occurs during embryoid body formation, leading to the organization of vascular structures, via successive maturation steps. Therefore this in vitro *model appears to be useful for the identification of factors and/or genes which may be potentially involved in the regulation of vasculogenesis.*

Vasculogenesis, the formation of blood vessels by *in situ* differentiation of endothelial cells from their angioblastic precursors, is one of the fundamental process which leads to the development of a primary vasculature in the embryo. During murine embryogenesis, precursor cells of the endothelial lineage are known to arise early within the mesoderm layer; both inside the embryo proper where they are first detected in paraxial and lateral plate mesoderm, and within the yolk sac extraembryonic mesoderm where they constitute part of blood islands [1,2]. However, the sequence of events and molecular mechanisms involved in the regulation of murine vasculogenesis still remain unclear.

Murine embryonic stem (ES) cell lines have previously been established from the pluripotential inner cell mass of blastocysts. These normal cells provide an excellent *in vitro* system to study molecular events involved in lineage determination and differentiation. Indeed, ES cells have been shown to have the potential to generate all embryonic cell lineages when they undergo differentiation [3]. ES cells can be maintained in an undifferentiated state by coculture with an embryonic fibroblast feeder layer or in the presence of LIF which inhibits their differentiation. In the absence of a feeder layer or when LIF is withdrawn, these cells spontaneously undergo differentiation and form embryoid bodies (EBs) containing derivatives of the three primitive germ layers [3].

A few studies have outlined that ES cells may represent a suitable *in vitro* model to study molecular events involved in vascular development. The appearance of blood islands that consist in immature hematopoietic cells surrounded by endothelial cells have been reported on the surface of cystic EBs resulting from the differentiation of many ES cell lines [4]. ES-derived EBs, when transplanted into the peritoneal cavity of syngeneic mice were also shown to develop a primary capillary plexus [5]. More recently, additional data have also given evidence for the development of vascular channels within mature EBs originating from the differentiation of the ES-D3 cell line [6], then suggesting that both primary endothelial differentiation and further vascular maturation were intrinsic to the ES cell culture system.

Unfortunately, analysis of the events leading to vascular development have been hampered by the lack of specific antigenic markers for murine embryonic endothelial cells. Such markers have now been identified and cloned [7-9], and antibodies reacting with presumptive endothelial cell precursors generated [10].

In order to have an experimental *in vitro* system suitable for the analysis of vasculogenesis regulation, we have then further characterized *in vitro* endothelial differentiation from ES cell lines, by looking at the kinetics of expression of specific murine endothelial markers during ES cell in vitro differentiation.

Murine endothelial markers

Several antigenic markers of the murine endothelial cell lineage have recently been characterized *(Table I)*. They allowed extensive analysis of the development of the blood vascular system in murine embryos and related models.

PECAM (CD31), whose murine cDNA has been cloned [8] is an adhesion molecule promoting cell-cell adhesion, which is expressed by the entire vascular endothelium in the adult [11]. In spite of being slightly expressed on cells of various hematopoietic lineages, it has been demonstrated to be one of the earliest marker expressed during endothelial cell differentiation [12].

Several protein tyrosine kinases were also identified, whose expression was restricted primarily to cells of the endothelial lineage. Their spatial and temporal expression during development has suggested that they may play different functional roles within the endothelial lineage. They include Flk-1, which has been characterized to be the functional receptor for VEGF and which is expressed in both the extraembryonic and embryonic mesoderm in regions thought to give raise to the embryonic vasculature [13,14]. tie-1 and tie-2, whose ligand are still unknown defi-

Table I. Antigenic markers expressed by murine endothelial cells and their presumptive precursors.

Markers	cDNA cloned	Antibody	Cellular distribution
PECAM (CD 31)	+	MEC 13-3 (mAb)	endothelial cells (++), platelets (+) myeloid and B lymphoid cells (±) megakaryocytes (±)
Flk1 (VEGF receptor)	+	Polyclonal	endothelial cells
tie 2	+	–	endothelial cells
tie 1	+	–	endothelial cells (+) erythromegakaryoblastic and myeloid leukemic cell lines (±)
VE-Cadherin	+	Polyclonal	endothelial cells
MEC 14-antigen (unknown)	–	MEC 14-7 (mAb)	endothelial cells (capillaries)
MECA 32-antigen (endopeptidase)	–	MECA 32 (mAb)	endothelial cells

ne another class of receptor tyrosine kinase genes expressed in early embryonic vascular system and in maternal decidual vascular endothelial cells where the vasculature undergoes an active angiogenesis [9]. During mouse development, expression of tie-2 was reported to be specifically restricted to cells of the endothelial lineage [15]. In addition, a targeted disruption of the tie-2 gene by homologous recombination has revealed an important functional role of tie-2 during the murine vascular development, since it led to profound and lethal defects in the embryo vasculature [16].

Vascular endothelial (VE)-cadherin or cadherin-5 is a member of the large and growing cadherin family mediating calcium dependent homotypic cell adhesion. VE-cadherin has been found to be specifically located at endothelial cells intercellular boundaries in all vascular beds [17]; and recent data has demonstrated that VE-cadherin is an early marker of endothelial cell differentiation *in vivo* [unpublished observation].

Few monoclonal antibodies reacting with murine endothelial cells and their presumptive precursors have also been generated. They are of great potential use to identify early endothelial cells. Among them two monoclonal antibodies, MEC 13-3 and MEC 14-7, obtained by immunizing a Lewis rat with the murine polyoma middle T transformed endothelial line t-end-1, which presented a specific reactivity with mouse endothelial cells [18; C. Garlanda, personal communication]. MECA-32 antibody which is derived from rats immunized with murine lymph node stroma, was found to be reactive with a specific mouse endothelial cell surface antigen in most embryonic and adult tissues [10].

Endothelial markers expression during *in vitro* ES cell differentiation

Analysis of the kinetics of expression of endothelial markers during *in vitro* ES cell differentiation was accomplished by using both reverse transcriptase-coupled polymerase chain reaction

(RT-PCR) and immunofluorescence studies. Two ES cell lines were used during the course of our experiments: ES-CCE [19] and ES-CJ7 [20], which have given similar results.

RT-PCR results showed that distinct genes are induced at different time points during ES cell differentiation. Flk-1 gene expression was rapidly upregulated during EBs development since it can be detected as soon as day 3. PECAM and tie-2 genes were found to be already expressed in undifferentiated ES cells. Although such a tie-2 expression was previously reported in the ES-D3 cell line [14], this was rather unexpected for PECAM. Thereafter, when the cells are induced to differentiate by removing LIF from the culture medium, both genes appeared to be temporarily shut off before reexpression within EBs by day 4. VE-cadherin and tie-1 transcripts cannot be detected before day 5; after which time expression of all these marker genes appeared rather sustained up to day 11.

Immunofluorescence studies were consistent with the RT-PCR results. PECAM immunostaining was observed on undifferentiated ES cells and by day 4 of differentiation mainly located at intercellular junctions of some cell clusters within some bodies.

Double staining experiments showed that the same cells were also expressing Flk-1. Expressions of PECAM and Flk-1 were observed to peak by day 6, where a great proportion of EBs were found to be positive for both markers. Their commitment towards the endothelial lineage was confirmed by MECA-32 antigen expression, which is first detected within some EBs by day 5 and which presented a similar distribution pattern than PECAM and Flk-1 by day 6. At this stage, both VE-cadherin and MEC-14 antigen expression could be detected; and after day 8 at least 30 to 40% EBs were observed to have engaged a spontaneous differentiation towards the endothelial lineage. The presence of vascular-like structures expressing all these markers was evident in day-11 EBs, where flattened and elongated processes closely ressembling primitive vascular channels can be seen both at the periphery and inside EBs. Serial sections of EBs stained by PECAM or MECA-32 antibodies showing such structures are illustrated in *Figure 1*.

Results of the kinetics of endothelial marker expression during *in vitro* ES cell lines differentiation, obtained by both RT-PCR and immunofluorescence analysis indicate that vasculogenesis seem to proceed through successive maturation stages. PECAM, Flk-1 ant tie-2 expressions

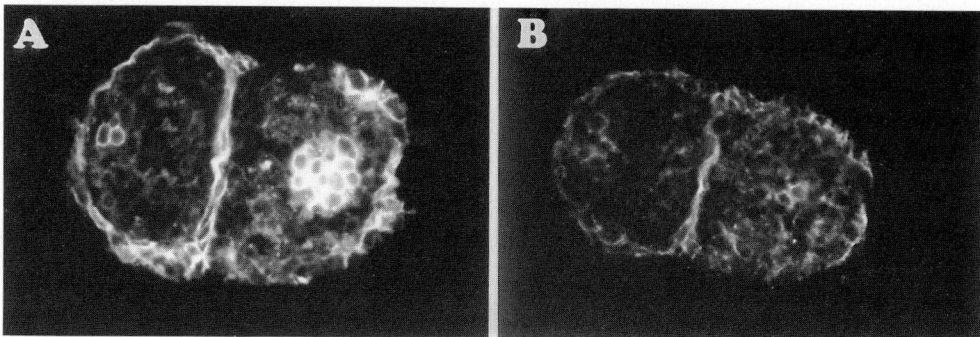

Figure 1. Immunofluorescent staining of serial sections of CJ7-ES-derived EBs. EBs formed 11 days after seeding 2,500 ES cells/ml in semi-solid culture medium (1% methylcellulose in IMDM) supplemented with 15% fetal calf serum were collected. Cryostat sections (10µm) of sucrose-embedded EBs were stained either with an anti-murine PECAM monoclonal antibody (A), or with MECA-32 antibody (B) which specifically reacts against a murine endothelial surface marker. Fixation of first antibodies was revealed by FITC-Goat anti rat IgG, and slides were mounted in antiquench mixture containing DABCO before examination by fluorescence microscopy.

appear to reflect early commitment towards the endothelial lineage, whereas MECA-32 antigen, MEC-14 antigen, tie-1 and VE-cadherin expression seems to correspond to a later maturation stage occurring before the assembly of developing vascular structures.

Conclusions and prospects

By looking at specific endothelial markers expression during ES cell lines differentiation, we have confirmed that ES cells efficiently and spontaneously differentiate into the endothelial lineage, leading to the organization of vascular-like structures, with a reproducible kinetic pattern. In addition, we got evidence for successive developmental stages within the endothelial lineage. Then, this *in vitro* model, seems to recapitulate the initial steps of *in vivo* vasculogenesis, and appears useful to analyze regulation of expression of endothelial specific genes, and to identify genes or factors which may be involved in the regulation of early vasculogenesis.

References

1. Risau W. Embryonic angiogenesis factors. *Pharmac Ther* 1991; 51: 371-376.
2. Coffin JD, Harrison J, Schwartz S, Heimark R. Angioblast differentiation and morphogenesis of the vascular endothelium in the mouse embryo. *Dev Biol* 1991; 148: 51-62.
3. Smith AG. Mouse embryo stem cells; their identification, propagation and manipulation. *Semin Cell Biol* 1992; 3: 385-399.
4. Doetschman TC, Eistetter H, Katz M, Schmidt W, Kemler R. The *in vitro* development of blastocyst-derived embryonic stem cell lines: formation of visceral yolk sac, blood islands and myocardium. *J Embryol Exp Morph* 1985; 87: 27-45.
5. Risau W, Sariola H, Zerwes HG, Sasse J, Ekblom P, Kemler R, Doetschman T. Vasculogenesis and angiogenesis in embryonic-stem-cell-derived embryoid bodies. *Development* 1988; 102: 471-478.
6. Wang R, Clark R, Bautch VL. Embryonic stem cell-derived cystic embryoid bodies form vascular channels: an *in vitro* model of blood vessel development. *Development* 1992; 114: 303-316.
7. Oelrichs RB, Reid HH, Bernard O, Ziemiecki A, Wilks AF. NYK/FLK-1: A putative receptor protein tyrosine kinase isolated from E10 embryonic neuroepithelium is expressed in endothelial cells of the developing embryo. *Oncogene* 1993; 8: 11-18.
8. Xie Y, Muller WA. Molecular cloning and adhesive properties of murine platelet/endothelial cell adhesion molecule 1. *Proc Natl Acad Sci USA* 1993; 90: 5569-5573.
9. Sato TN, Qin Y, Kozak CA, Audus KL. Tie-1 and tie-2 define another class of putative receptor tyrosine kinase genes expressed in early embryonic vascular system. *Proc Natl Acad Sci USA* 1993; 90: 9355-9358.
10. Leppink DM, Bishop DK, Sedmak DD, Henry ML, Ferguson RM. Inducible expression of an endothelial cell antigen on murine myocardial vasculature in association with interstitial cellular infiltration. *Transplantation* 1989; 48:874-877.
11. Delisser HM, Newman PJ, Albelda SM. Molecular and functional aspects of PECAM-1/CD31. *Immunol Today* 1994; 15: 490-495.
12. Baldwin HS, Shen HM, Yan HC, Delisser HM, Chung A, Mic Kanin C, Trask T, Kinschbaum NE, Newman PJ, Albelda SM, Buck CA. Platelet endothelial cell adhesion molecule-1 (PECAM-1/CD31): alternatively spliced, functionally distinct isoforms expressed during mammalian cardiovascular development. *Development* 1994; 120: 2539-2553.
13. Millauer B, Wizigmann-Voos S, Schnürch H, Martinez R, Moller NPH, Risau W, Ullrich A. High affinity VEGF binding and developmental expression suggest Flk-1 as a major regulator of vasculogenesis and angiogenesis. *Cell* 1993; 72: 835-846.
14. Yamaguchi TP, Dumont DJ, Conlon RA, Breitman ML, Rossant J. Flk-1, an flt-related receptor tyrosine kinase is an early marker for endothelial cell precursors. *Development* 1993; 118: 489-498.

15. Schnürch H, Risau W. Expression of tie-2 a member of a novel family of receptor tyrosine kinases, in the endothelial cell lineage. *Development* 1993; 119: 957-968.
16. Dumont DJ, Gradwohl G, Fong GH, Pari MC, Gertsenstein M, Auerbach A, Breitman ML. Dominant-negative and targeted null mutations in the endothelial receptor tyrosine kinase, tek, reveal a critical role in vasculogenesis of the embryo. *Genes & Dev* 1994; 8: 1897-1909.
17. Lampugnani MG, Resnati M, Raiteri M, Pigott R, Pisacane A, Houen G, Ruco LP, Dejana E. A novel endothelial-specific membrane protein is a marker of cell-cell contacts. *J Cell Biol* 1992; 118: 1511-1522.
18. Vecchi A., Garlanda C, Lampugnani MG, Resnati M, Matteucci C, Stoppaciaro A, Schnurch H, Risau W, Ruco L, Mantovani A, Dejana E. Monoclonal antibodies specific for endothelial cells of mouse blood vessels. Their application in the identification of adult and embryonic endothelium. *Eur J Cell Biol* 1994; 63:247-254.
19. Robertson E, Bradley A, Kuehn M, Evans M. Germ-line transmission of genes introduced into cultured pluripotential cells by retroviral vector. *Nature* 1986; 323: 445-448.
20. Swiatek PJ, Gridley T. Perinatal lethality and defects in hindbrain development in mice homozygous for a targeted mutation of the zinc finger gene Krox20. *Gene & Dev* 1993; 7: 2071-2084.

Résumé

Les mécanismes impliqués dans la régulation de la vasculogenèse sont mal connus. Plusieurs études récentes ont indiqué que la différenciation *in vitro* des cellules souches embryonnaires (ES) pourrait représenter un bon modèle pour l'analyse des événements moléculaires impliqués lors du développement vasculaire. Des travaux ont en effet rapporté la formation d'îlots sanguins et le développement de tubules vasculaires dans les corps embryonnaires (EBs) issus de la différenciation des cellules ES. Bien que les phases du développement vasculaire dans les EBs n'aient pas été caractérisées, ces études ont indiqué que les cellules ES avaient la capacité de se différencier spontanément vers le lignage endothélial aboutissant à l'organisation d'un réseau vasculaire primitif.

Afin d'avoir un modèle expérimental *in vitro* permettant l'analyse des facteurs et des mécanismes qui régulent la vasculogenèse, nous avons cherché à caractériser plus avant la différenciation des cellules ES dans le lignage endothélial. Dans ce but, nous avons analysé la cinétique d'expression de plusieurs marqueurs antigéniques des cellules endothéliales murines au cours de cette différenciation.

Les résultats, provenant des analyses par RT-PCR et par immunofluorescence, de l'expression de ces antigènes permettent de distinguer des stades successifs de maturation précoce des cellules de la lignée endothéliale. PECAM, Flk-1 et tie-2 sont exprimés dès le jour 4. A ce stade les expériences de double marquage révèlent que PECAM et Flk-1 sont exprimés par les même cellules. Les expressions de tie-1, de l'antigène reconnu par l'anticorps MECA-32 et de la VE-cadhérine ne sont observées qu'au jour 6, et la présence de structures vasculaires n'apparaît de façon évidente qu'au jour 11 de la différenciation.

Ces études confirment le potentiel des cellules ES à se différencier spontanément dans le lignage endothélial. De plus, l'analyse de l'expression de marqueurs spécifiques permet de distinguer plusieurs stades de développement du système endothélial, qui paraissent récapituler les événements initiaux de la vasculogenèse. La différenciation *in vitro* des cellules ES semble donc constituer un excellent modèle pour l'étude du développement vasculaire.

Primitive hematopoietic stem cells and endothelial cells in the mouse yolk sac

Li-Sheng Lu, Shur-Jen Wang and Robert Auerbach

Laboratory for Developmental Biology, University of Wisconsin, 1117 West Johnson Street, Madison, WI 53706 USA, tel.: (212) 327 7533, fax: (212) 327 8232

Overview

The yolk sac is the first site of hematopoiesis during mammalian development. The yolk sac is also the first site of blood vessel formation. Development of the blood islands in the yolk sac is an integrated process in which these two developmental events, hematopoiesis and vasculogenesis proceed in concert. In this brief review of the studies of yolk sac development carried out in our own laboratory we will describe our experiments that address separately the identification, isolation and differentiation of the hematopoietic stem cells and of the vascular endothelial cell precursors [1-6], and we will then consider our hypothesis that the two processes, vasculogenesis and hematopoiesis, are intimately related and causally interdependent. To gain a proper perspective on our studies, the reader is referred to parallel research carried out in other laboratories [7-10].

Within the mouse yolk sac, the primitive hematopoietic stem cell population present on day 8+ of embryonic development can be identified on the basis of the expression of specific phenotypic markers. These include: 1) the expression on the cell surface of glycoconjugates that are recognized by the lectin wheat germ agglutinin; 2) a buoyant cell density lower than that of the preponderant cell population found in the yolk sac (density <1.077); 3) the expression of a cell surface antigen recognized by antibody AA4.1; 4) the absence of cell surface properties that promote adhesion to plastic; and 5) a characteristic profile of forward and side scatter signals when examined by flow cytometry. A still more primitive precursor cell is also present in the yolk sac. This cell appears to be moderately adherent to plastic and does not yet express the AA4.1-reactive cell surface antigen (R. Snodgrass, personal communication). Whether this cell has the ability to generate not only the hematopoietic lineages but endothelial cell lineages as well, i.e. whether this cell is a true hemangioblast, is not known but is currently under investigation.

The earliest endothelial cell precursors have also been identified at day 8+ of yolk sac development. As vasculogenesis proceeds, endothelial cells acquire their own panel of markers. These include 1) presence of a receptor for acetylated low density lipoprotein (acLDL); 2) expression of a characteristic pattern of cell surface glycoconjugates, including those recognized by the Griffonica simplifolia agglutinin and (for certain strains) the Dolichos biflorus agglutinin;

3) expression of cell surface antigens recognized by MECA-99 and H513E3 antibodies; 4) the presence of the vascular cell adhesion molecule VCAM-1; 5) the presence of cell surface-associated angiotensin-converting enzyme; and 6) the presence of von Willebrand factor-associated antigen (vWF-Ag) [ref. 6 and unpublished observations]. When first detectable, endothelial cell precursors are adherent cells, and adherence to plastic is a prime means of early separation of vascular endothelial cells from hemato-poietic stem cells.

Hematopoietic stem cells in the yolk sac

In our earlier studies of unfractionated non-adherent yolk sac cells we were able to document transient differentiation of cells obtained from 9-12 day embryos to generate Thy 1+ and IgM producing lymphocytes as well as macrophages and mast cells *in vitro* [1]. Subsequently, we were able to demonstrate that unfractionated yolk sac cells obtained as early as on embryonic day 8 (4-10 somites) could be induced to enter stem cell-depleted thymus rudiments and there differentiate into the various definitive T-cell subsets. These experiments were consistent with the view that within the yolk sac there might be primitive multipotential progenitor cells capable of giving rise to several different blood cell lineages.

Using protocols initially developed for the study of fetal liver hematopoiesis, Huang and Auerbach were able to identify a small minority of cells which contained the principal if not only precursor cells with the capability of developing into the various blood cell lineages. These protocols, which included density gradient separation, immunocytoadherence, adherence to plastic and cell sorting on the basis of lectin-binding properties yielded a population of cells among which >2% were able to generate B cells when grown on an S17 stromal feeder layer, a similar number could generate T cells when provided with a thymic microenvironment, and >20% could undergo myelopoiesis when grown in methyl cellulose. The same population of cells also could yield nucleated erythroid colonies, with the subsequent generation of mature, non-nucleated erythrocytes (Huang and Auerbach, unpublished observations).

Clonal proliferation of multipotential hematopoietic stem cells

These experiments did not, however, provide conclusive evidence for a single multipotential hematopoietic progenitor cell. To address this question directly, we undertook cloning experiments in which purified yolk sac cells were deposited singly into microwell culture plates to achieve single cell cloning. A combination of growth factors was used to promote *in vitro* differentiation. Using this approach, we were able to obtain predominantly (>90%) mixed myeloid (granulocyte/macrophage) colonies. However, only 2 of 30 colonies contained cells that could be transferred for further subculture.

Endothelial cells in the yolk sac

When plastic-adherent cells are isolated from the embryonic yolk sac they rapidly generate cultures that are comprised almost entirely of macrophages and mast cells. Although it is possible by careful selection and choice of growth factors to obtain some endothelial cell isolates, we decided to take advantage of a gain-of-function proto-oncogene *(fps/fes)* that increases the vascularity of the developing embryo. Several clonal cell lines that express the appropriate endothelium-specific markers and that can form three-dimensional structures *in vitro* have been obtained (Wang and Auerbach, submitted).

Role of endothelial cells in the regulation of hematopoiesis

Within the yolk sac, hematopoietic stem cell proliferation normally takes place in the blood islands, where there is a close proximity between the cells comprising the primitive vasculature and those destined either to differentiate into erythroid cells or to migrate to sites of subsequent hematopoiesis such as the thymus, liver, spleen or lymph nodes. Thus it seemed logical to consider the possibility that the endothelial cells which comprise the yolk sac microenvironment might have a specialized function in promoting stem cell proliferation. Having previously established clonally derived, stable yolk sac endothelial cell lines, we tested the ability of several of these to support yolk sac stem cell maintenance and proliferation.

The results of these studies show a selectivity even among yolk sac cell lines, and to date only one clonal cell line has been shown to support long term maintenance of stem cells. In the absence of added growth factors at least some of the stem cells can be maintained for at least three passages while retaining the ability to differentiate subsequently when placed in an appropriate microenvironment (e.g. the ability to generate B220+, µchain+ B cell precursors when grown on S17 feeder layers).

Potential importance of yolk sac hematopoietic stem cells

One of the striking differences between stem cells from the yolk sac and those derived from later stages of embryogenesis is that yolk sac cells lack many of the cell surface antigens, including those of the major histocompatibility complex, that elicit graft rejection. Thus they may be the best source of cells for transplantation. We already know that fewer than 100 cells isolated and purified from the mouse yolk sac and injected into histocompatible hosts, can, in time, generate hematopoietic cells in the blood, spleen, thymus and peritoneal cavity. With the ability we now have to maintain and expand this primitive yolk sac stem cell population we are in a position to exploit techniques of genetic manipulation. Thus the yolk sac cells may be able to serve as a vector for gene transfer. Moreover, there are good reasons to believe that the techniques that we have developed for the study of mouse yolk sac hematopoietic stem cells will be applicable to other mammalian species including humans.

References

1. Globerson A, Woods V, Abel L, Morrissey L, Cairns JS, Kukulansky T, Kubai L and Auerbach R. *In vitro* differentiation of embryonic yolk sac cells. *Differentiation* 1987; 36:185-193.
2. Liu C-P, Auerbach R. Ontogeny of murine T cells: Thymus regulated development of T cell receptor-bearing cells derived from embryonic yolk sac. *Eur J Immunol* 1991; 21:1849-1855.
3. Liu C-P, Auerbach R. *In vitro* development of murine T cells from pre-thymic and pre-liver embryonic yolk sac hematopoietic stem cells. *Development* 1991; 113:1315-1323.

4. Huang H, Auerbach R. Identification and characterization of hematopoietic stem cells from the yolk sac of the early mouse embryo. *Proc Natl Acad Sci* USA 1993; 90:10110-10114.
5. Huang H, Zettergren LD, Auerbach R. *In vitro* differentiation of B cells and myeloid cells from the early mouse embryo and its extraembryonic yolk sac. *Exp Hematol* 1994; 22:19-25.
6. Wang S-J, Greer P, Auerbach R. Isolation and propagation of yolk sac-derived endothelial cells from a hypervascular transgenic mouse expressing a gain-of-function fps/fes proto-oncogene. *Amer J Pathol* 1995 (submitted).
7. Cumano A, Furlonger C, Paige CJ. Differentiation and characterization of B-cell precursors detected in the yolk sac and embryo body of embryos beginning at the 10- to 12- somite stage. *Proc Natl Acad Sci* USA 1993; 11:593-601.
8. Medvinsky AL, Samoylina NL, MÅller AM, Dzierak EA. An early pre-liver embryonic source of CFU-S in the developing mouse. *Nature* 1993; 364:64-67.
9. Palacios R, Imhof BA. At day 8-8.5 of mouse development the yolk sac, not the embryo proper, has lymphoid precursor potential *in vivo* and *in vitro*. *Proc Natl Acad Sci* USA 1993; 90:6581-6585.
10. Godin I, Dieterlen-Lievre F, Cumano A. Emergence of multipotent hemopoietic cells in the yolk sac and paraortic splanchnopleura in mouse embryos, beginning at 8.5 days postcoitus. *Proc Natl Acad Sci* USA 1995; 92:773-777.

Résumé

Ce travail pose le problème de la potentialité des progéniteurs hématopoïétiques présents dans la vésicule vitelline d'embryons de souris. Plusieurs études antérieures de cette équipe ont identifié dans la vésicule vitelline des progéniteurs capables de différenciation dans les lignées myéloïdes (test en milieu semi-solide), lymphoïde B (coculture sur des cellules stromales S17) et lymphoïde T (coculture dans un environnement thymique). Dans l'étude actuelle, les auteurs ont enrichi les progéniteurs de la vésicule vitelline par des étapes successives de séparation sur gradient de densité, immunoadhérence (antigène AA4.1) et tri au cytofluoromètre et ont analysé à l'échelon unicellulaire la capacité de ces progéniteurs à se différencier dans les différentes lignées myéloïdes en présence de combinaisons de cytokines. Par aillleurs, des lignées de cellules endothéliales ont été obtenues à partir de la vésicule vitelline d'animaux transgéniques pour l'oncogène *fps/fes* et leur capacité à stimuler l'expression des propriétés de cellules souches hématopoïétiques de la vésicule vitelline a été testée. Une de ces lignées semble être capable de permettre une certaine amplification de progéniteurs immatures ayant conservé une potentialité lymphoïde B.

Embryonic and early fetal development of the human hematopoietic system in the yolk sac, dorsal aorta, liver and bone marrow

Manuela Tavian[1], Pierre Charbord[2], Laurent Humeau[1], Laure Coulombel[3], Dominique Luton[1], Françoise Dieterlen-Lièvre[1] and Bruno Péault[1]

[1] Institut d'Embryologie Cellulaire et Moléculaire du CNRS et du Collège de France, CNRS UMR 9924, Nogent-sur-Marne, France, tel.: (33 1) 48 73 60 00, fax: (33 1) 48 73 43 77; [2] Laboratoire d'Étude de l'Hématopoïèse, Établissement de Transfusion Sanguine, Besançon, France; [3] Laboratoire Hématopoïèse et Cellules Souches, INSERM U 362, Villejuif, France

Abstract

The embryonic and early fetal development of the human hematopoietic system has been examined from 3 to 28 weeks of gestation. Immunohistochemistry was used to detect markers for the vascular, stromal and myeloerythroid cell compartments in developing blood-forming tissues. High CD34 expression was ubiquitous on vascular endothelial cells from the earliest stage tested, at the exception of embryonic liver blood vessels whose endothelium was weakly labeled to negative. In contrast, scattered, round hematopoietic $CD34^+$ cells were consistently detected from week 4 to 5 and onwards in the liver rudiment where foci of erythroblasts and monocytes appeared simultaneously. The early development of the bone marrow was marked by the rapid and simultaneous invasion, at 8 weeks, of the cartilaginous long bone rudiments by $CD68^+$ osteoclast precursors, $CD34^+$ vascular sprouts and osteoblast precursors, leading to the establishment of large vascular sinuses between ossifying trabeculae. Primary marrow logettes, always centered by an arteriole, were formed in the diaphysis. Endogenous erythro- and granulopoiesis developed within these logettes from week 11 between the media of the arterioles and the endothelial cells bordering the large sinuses. Unexpectedly, no $CD34^+$ hematopoietic precursors were detected in the early developing marrow.

Strikingly, a dense population of hematopoietic $CD34^+$ cells was observed to develop in association with the ventral wall of the aorta during the fifth week of gestation. These exhibited a similar anatomic localization as the intraembryonic stem cells identified in the avian and murine embryo as the forerunners of the whole adult blood system.

In the early ontogeny of amniote vertebrates, hematopoiesis begins before the onset of organogenesis in an extraembryonic appendage, the yolk sac, then transiently proceeds in some abdominal viscera, the liver and spleen before getting stabilized for the lifetime in the bone marrow and thymus [1]. At these early stages, the organization of the hematopoietic hierarchy is essentially similar to its adult counterpart; yet, the study of human embryonic and fetal blood-forming tissues presents several practical advantages: regular procurement of precisely staged, healthy tissues is possible; these rudiments are usually easier to grow in organ or cell culture, and definitely much more amenable for engraftment into immunodeficient animal hosts [2] than adult tissues. More fundamentally, some key aspects of blood stem cell emergence, expansion and differentiation may be more easily studied during the highly dynamic process of embryonic development than in the model of steady-state adult hematopoiesis. It may be reasonably assumed, for example, that the settlement of hematopoiesis in the developing bone cavities is preceded by a phase of active stem cell recruitment and proliferation, which yet takes place inside a stromal structure that should be easier to describe than that of the blood cell-packed adult marrow. Thus, analysis of the early fetal bone marrow might give clues to the relationship between hematopoietic stem cells and their regulating microenvironment.

However attractive the model of embryonic hematopoiesis can be, very few studies are yet available on the early ontogeny of the human blood system. We have attempted to circumvent that limitation, in order to establish a firm basis for further studies making use of embryonic and fetal blood-forming tissues, by using markers of human hematopoietic, endothelial, smooth muscle, stromal cells and fibroblasts to describe the onset of hematogenesis on tissue sections of the yolk sac, embryonic liver and fetal bone marrow from 3 to 28 weeks of gestation.

Vitelline and hepatic early hematopoiesis

The yolk sac is the primal site of blood cell formation in vertebrates; it is also the only hematopoietic tissue that generates its own stem cells in situ from the pluripotential mesodermal "hemangioblasts" [3].

The earliest blood cell development, i.e. the appearance at the contact of yolk sac endoderm of solid hemangioblastic cell clusters followed by their transformation into blood island-containing vessels, is almost impossible to study in man since it happens during the third week of gestation. In the earliest yolk sac sample we could obtain, at 23 days of gestation (i.e. post-conception), blood vessels were already differentiated and hollow. Of note, all endothelial cells at that stage were already brightly CD34-positive which confirms recently published results on the early ontogeny of the CD34 antigen in the mouse [4]. Occasionally, a few round $CD34^+$ cells identified as hematopoietic precursors were seen, adherent to the endothelium. As expected, the only differentiated blood cells encountered in the yolk sac at that stage were primitive erythrocytes, expressing glycophorin A.

As early as 4.5 weeks, extravascular erythroid cell clusters were also detected in the hepatic rudiment, together with disseminated $CD68^+$ cells. At that same stage and onwards, $CD34^+$ round hematopoietic precursor cells were visible in the embryonic liver, intermingled as single cells in the developing cords of hepatocytes. However, in striking contrast with all the other embryonic and fetal blood-forming tissues, hepatic endothelial cells were consistently CD34-negative, or very faintly stained.

Further hematopoietic development in the embryonic liver was marked by the considerable expansion of the erythroid lineage, and by the establishment of the $CD68^+$ Kupffer cell compartment.

Early ontogeny of the bone marrow

Our interest has been mainly focused on the initial development of the marrow cavities in long bones. Bone marrow, the chief blood-forming tissue in the adult mammal, is also the last one that develops in ontogenesis, when hematopoiesis is already extinct in the yolk sac, transiently proceeding in the liver and actively developing in the thymus [1]. The early ontogeny of the bone marrow cavity has been described in several histologic studies in the animal [5-7] and human embryo [8,9]. In the process of endochondral ossification, surrounding mesenchymal cells and blood vessels rapidly invade the calcified cartilage of the diaphyseal region of long bone rudiments. Cartilage resorption is paralleled with the establishment of the bone-modeling osteoblast and osteoclast cell populations, leading to the formation of bony trabeculae separated by vascular spaces and loose mesenchymal areas. The analysis of blood cell development in avian embryo chimeras has revealed that embryonic bone marrow, like other blood-forming tissues but the yolk sac, is colonized by circulating hematopoietic cells [10] that include the forerunners of the osteoclast cell population [11]. We have explored that phase of human development in deeper detail by performing the immune detection, on tissue sections of long bone rudiments between 6 and 28 weeks of gestation, of the hematopoietic, vascular and stromal cell compartments identified with specific markers [12].

The development of the human long bone marrow could be subdivided into 5 successive steps:

The uncolonized cartilaginous bone rudiment (week 6 to 8.5)

As early as week 6, the epiphyseal and diaphyseal regions of long bone rudiments were already demarcated, yet constituted solely of dilated chondrocytes. The presumptive shaft of the bone was closely surrounded by numerous capillary vessels – lined with $CD34^+$ endothelial cells – and by $CD68^+$ monocytic cells.

Bone marrow cavities appear from week 8.5 to 9

Bone marrow spaces appeared as a result of a very rapid chondrolysis/cell colonization process. Osteoblasts closely surrounded the remaining cartilage islets, as did $CD68^+$ osteoclasts, some of them already multinucleated. No other hematopoietic cells could be detected at that stage.

Development of the hematopoietic stroma (week 9-10.5)

As cartilage withdrew and ossification started, large vascular sinuses and a loose connective tissue developed, that included the "logettes" where hematopoiesis later proceeds. These structures which connect to the ossifying trabeculae through short pedicles, and thus appear on sections as peninsulas extending inside the sinuses, are framed by a loose network of $CD45^-$ cells containing fibrillar material. They always include a central arteriole whose endothelial cells, as those which limit the sinusal space, brightly express CD34. No hematopoietic cells but osteoclasts were detected at these stages either.

Onset of medullary hematopoiesis (week 10.5 to 15)

At week 10.5, medullary logettes have enlarged and are then organized around a differentiated central artery surrounded by a thick layer of smooth muscle actin (αSM)-positive muscle cells. Dendritic-like αSM^+ myoid cells are also interspersed in the logette stroma, into which they extend long winding tails that contact already numerous hematopoietic cells. The earliest blood cells that develop within the bone marrow include $CD15^+$ myelocytes and, to a lesser extent, glycophorin A^+ erythroblasts that span, at least, the E1 and E2 differentiation stages. Monocytic cells, as well as megakaryocytes, are very rare. At week 15, hematopoietic logettes are replete with granulocytes and erythroblasts while the surrounding sinuses are still virtually devoid of hematopoietic cells. It is important to notice again that this early settlement of hematogenesis within the bone cavity proceeds in the complete absence of CD34$^+$ hematopoietic precursor cells.

From week 16 onwards, long bones evolve towards their definitive pattern

Solid bone replaces progressively the hematopoietic areas of the diaphysis, which are displaced towards the meta- and epiphyseal regions.

An intraembryonic site of CD34$^+$ hematopoietic cell production

According to the classic "hematogenous" theory of blood cell development [10], hematopoietic stem cells are produced at one stage and in one site only, the extraembryonic mesoderm of the yolk sac, from which they egress to seed the rudiments of all other blood-forming tissues. Such a central role of the yolk sac had to be, however, reconsidered to accommodate the results of experiments in which heterospecific associations of yolk sacs and embryo bodies were performed in the quail/chicken model. In such chimeras, the yolk sac was observed to solely contribute primitive erythrocytes, whereas all other blood cell lineages through adult life were the progeny of stem cells derived from the embryo itself, that were later allocated to progenitor cell clusters developing in the vicinity of the floor of the dorsal aorta (reviewed in [13]). More recently, the homologous embryonic territory in the mouse, the paraaortic splanchnopleura and derived aorta/gonad/mesonephros region was also shown to be the source of pluripotential hematopoietic stem cells [14-17]. In striking correlation with these studies on animal embryos, we have observed the presence of a dense population of round CD34$^+$ cells closely associated with the endothelium of the ventral wall of the aorta, from 5 weeks of gestation, in the immediate preumbilical region of the human embryo (i.e. just underneath the anterior limb rudiment), on a length spanning one to two somites. These CD34$^+$ cells are hematopoietic and not endothelial, since they are CD45$^+$, Ulex europaeus-. They express none of the differentiation markers tested: CD15, CD68 and glycophorin A.

These intraaortic clusters of several hundred hematopoietic CD34$^+$ cells have been observed in 6 out of 7 5-week embryos, but were never detected at earlier stages. Most suggestively, those cells develop in the same anatomic location, and at an equivalent developmental stage as the intraembryonic aorta-associated hematopoietic stem cells which have been shown in birds and in the mouse to be at the origin of the whole definitive blood system. By extrapolation, we propose that those aorta-associated CD34$^+$ cells are the real stem of human hematopoiesis [18].

These observations have to be paralleled with the recent demonstration, in the group of one of us, of the existence of a population of pluripotential HPP-CFC in the 5-week eviscerated human embryo, whereas the yolk sac and hepatic rudiment at the same stage contain committed myeloid precursors only [19].

Conclusion

The main purpose of our descriptive study of embryonic and early fetal hematopoietic development in man was the identification of anatomical sites of blood stem cell generation, expansion and differentiation. At all stages tested, CD34$^+$ hematopoietic cells were rare and scattered in the yolk sac and liver rudiment, where they did not seem to be associated with a privileged stromal environment. Moreover, very surprisingly and in contrast with our working hypothesis, establishment of hematopoiesis in the marrow cavity was not preceded by an influx of CD34$^+$ hematopoietic cells. We could in fact never detect such presumptive stem cells in the developing logettes, which can be interpreted in different ways: i) extremely few CD34$^+$ cells colonize the marrow rudiment and/or their expression of CD34 is so transient that we always missed them; ii) more provocatively, hematopoietic stem cells are intrinsic in origin to the early marrow environment, a candidate source for those being the numerous CD34$^+$ immature endothelial cells present at that stage in the bone rudiment.

Vascular cells (endothelium and abluminal myoid cells) are actually the main cellular compartments of the environment where medullary hematopoiesis initially develops. We could describe that stroma with some accuracy before high numbers of blood cells obscured it. It is framed by loosely arranged non hematopoietic mesodermal cells into which long dendritic processes from smooth muscle actin-containing myoid cells are intermingled. The respective roles of these distinct stromal cell populations are under current *in vitro* study.

Finally, and most unexpectedly, we have identified a compact accumulation of hematopoietic CD34$^+$ cells associated with the floor of the dorsal aorta, in a precise time- and site-dependent manner. This clearly represents the densest local concentration of hematopoietic CD34$^+$ cells observed throughout ontogeny and adult life, and calls forth the characterization of the factors involved in the production, expansion, adherence and differentiation of these early stem cells which, if we extrapolate recent findings in animal embryos, might represent the source of the definitive human hematopoietic system.

Work supported by a grant from Systemix Inc., by a Contrat de Recherches INSERM, Direction des Études et Techniques (DRET n° 92-132) and by the Fonds d'Organisation pour la Recherche en Transfusion Sanguine.

References

1. Metcalf D, Moore MAS. Embryonic aspects of haematopoiesis. In: Neuberger A, Tatum EL, eds. *Haemopoietic Cells. Amsterdam: North Holland Publ,* 1971: 172-271.
2. Péault B, Namikawa R, Krowka J, McCune JM. Experimental human hematopoiesis in immunodeficient SCID mice engrafted with fetal blood-forming organs. In: Edwards RG, ed. *Fetal Tissue Transplants in Medicine. Cambridge: Cambridge University Press,* 1992: 77-95.
3. Sabin FR. Studies on the origin of blood vessels and of red blood corpuscules as seen in the living blastoderm of chicks during the second day of incubation. *Contrib Embryol Carnegie Institute Pub* 9-36 1920; 214-62.
4. Young PE, Baumhueter S, Lasky LA. The sialomucin CD34 is expressed on hematopoietic cells and blood vessels during murine development. *Blood* 1995; 85: 96-105.
5. Bloom W. The embryogenesis of mammalian blood. In: Downey H, ed. *Handbook of Hematology,* vol II. *London: Harper and Row,* 1938: 865.
6. Sabin FR, Miller FR. Normal bone marrow. In: Downey H, ed. *Handbook of Haematology,* Vol III. *New York: Hoeber,* 1938: 1791.
7. Hamilton HL. Lillie's development of the chick. *New-York: Henry Holt & Company,* 1952.
8. Streeter GL. Developmental horizons in human embryos. A review of histogenesis of cartilage and bone. *Contrib Embryol* 1949; 220: 151-67.
9. Chen LT, Weiss L. The development of vertebral bone marrow of human fetuses. *Blood* 1975; 46: 389-408.
10. Moore MAS, Owen JJT. Stem cell migration in developing myeloid and lymphoid systems. *Lancet* 1967; 2: 658-59.

11. Jotereau FV, Le Douarin NM. The developmental relationship between osteocytes and osteoclasts: a study using the quail-chick nuclear marker in endochondral ossification. *Dev Biol* 1978; 63: 253-65.
12. Charbord P, Tavian M, Humeau L, Péault B. Early ontogeny of the human marrow from long bones: an immunohistochemical study of hematopoiesis and its microenvironment. Submitted for publication.
13. Dieterlen-Lièvre F, Le Douarin NM. Developmental rules in the hemopoietic and immune systems of birds: how general are they? *Sem Dev Biol* 1993; 4: 325-32.
14. Medvinsky AL, Samoylina NL, Müller AM, Dzierzak EA. An early pre-liver intraembryonic source of CFU-S in the developing mouse. *Nature* 1993; 364: 64-67.
15. Godin IE, Garcia-Porrero JA, Coutinho A, Dieterlen-Lièvre F, Marcos MA. Para-aortic splanchnopleura from early mouse embryos contains B1a-cell progenitors. *Nature* 1993; 364: 67-70.
16. Godin I, Dieterlen-Lièvre F, Cumano A. Emergence of multipotent hemopoietic cells in the yolk sac and paraaortic splanchnopleura in mouse embryos, beginning at 8.5 days postcoitus. *Proc Natl Acad Sci USA* 1995; 92: 773-77.
17. Muller AM, Medvinsky AL, Strouboulis J, Grosveld F, Dzierzak EA. Development of hematopoietic stem cell activity in the mouse embryo. *Immunity* 1994; 1: 291-301.
18. Tavian M, Coulombel L, Luton D, San Clemente H, Dieterlen-Lièvre F, Péault B. Aorta-associated CD34+ hematopoietic cells in the early human embryo. Submitted for publication.
19. Huyhn A, Dommergues M, Katz A, Izac B, Vainchenker W, Coulombel L. Characterization of hematopoietic progenitors and identification of cytokine gene expression in human extraembryonic yolk sacs and embryos. Submitted for publication.

Résumé

Le développement embryonnaire et fœtal précoce du système sanguin humain a été analysé par détection immunohistochimique de marqueurs des compartiments vasculaire, stromaux et myéloérythroïdes sur coupes de tissus hématopoïétiques entre les 3e et 28e semaines de la gestation. L'antigène CD34 est exprimé de façon ubiquitaire sur les cellules endothéliales à tous les stades, à la seule exception du foie embryonnaire dont l'endothélium vasculaire est négatif ou très faiblement marqué. En revanche, des cellules hématopoïétiques CD34+ ont été détectées, dispersées dans l'ébauche hépatique, à partir de 4-5 semaines et au-delà alors qu'apparaissaient simultanément des colonies d'érythroblastes et de monocytes. Le développement précoce de la moelle des os longs est marqué par l'envahissement, à partir de la 8e semaine, de l'ébauche cartilagineuse de l'os par les précurseurs ostéoclastiques CD68+, par les précurseurs des ostéoblastes et par des bourgeons vasculaires CD34+, menant à l'établissement de larges sinus vasculaires séparant des travées en cours d'ossification. Les logettes où s'établira l'hématopoïèse se développent dans la diaphyse osseuse, toujours organisées autour d'une artériole centrale. Des colonies endogènes d'érythro- et de granulopoïèse y apparaissent à partir de la 11e semaine, entre la paroi artérielle et les cellules endothéliales bordant le sinus. De façon inattendue, nous n'avons pas détecté de cellules CD34+ hématopoïétiques dans la moelle osseuse en cours de développement.

En revanche, nous avons observé une population très dense de cellules hématopoïétiques CD34+ associées à la paroi ventrale de l'aorte embryonnaire à partir de la 5e semaine de la gestation. Ces cellules présentent une distribution anatomique identique – et se développent à un stade équivalent – à celle des cellules souches hématopoïétiques intraembryonnaires qui ont été identifiées, chez l'oiseau et chez la souris, comme étant à l'origine de l'ensemble du système sanguin définitif.

Characterization of hematopoietic progenitor cells in the human extraembryonic yolk sac and in the human embryo

Laure Coulombel[1], Anne Huyhn[1], Marc Dommergues[2], Brigitte Izac[1], André Katz[1], William Vainchenker[1]

[1] INSERM U 362, Institut Gustave-Roussy, 94800 Villejuif, France; [2] Maternité Port-Royal, Paris, France, tel.: (33 1) 45 59 42 33, fax: (33 1) 46 77 84 37

Abstract

In a search for assays that might facilitate identification of pluripotent stem cells with extended potentialities, we analysed the properties of hematopoeitic progenitor cells detected in the extra-embryonic yolk sac and in the intraembryonic part of human embryos between approximately 28 and 45 days of development. Cells from the yolk sac, the liver rudiment and the remainder of the embryo were plated in semi solid methylcellulose colony-assays supplemented with combinaisons of cytokines. Large BFU-E-derived colonies as well as granulocytic colonies were detected in every yolk sac sample. Interestingly, progenitor cells were also detected in the intraembryonic part, outside the liver and a subclass of these progenitors were detected that generated large granulomacrophagic colonies capable of generating secondary colonies when replated. These were preferentially located in the embryo. Colony-assays initiated with CD34$^+$ cells sorted from the different tissues confirmed these data. These results first indicate that embryonic progenitors exhibit unique phenotypic features, and second, analysis of the distribution of progenitors between the different tissues may suggest the existence of other sites of hematopoietic production. More detailed analysis of the potentialities of these progenitors should now be assessed in vitro in cocultures assays and in vivo by reconstituting immunodeficient mice.

Classically, the sequence of events occuring during hematopoietic development involves first the emergence of hematopoietic stem cells in extraembryonal mesoderm of the yolk sac, followed by migration of stem cells which colonize tissues endowed with hemaopoietic activity such as the liver rudiment and later the bone marrow [1]. Evidence that stem cells do not originate exclusively in the yolk sac but can also be produced in the embryo proper was first proposed twenty years ago in birds following analysis of experimental chimeras [2, 3]. More recently, elegant studies have demonstrated that these observations also applied to mammals and hematopoietic stem cells have been mapped to the splanchnopleura [4] or to the aorta-gonad-mesonephros region (AGM) of mouse embryo at days 9-10 [5]. It is therefore likely that several distinct sites of hematopoiesis exist in the developing mouse embryo which might function sequentially at very precise stages of development and that the hematopoietic activity of one given tissue results from its colonization by stem cells of different origins. The real potential of stem cells from these different sites has been recently characterized: individual cells from the splanchopleura region in the mouse can generate cells from all lineages *in vitro* [6] and cells from the AGM region have in vivo long-term repopulating capabilities [7] which confirm that these progenitor cells represent indeed "true" stem cells.

Similar studies on the onset of hematopoiesis in the humans have not been possible until very recently (see [8] and also Péault, this volume) due to obvious limitations in the collection of samples. Very few data exist on hematopoiesis in the yolk sac or in the liver rudiment during the first weeks of human development and they are restricted to the identification of relatively mature clonogenic progenitors (*i.e.* forming colonies) committed to the myeloid lineages [8-10]. These CFU-E and BFU-E and also CFU-GM have been quantified by standard colony-assays in the human extraembryonic yolk sac around week 5-6 of development. Kinetics analysis were attempted in this initial work to correlate a decrease in hemopoietic potential of the yolk sac and the onset of liver hematopoiesis. Such committed progenitors have also been detected in mouse yolk sac [11-13]. Contrasting with these scarce data early in life, the phenotype and potentialities of progenitor cells in fetal bone marrow and liver beyond 18 weeks have been studied in more details. The most interesting observations pertain to the differences observed in the hematopoietic potential between adult and embryonic and fetal progenitor cells [14,15]. These data have given credit to the hypothesis that the hematopoietic potential of stem cells found during fetal life may be much larger than that of adult marrow-derived stem cells. This was based on several sets of data: (1) a high proportion of individual progenitor cells with a primitive phenotype ($CD34^+$/$Thy1^+$) isolated from bone marrow of 16-18 weeks old human fetuses generate myeloid and B lymphoid cells, whereas the potential of adult marrow cells maintained in similar culture conditions is usually restricted to the myeloid lineages [16]. (2) Reconstitution of the T lymphoid lineage in thymic lobes either after in vitro organotypic cultures [17] or after injection of thymic tissue in SCID mice has been successful only by using $CD34^+$ cells from fetal organs [18]. Higher numbers of $CD34^+$ cells were generated from liquid cultures initiated with cord blood and fetal liver $CD34^+$ than with adult marrow $CD34^+$cells [14]. This suggests that fetal hematopoietic stem cells may have a higher proliferative potential (perhaps a self-renewal capacity) and a less restricted potential than their adult counterparts (see Lansdorp, this colume). Particularly important in a clinical context is the observation that amplification of $CD34^+$ cells might be possible in hematopoietic tissues of fetal origin.

We reasoned that identification of "true" stem cells with extended potentialities and proliferation potential might be facilitated by the use of embryonic hematopoietic stem cells. To that purpose, we started a research project on human embryonic hematopoiesis. In a first approach, we characterized clonogenic progenitor cells isolated from the extraembryonic yolk sac, and investigated whether progenitor cells were also found in the embryo proper. We collected abortion products between approximately 30 and 50 days of development, and separated the yolk sac from the embryo proper. Whenever it was possible the liver rudiment was isolated from the remainder of the embryo. All tissues were digested by incubation with 0.1% collagenase and cells were subsequently plated in standard methylcellulose colony-assays supplemented with human (rhu) cytokines, rhu erythropoietin (Epo), rhu interleukin-3 (rhu IL-3), rhu stem cell factor (SCF), rhu granulocyte colony-stimulating factor (G-CSF). Colonies were scored at days 10-15 according to standard criteria.

Both erythroid and non-erythroid colonies were detected in the yolk sac, in the embryo and in the liver rudiment. Interestingly, yolk sac-and embryo-derived BFU-E generated colonies with a phenotype different from that observed for erythroid colonies derived from adult marrow BFU-E. Comparison of the response of yolk sac-derived and liver-derived BFU-E revealed that a high proportion of BFU-E from the liver rudiment grew with only 2 units/ml of Epo, whereas most of yolk sac-derived BFU-E required a second cytokine and grew best in SCF + IL-3. Analysis of the absolute numbers of BFU-E and CFU-GM detected in the yolk sac and in the embryo proper from approximately 28 to 45 days of development revealed the followings:

– The content of yolk sac in erythroid progenitors was rather constant between 30-45 days of development and we did not observed the decrease in erythroid colonies observed by Migliaccio in yolk sac beyond 6 weeks. A second difference with this study was that we detected very few CFU-E in colony-assays established from yolk sacs. In contrast, the number of granulopoietic progenitor cells (CFU-GM), which was similar to that of BFU-E at early stages decreased in yolk sacs from samples beyond day 35 of development.

– At every stage, progenitor cells were detected in the embryo proper and analysis of the distribution of progenitors between the extraembryonic yolk sac and the embryo revealed an equal distribution in erythroid progenitors (BFU-E), whereas higher numbers of granulopoietic progenitor cells (CFU-GM) were found in the embryos beyond day 35. Interestingly, we detected progenitors with an HPP-CFC (high-proliferative potential colony-forming cell) like [16] phenotype in colony-assays established with cells isolated from the embryos. These colonies, mostly ganulomacrophagic, were characterized by a very large size, and the response of the progenitor to rhuSCF and rhu IL-3. Some exhibited high replating capacity and the existence of both erythroid and granulocytic colonies in some secondary plates suggested that these HPP-CFC-like progenitors were pluripotent.

– In four experiments, cells expressing the CD34 antigen were sorted from the yolk sac, the embryo and the liver rudiment and plated in colony-assays. Two comments should be done about these experiments: (1) the plating efficiency of these $CD34^+$ was below the cloning efficiency of adult marrow-derived $CD34^+$cells. This is probably explained by the contamination of embryonic hematopoietic cells by a high number of developing endothelial cells [17]. (2) Unique features in the phenotype of erythroid and non-erythroid colonies grown from unfractionated cells from yolk sac, embryos or liver rudiment were also seen in plates seeded with $CD34^+$ cells from these tissues. This argues against the possibility that the particular phenotype of colonies in assays performed with unfractionated cells reflected the presence of accessory cells, possibly secreting additional cytokines.

Finally, in order to understand which cytokines were active *in vivo* at that stage of development, we performed RT-PCR on the different tissues. RNAs encoding Epo, SCF, IL-3 and GM-CSF were investigated. Interestingly, only RNAs coding for Epo and SCF were consistently found in extracs from yolk sacs and embryos, and liver rudiments.

Conclusion

In this study we provide new informations on the functional characterization of clonogenic progenitor cells in extraembryonic yolk sac and embryos in the human species, from 30-45 days of development. Analysis of the phenotype of colonies and of their response to cytokines reveal functional differences with adult marrow-derived progenitors, but the most striking finding was the exstence of high numbers of progenitor cells in the embryos. Several interpretations can be proposed: (1) these cells can represent a circulating pool of progenitors which are produced in the yolk sac. At that stage the embryos are vascularized and it is impossible to quantitate circulating cells. (2) It is also tempting to speculate that they originate from intra-embryonic hematopoietic sites outside the liver. This is further suggested by the presence of HPP-CFC like progenitor cells nearly exclusively in the intraembryonic part, whereas they were absent from the liver rudiment. However, this study was focued on clonogenic cells and further work is now undertaken to identify more immature stem cells using namely in vitro approaches such as LTC-IC assays and also reconstitution of immunodeficient mice.

References

1. Moore M, Metcalf D. Ontogeny of the hemopoietic system: yolk sac origin of in vivo and in vitro colony-forming cells in the developing mouse embryo. *Br J Haematol* 18: 279, 1970
2. Dieterlen-Lievre F. On the origin of haemopoietic stem cells in the avian embryo: an experimental approach. *J Embryol Exp Morph* 33: 607, 1975
3. Dieterlen-Lievre F. Emergence of intraembryonic blood stem cells in avian chimeras by means of monoclonal antibodies. *Dev Comp Immunol* 3: 75, 1984
4. Godin I, Garcia-Perero J, Coutinho A, Dieterlen-Lievre F, Marcos M. Para-aortic splanchnopleura from early mouse embryos contains B1a cell progenitors. *Nature* 364: 67, 1993
5. Medvinski A, Samoylina L, Muller A, Dzlerzak E. An early pre-liver intraembryonic source of CFU-S in the developing mouse. *Nature* 364: 64, 1993
6. Godin I, Dieterlen-Lievre F, Cumano A. Emergence of multipotent hemopoietic cells in the yolk sac and paraaortic splanchnopleura in mouse embryos, beginning at 8.5 dpc. *Proc Natl Acad Sci* USA 92: 773, 1995.
7. Müller AM, Medvinsky A, Strouboulis J, Grosveld F, Dzierzak E. Dezvelopment of hematopoietic stem cell activity in the mouse embryo. *Immunity* 1: 291, 1994.
8. Migliaccio G, Migliaccio A, Petti S, Mavilio F, Russo G, Lazzaro D, Lazzaro D, Testa U, Marinucci M, Peschle C. Human embryonic hemopoiesis. Kinetics of progenitors and precursors underlying the yolk sac liver transition. *J Clin Inv* 78: 51, 1986
9. Emerson S, Thoma S, Ferrar J, Greenstein J. Developmental regulation of erythropoiesis by hematopoietic growth factors: analysis on populations of BFU-E from bone marrow, peripheral blood and fetal liver. *Blood* 74: 49, 1989
10. Valtieri M, Gabbianelli M, Pelosi E, Bassano E, Petti S, Russo G, Testa U, Peschle C. Erythropoietin alone induces erythroid burst formation by human embryonic but not adult BFU-E in unicellular serum-free cultures. *Blood* 74: 460, 1989
11. Wong P, Chung S, Chui D, Eaves C. Properties of the earliest clonogenic precursors to appear in the developing murine yolk sac. *Proc Natl Acad Sci* USA 83: 3851, 1986
12. Huang HH, Auerbach R. Identification and characterization of hematopoietic stem cells from the yolk sac of the early mouse embryo. *Proc Natl Acad Sci* USA 90: 10110, 1993
13. Johnson G, Barker D. Erythroid progenitor cells and stimulating factors during murine embryonic and fetal development. *Exp Hematol* 13: 200, 1985
14. Lansdorp P, Dragowska W, Mayani H. Ontogeny-related changes in proliferative potential of human hematopoietic cells. *J Exp Med* 178: 787, 1993
15. Lansdorp PM. Developmental changes in the function of hematopoietic stem cells. *Exp Hematol* 23: 187, 1995.
16. Baum C, Weissman I, Tsukamoto A, Buckle A, Peault B. Isolation of a candidate human hematopoietic stem cell population. *Proc Natl Acad Sci* USA 89: 2804, 1992
17. Plum J, DeSmedt M, Defresne MP, Leclercq G, Vanderkerkhove B. Human CD34$^+$ fetal liver stem cells differentiate to T cells in a mouse thymic microenvironment. *Blood* 84, 1587, 1994.
18. Péault B, Weissman IL, Baum C, McCune J, Tsukamoto A. Lymphoid reconstitution of the human fetal thymus in SCID mice with CD34^{++} precursor cells. *J Exp Med* 174: 1287, 1991.
19. MacNiece I, Stewart F, Deacon D, Temeles D, Zsebo K, Clark S, Quesenbery P. Detection of human CFC with a high proliferative potential. *Blood* 74:609, 1989.
20. Young P, Baumhueter S, Lasky L. The sialomucin CD34 is expressed on hematopoietic cells and blood vessels during murine development. *Blood* 85: 96, 1995.

Résumé

Le schéma classique du développement de l'hématopoïèse désigne le mésoderme du sac vitellin comme site d'émergence des premières cellules souches hématopoïétiques, les autres organes, foie et moelle osseuse, étant colonisés par des cellules souches migrant à partir de ce site initial. Dans cette étude, nous avons caractérisé et quantifié, dans un système de formation de colonies, les progéniteurs érythroïdes, granuleux et pluripotents présents dans la vésicule vitelline, organe extraembryonnaire mais aussi dans l'ébauche hépatique et l'embryon entre 28 et 45 jours de développement. Nous avons également analysé la réponse de ces progéniteurs à différentes cytokines, facteur steel, interleukine-3 et érythropoïétine. Les résultats révèlent que le phénotype des progéniteurs embryonnaires et leur réponse aux cytokines sont différents de ceux des progéniteurs de la moelle osseuse adulte et qu'existe une distribution très particulière de ces cellules dans les tissus embryonnaires. L'analyse en RT-PCR de l'expression des gènes codant pour différentes cytokines montre que seuls le facteur Steel et l'érythropoïétine sont transcrits spontanément dans la vésicule vitelline et l'embryon.

Proliferative and differentiation potential of neonatal and fetal hematopoietic stem cells

Peter M. Lansdorp[1], V.I. Rebel[2], W. Dragowska[2], M.T.E. Little[2],
T.E. Thomas[2], R.K. Humphries[2], C.J. Eaves[2] and H. Mayani[1]

[1] BRU/Oncology Hospital, National Medical Center, Mexico City, Mexico; [2] Terry Fox Laboratory for Hematology/Oncology, British Columbia Cancer Agency and Department of Medicine and Medical Genetics, University of British Columbia, Vancouver, Canada, tel.: (604) 877 6070, fax: (607) 877 0712

Abstract

Recent studies in our laboratory have shown significant ontogeny-related changes in the functional properties of primitive hematopoietic cells which coincide with the loss of telomeric DNA from the end of human chromosomes. These findings are best explained by assuming that the self-renewal and replicative potential of hematopoietic stem cells decrease with age and are under tight developmental and genetic control. Studies in mice have shown that in the absence of a transplantation barrier (irradiated syngeneic recipient mice), limiting numbers of fetal stem cells out can compete their adult counterparts, indicating that fetal cells can function in an «adult» microenvironment. Many clinical and preclinical transplantation studies have shown that in the presence of minor or major histocompatibility differences, the number of transplanted hematopoietic cells is an important parameter in predicting engraftment (donor cell repopulation). The major challenges for clinical use of fetal and neonatal hematopoietic cells thus appear to be related to the identification and elimination of the various host factors that may represent an immunological barrier towards the transplanted cells.

Functional changes in primitive hematopoietic cells

Although many studies have provided indirect support for the notion that functional properties of primitive hematopoietic cells may change during development, few studies have provided direct proof for this notion [1]. Ikuta and colleagues have provided a clear demonstration that the lymphoid potential of murine fetal hematopoietic stem cells (HSC) is different from their adult counterparts [2]. Day 14 fetal liver HSCs, isolated by antibody staining and fluorescence activated cell sorting (FACS), developed as T lymphocytes expressing the Vγ3 T cell receptors, whereas adult HSC were incapable of developing into a similar manner in organ cultures in fetal thymic lobes. Interestingly, fetal HSC nor adult HSC could produce Vγ3 T cells upon culture in adult thymic lobes, indicating that developmental changes in the function of cells are not restricted to hematopoietic cells, but can also be demonstrated in other tissues including the thymus. The latter is in agreement with a recent paper describing age-related restrictions in thymic regeneration after high dose therapy [3].

Extensive differences in various functional properties between "candidate" human HSC purified from fetal liver, cord blood and adult bone marrow were described previously [4]. In these studies $CD34^+$ $CD45RA^{low}$ $CD71^{low}$ cells purified by FACS were cultured in cytokine supplemented serum-free cultures. Large differences in the number of mitotic cells (adult: minority; fetal liver/cord blood: all), the turn-over rate of the responding cells (fetal liver > cord blood > adult bone marrow) and, most importantly, the production of $CD34^+$ progenitor cells were observed. If cultures were initiated with cells from adult marrow the absolute number of $CD34^+$ cells was maintained [5, 6], but in cultures initiated with purified cord blood cells several hundred-fold and in fetal liver cell cultures several thousand-fold increases in the number of $CD34^+$ cells were observed [4]. Interestingly, cells with long-term lympho-myeloid repopulation potential from murine adult bone marrow were also maintained in number (*i.e.* no expansion or loss) in similar cultures [7]. Because the culture conditions for all cell types were identical, these observations suggest that self-renewal properties are primarily controlled intrinsicly and cannot be readily manipulated by cytokines and other factors of the microenvironment [8]. According to this notion it should, in theory, be possible to increase the number of transplantable HSC in fetal liver and cord blood cultures, be it that such expansion may be at the expense of the replicative potential of the cells before the culture *(see below)*. Experimental verification of this prediction has however not yet been reported, perhaps because not all cytokines [9] and/or microenvironmental signals from the fetal liver have been completely characterised or tested.

Loss of telomeric DNA in hematopoietic cells

An exciting avenue for further studies on the replicative potential and self-renewal properties of HSC is the recent observation that hematopoietic cells, including purified $CD34^+$ $CD38^-$ cells have shorter telomeres then their counterparts from fetal liver and cord blood [10]. Telomeres are the physical ends of chromosomes and consist of T_2AG_3 repeat sequences together with associated proteins [11]. In the absence of the enzyme telomerase 10-30 T_2AG_3 repeats are lost upon replication from the 3' end of each chromosome with each cell division, limiting the overall replicative potential to an estimated 50-80 divisions [12]. Shortening of telomeres has been observed in all somatic cells studied to date including fibroblasts and lymphocytes [13,14]. Telomere shortening is not observed in immortal cell lines and certain cancers which express the enzyme of telomerase [15]. The role of telomeres in the biology of hematopoietic cells was recently reviewed [16]. Shortening of telomeres in leukemic cells relative to residual normal hematopoietic cells was described by at least two groups [17-19] and studies on the expression of telomerase in normal and malignant hematopoietic cells are eagerly awaited. The results obtained so far are compatible with the notion that HSC lack functional telomerase activity, have a finite replicative potential and thus lack true self-renewal properties. Conservation of a limited replicative potential also explains why the large majority of HSC in mice and man are not actively cycling during steady state hematopoiesis.

Transplantation of adult recipients with fetal and neonatal hematopoietic cells

Given the superior functional expansion potential and telomere related genetic replication potential of fetal and neonatal cells discussed above, one might expect wide-spread clinical use of such cells for reconstruction of hematopoiesis in myeloablated individuals including adults. However especially the latter has proven problematic over the last several decades and is not common practice. Several explanations for the frequent failures of for example fetal liver transplants have been proposed including the inability of fetal cells to function in an "adult" microenvironment. This concern does not appear to be valid at least in a murine model, as limiting numbers of purified fetal liver stem cells in fact outcompete similar cells from adult bone marrow [20]. A more likely explanation is that the relatively small number of fetal or neonatal cells available for transplantation are unable to overcome host resistance towards «foreign» cells, especially in the case of major or minor histocompatibility differences between donor and recipient. Host immune barriers towards transplanted cells may include (natural) antibodies (which could eliminate the transplanted cells via the complement system or antibody dependent cytotoxicity), natural killer cells and residual T cell immunity after the immunosuppression that is typical part of the transplant conditioning regimen. Unfortunately the relative contributions of each of these three most obvious host defense mechanisms towards the transplanted fetal or neonatal cells are not known and are furthermore likely to vary in different donor-recipient combinations. Complicating factors for studies in this general area are the lack of suitable (outbred) animal models and the likelihood that different mechanisms may operate depending on the matching between donor and recipient for known and unknown major and minor histo-compatibility differences. Because it seems likely that, whatever the exact mechanism, host resistance can eventually be overcome by infusion of larger number of donor cells, the possibility to increase the number of fetal or neonatal cells prior to transplantation should urgently be examined. The superior expansion and replicative potential of such cells discussed above support the feasibility of this approach.

Acknowledgments

We wish to thank Mike Strong and Ted Bisley (North West Tissue Center Seattle, WA) for making organ donor bone marrow cells available for these studies. Gayle Thornburg helped with flow cytometry and cell sorting. These studies were supported by NIH grant AI29524, and by grants from the Medical Research Council and the National Cancer Institute of Canada. The manuscript was typed by Wanda Winkel and Caroline Snethlage.

References

1. Lansdorp PM. Developmental changes in the function of hematopoietic stem cell. *Exp Hematol* 1995; 23: 187-191.
2. Ikuta K, Kina T, MacNeil I, Uchida N, Peault B, Chen Y-H, and Weissman IL. A developmental switch in thymic lymphocyte maturation potential occurs at the level of hematopoietic stem cells. *Cell* 1990; 62: 863.
3. Mackall CL, Fleisher TA, Brown MR, Andrich MP, Chen CC, Feuerestein IM, Horowitz ME, Magrath IT, Shad AT, Steinberg SM, Wexler LH, Gress RE. Age, thymopoiesis, and $CD4^+$ T-lymphocyte regenration after intensive chemotherapy. *New Eng J Med* 1995; 19: 143-149.

4. Lansdorp PM, Dragowska W, Mayani H. Ontogeny-related changes in proliferative potential of human hematopoietic cells. *J Exp Med* 1993; 178: 787-791.
5. Lansdorp PM, Dragowska W. Long-term erythropoiesis from constant numbers of CD34$^+$ cells in serum-free cultures initiated with highly purified progenitor cells from human bone marrow. *J Exp Med* 1992; 175: 1501.
6. Lansdorp PM, Dragowska W. Maintenance of hematopoiesis in serum-free bone marrow cultures involves sequential recruitment of quiescent progenitors. *Exp Hematol* 1993; 21: 1321-1327.
7. Rebel VI, Dragowska W, Eaves CJ, Humphries RK, and Lansdorp PM. Amplification of Sca-1$^+$ Lin$^-$ WGA$_+$ cells in serum-free cultures containing Steel factor, interleukin-6, and erythropoietin with maintenance of cells with long-term *in vivo* constituting potential. *Blood* 1994; 83: 128-136.
8. Lansdorp PM. Properties of purified stem cells. *Exp Hematol* 1994; 22: 714
9. Lyman SD, James L, Vanden Bos T, de Vries P, Brasel K, Gliniak B, Hollingsworth LT, Picha KS, McKenna HJ, Splett RR, Fletcher FA, Maraskovsky E, Farrah T, Foxworthe D, Williams DE and Beckmann MP. Molecular cloning of a ligand for the flt3/flk-2 tyrosine kinase receptor: A proliferative factor for primitive hematopoietic cells. *Cell* 1993; 75: 1157-1167.
10. Vaziri H, Dragowska W, Allsopp RC, Thomas TE, Harley CB, and Lansdorp PM. Evidence for a mitotic clock in human hematopoietic stem cells: loos of telomeric DNA with age. *Proc Natl Acad Sci* 1994; 91: 9857-9860.
11. Blackburn EH. Telomeres: No end in sight. *Cell* 1992; 77: 621-623.
12. Harley CB, Vaziri H, Counter C, and Allsopp RC. The telomeric hypothesis of cellular aging. *Exptl Geront* 1992; 27: 375-382.
13. Counter CM, Avilio AA, LeFeuvre CE, Stewart NG, Greider CW, Harley CB, and Bacchetti S. Telomere shortening associated with chromosome instability is arrested in immortal cells which express telomerase activity. *EMBO J* 1992; 11: 1921-1929.
14. Vaziri H, Schachter F, Uchida I, Wei L, Zhu X, Effors R, Cohen D and Harley CB. Loss of telomeric DNA during aging of normal and trisomy 21 human lymphocytes. *Am J Hum Genet* 1993; 52: 661-667.
15. Kim NW, Proswe KR, Ho PLC, Coviello GM, Harley CB, Piatyszek MA, Shay JW, Wright WE, and Weinreich SL. Telomerase activity is specifically associated with human cell immortality (sbumitted).
16. Lansdorp PM. Telomere length and proliferation potential of hematopoietic stem cells. *J Cell Sci* 1995; 108: 1-6.
17. Yamada O, Oshimi K, and Mizoguchi H. Telomere reduction in hematologic cells. *Int J Hematol* 1993; 57: 181-186.
18. Adamson DJ, King DJ, and Haites NE. Sginificant telomere shortening in childhood leukemia. *Cancer Genet Cytogenet* 1992; 61: 204-206.
19. Yamada O, Oshimi K, Motoji T, and Mizoguchi H. Telomeric DNA in normal and leukemic blood cells. *J Clin Invest* 1995; 95: 1117-1123.
21. Rebel V, Miller C, Eaves CJ and Lansdorp PM. The *in vivo* proliferative activity of single fetal liver repopulating units exceeds that of their adult bon marrow counterparts. *Exp Hematol* 1994; 22: 724.

Résumé

Des résultats récents obtenus dans le laboratoire ont montré que les propriétés fonctionnelles des cellules hématopoïétiques primitives dépendaient de l'âge de l'individu, ce qui coïncidait avec la perte de matériel génétique au niveau des télomères des chromosomes humains. Ces données sont en accord avec l'hypothèse d'une restriction progressive de la capacité d'autorenouvellement des cellules souches au cours du développement, ces événements étant certainement contrôlés à la fois au niveau génétique et en fonction de l'âge. Des expériences chez la souris en situation syngénique ont montré que des cellules fœtales, même greffées en petit nombre, se développent dans un environnement adulte et acquièrent un avantage prolifératif par rapport aux cellules adultes. Dans beaucoup de situations de transplantation où existent des différences dans les groupes majeurs ou mineurs d'histocompatibilité, le nombre de cellules transplantées est un paramètre important de prédiction du succès de la greffe. Il est donc essentiel pour que se développe un usage clinique de cellules fœtales et néonatales d'identifier les facteurs d'origine receveur qui compromettraient la prise de greffe et de les maîtriser.

Differential role of Steel factor on hematopoietic stem cells during ontogeny, in adults and after bone marrow transplantation

C.L. Miller, V.I. Rebel, C.D. Helgason, M.E. Lemieux, R.K. Humphries, P.M. Lansdorp and C.J. Eaves

Terry Fox Laboratory, British Columbia Cancer Agency, Vancouver, BC, Canada, V5Z 1L3, tel.: (604) 877 6070, fax: (604) 877 0712

Summary

Steel factor (SF) is a pleiotropic cytokine which acts directly on a variety of cell types within the hematopoietic system. The receptor for SF is encoded by the c-kit protooncogene originally identified as the murine white spotting (W) locus. Germline mutations affecting either SF or its receptor have been recognized in mice for many years for their ability to cause a macrocytic anemia as well as changes in coat color and fertility. Previous studies have also suggested that mutations at these loci may compromise the activity in vivo *of pluripotent hematopoietic stem cells, although conflicting data in this regard have been reported. To obtain more precise information about the role of SF as an endogenous regulator of hematopoietic stem cells in vivo, we compared the number and activity of these cells in fetal liver as well as in adult marrow of normal and W^{41}/W^{41} mice. The results suggest that a normal number of hematopoietic stem cells can be generated and maintained throughout fetal development and adult life in the absence of a fully functional SF response. Moreover, when stimulated* in vitro *under conditions that do not involve SF, W^{41}/W^{41} stem cells exhibit a normal proliferative capacity. On the other hand, the hematopoietic stem cell expansion that occurs in adult mice undergoing hematologic recovery after myeloablative therapy appears to be much more dependent on SF stimulation than the relatively SF-independent stem cell expansion that occurs during fetal development. This change in the role of SF during ontogeny is paralleled by a corresponding decrease in the ability of the hematopoietic stem cells present in the adult to be regulated by alternative mechanisms which are more important in controlling stem cell proliferation in fetal life.*

The last three decades have seen considerable progress in understanding the complex process by which multiple types of mature blood cells develop from a common self-maintaining population of pluripotent hematopoietic stem cells. Such stem cells emerge early in embryogenesis [1, 2] and persist throughout adult life although the precise differentiation steps they undergo in the adult are not identical to those that occur during the initial expansion of the hematopoietic system in the fetus. It might be anticipated, therefore, that endogenous molecular mechanisms regulating the recruitment, self-renewal and differentiation of hematopoietic stem cells *in vivo* might also change during ontogeny.

One ligand-receptor system known to affect both fetal and adult hematopoietic cells is the interaction of Steel factor (SF) with its receptor (c-kit), a member of the tyrosine kinase transmembrane receptor superfamily [3]. The c-kit gene is located at the *white spotting* (W) locus and a large array of germline Steel and W mutations with specific effects on hematopoiesis have now been characterized at the molecular level [4]. When signaling through the SF receptor is completely blocked, the resultant deficiencies in red cell production are lethal to the developing embryo [5]. *In vitro,* SF has been shown to augment the formation of many types of hematopoietic colonies variously stimulated by IL-3, IL-6, IL-7, GM-CSF and erythropoietin [4]. Conversely, *in vivo* administration of an anti-c-kit monoclonal antibody has been shown to decrease *in vitro* colony-forming cell (CFC) numbers in the developing fetus [6] and both CFC and colony-forming unit-spleen (CFU-S) in adult mice [7]. The classic transplantation studies demonstrating a failure of spleen colony formation by W-mutant cells in normal recipients or by normal cells in Steel-mutant recipients [8, 9] were the first to suggest a role of this pathway in regulating hematopoietic stem cell recruitment in the adult. This prediction was also supported by the demonstration that relatively small numbers of normal stem cells when injected into certain strains of otherwise unmanipulated W mutant mice (*e.g.,* W/W^v or W^{41}/W^{41}) could outcompete the endogenous W-mutant stem cell population and take over all blood cell production [10, 11]. On the other hand, it was also recently shown that Steel mutant embryos of genotype Sl/Sl, which are incapable of producing Steel factor, have near normal numbers of CFU-S in spite of their anemia [12]. This apparent paradox could, however, be explained by a model of hematopoietic stem cell regulation in which alternative mechanisms of varying importance during ontogeny were involved in controlling the viability and turnover of these cells.

Experimental results

To further investigate this model, we undertook a series of experiments comparing the numbers and behaviour of hematopoietic cells from W^{41}/W^{41} mutant mice and their congenic wild-type C57BL/6J controls (+/+) [13]. The W^{41} mutation arises from a single nucleotide substitution resulting in the conversion of a valine to methionine at amino acid position 831 within the tyrosine kinase domain of the SF receptor [14]. Although the receptor is still expressed at normal levels on the surface of cells from W^{41} homozygotes, its kinase activity is markedly reduced [14] and the SF enhanced detection *in vitro* of mature BFU-E from these mice is similarly decreased *(Figure 1).* Nevertheless, the W^{41} mutation is not lethal in the homozygous state and although there is a persistent anemia, CFU-E numbers are near normal. In addition, normal numbers of B-lymphoid and myeloid progenitors (which do not require the presence of SF for their detection *in vitro*) are found in the marrow of adult W^{41}/W^{41} mice [13]. Thus, in spite of the fact that many W^{41}/W^{41} hematopoietic cells display c-kit on their surface ([14], C. Miller unpublished observations) and their normal counterparts can be shown to be SF responsive (*e.g. Figure 1*), for most lineages a reduction of this responsiveness can probably be compensated for *in vivo* by other mechanisms.

To examine the potential role of SF in the generation of hematopoietic stem cells *in vivo*, we first quantitated the number of cells with a phenotype characteristic of normal pluripotent stem cells that are present in the marrow of adult W^{41}/W^{41} mice or the liver of day 14.5 W^{41}/W^{41} fetuses. In the marrow of normal adult +/+ mice, functionally defined hematopoietic stem cells are contained primarily within the small subpopulation of cells that do not express any of the lineage markers recognized by the monoclonal antibodies Gr-1 (RB6-8C5; granulocytic), B220 (RA3-6B2; B-cells), Ly-1 (53-7.3; T-cells) and Mac-1 (M1/70; myelo-monocytic) but do express Ly-6 (Sca-1, E13-161.7) and bind wheat germ agglutinin (WGA) [15]. Flow cytometric analysis of W^{41}/W^{41} marrow cells has shown that cells with this Sca-1$^+$ Lin$^-$ WGA$^+$ phenotype are present [13] and at the same frequency as in the marrow of +/+ control mice [15]. Since the W^{41} mutation has no effect on the cellularity of the marrow, the total number of cells with this "stem cell phenotype" in W^{41}/W^{41} marrow must also be unchanged. In the fetal liver of normal day 14.5 embryos, the majority of stem cells have a similar (albeit not identical) phenotype (V. Rebel et al, submitted). Analysis of W^{41}/W^{41} fetal livers of the same gestational age again showed no difference in the frequency of cells with a Sca-1$^+$ Lin$^-$ (fetal stem cell) phenotype although, because the total cellularity of the W^{41}/W^{41} fetal liver is slightly reduced (~ 2-fold), the total number of Sca-1$^+$ Lin$^-$ cells present is correspondingly lower ([13], C. Miller *et al*, manuscript in preparation).

These findings are consistent with previous evidence that SF may not be a limiting regulator of stem cell turnover in the developing embryo [12] and provide the first quantitative data suggesting that this may also hold true in the normal adult. However, although hematopoietic stem cells are highly enriched within the Sca-1$^+$ Lin$^-$ (± WGA) subpopulations of both fetal liver and adult marrow cells, > 90% of these cells may not have the functional properties of stem cells ([15], V. Rebel, submitted), in which case significant effects on stem cell numbers would not necessarily be discernible as a change in the total number of cells with this phenotype. To evaluate stem cells directly, several functional assays are now available. These include both the competitive repopulating unit (CRU) and the longterm culture-initiating cell (LTC-IC) assays. The CRU assay allows totipotent hematopoietic stem cell populations to be quantitated based on

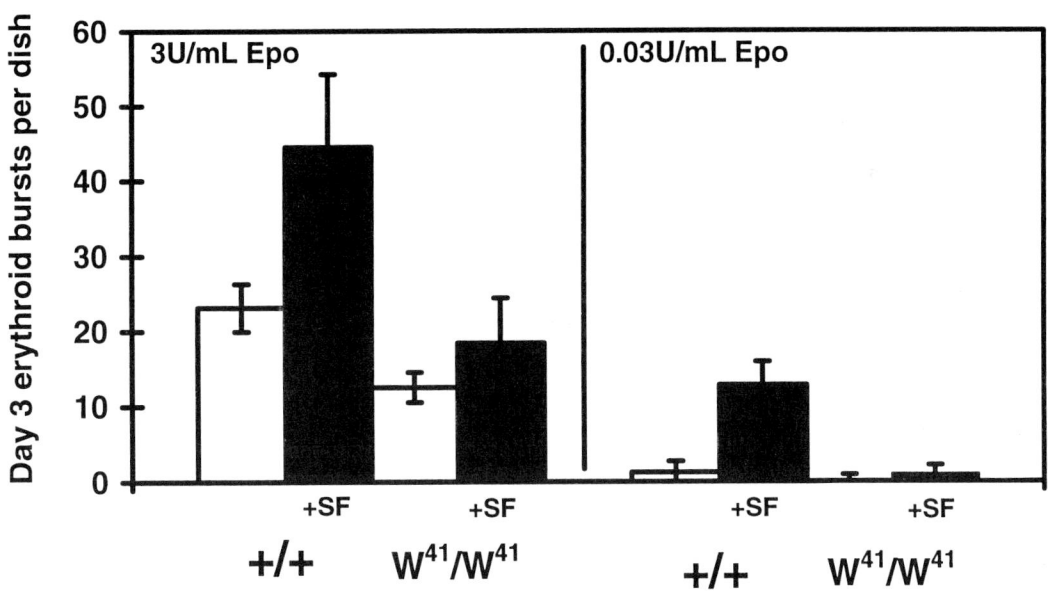

Figure 1. Near normal numbers of Day 3 (mature) BFU-E are found in the bone marrow of adult W^{41}/W^{41} mice but they do not show the enhanced plating efficiency in the presence of SF that is characteristic of their normal counterparts from +/+ mice. 8x10^4 marrow cells were plated per dish. Data redrawn from [13].

their ability to reconstitute both the lymphoid and myeloid compartments when transplanted at limiting dilution into irradiated recipients [16]. The LTC-IC assay is an *in vitro* assay which detects and quantitates the number of cells in a test cell suspension that, when stimulated by unknown factors produced by marrow fibroblast feeder layers, are able to generate *in vitro* CFC progeny for at least 4 weeks. LTC-IC are found in the same subpopulation of Sca-1^+ Lin$^-$ ($\pm$ WGA) fetal liver and adult marrow cells as are CRU [17], (C.D. Helgason, manuscript in preparation). Some LTC-IC can be shown to have both myeloid and lymphoid potential and, in the adult, LTC-IC show the same relative resistance to 5-fluorouracil as CRU (in contrast to most CFU-S and CFC) [17]. It therefore seems likely that LTC-IC and CRU are closely related, if not completely overlapping, cell populations. An advantage of the LTC-IC assay for studies of stem cells in W-mutant mice is the fact that their detection does not appear to depend on, or involve, a response to SF [18, 19]. Thus a deficient ability to mount such a response, as would be expected of a W^{41}/W^{41} stem cell, would not mask its ability to be detected as an LTC-IC. SF does appear to play a major role in the detection of CFU-S *in vivo* [8, 9] but its role in the *in vivo* detection of CRU had not been previously investigated.

Application of these different stem cell assays to bone marrow cells from adult +/+ or W^{41}/W^{41} mice [13] and day 14.5 fetal liver cells from +/+ or W^{41}/W^{41} embryos has shown the size of the LTC-IC population to be approximately 2-fold smaller in the W-mutant mice at both stages of development. The same finding has been obtained for Day 12 CFU-S. The proliferative behaviour (CFC output per LTC-IC) exhibited by the W^{41}/W^{41} LTC-IC also appears to be normal. Similarly, there is no difference in the size of the spleen colonies produced by +/+ and W^{41}/W^{41} fetal liver cells, although those produced by adult W^{41}/W^{41} marrow cells are somewhat smaller than those produced by their adult +/+ counterparts. This trend is even more exaggerated when +/+ and W^{41}/W^{41} CRU from these same sources are compared. The average number of CRU in W^{41}/W^{41} fetal liver is approximately two thirds of that measured in +/+ embryos whereas in the bone marrow of adult W^{41}/W^{41} mice, the number of cells detectable as CRU is only one twentieth of the +/+ value. The simplest interpretation of these findings is that SF is not required for the generation and maintenance of near normal numbers of hematopoietic stem cells at any stage of development but can become rate-limiting in the adult under conditions where rapid regeneration of the system is stimulated by myeloablative treatment. However, this critical role of SF is only revealed when the cells called upon are of adult origin.

Discussion

W^{41}/W^{41} mice represent a useful model system to investigate the role of SF in regulating hematopoietic stem cell activity and to examine potential changes in that role under the different conditions of demand for new blood cell production that may occur in the embryo and in the adult. The W^{41} mutation causes a significant reduction in the kinase activity of the c-kit receptor that is prerequisite for SF-induced signaling [14] and the effect of this at the biological level can be readily demonstrated *(e.g., see Figure 1)*. Nevertheless, W^{41}/W^{41} mutant mice are both viable and fertile which facilitates the maintenance of homozygous stocks for a variety of functional investigations.

A considerable literature has accumulated demonstrating the ability of many hematopoietic cell types to respond to SF. On the other hand, redundancy in the activities of cytokines is also now a well established principle for many target cells including members of the hematopoietic system. Identification of the precise mechanisms used to regulate hematopoiesis *in vivo* under different conditions has thus become a major challenge. Early studies of W- and Steel-mutant mice indicated a major role of SF in the recruitment of stem cells or their early progeny following their transplantation into irradiated recipients [8, 9]. Even in normal adult mice a role for SF in regulating stem cell recruitment was suggested by the fact that a defect in SF signaling makes adult stem cells less competitive [10, 11]. More recent experiments indicate that this is probably insufficient to affect the generation of a normal stem cell population during normal development, presumably because of the existence of other cytokines that can also stimulate stem cell self-renewal divisions and compensate for a defective SF response. On the other hand, under the conditions created following a lethal dose of total body irradiation, SF assumes a more critical role in enabling rapid hematopoietic recovery. It might, therefore, have been anticipated that the heightened stem cell turnover required for the rapid expansion of the hematopoietic system that occurs during fetal development might also be compromised in mice with a defective capacity to respond to SF. However, this has turned out not to be the case, as shown by studies of both Steel [12] and W-mutant embryos. Moreover, hematopoietic stem cells isolated from the fetal liver of W-mutant mice, unlike their derivatives subsequently found in adult marrow, can undergo rapid expansion *in vivo,* even in an adult microenvironment. Thus in two situations where there is a rapid proliferation of normal hematopoietic cells (early ontogeny and after myeloablative treatment of the adult), the differences observed are dependent in part on a difference in the environment/conditions to which the cells are exposed and in part on the ontological state of the target stem cells. Further delineation of conditions that are operative in the fetus and to which factors fetal stem cells appear more responsive may be useful for improving strategies for clinical procedures requiring the genetic modification and/or expansion ex vivo of fetal stem cells.

References

1. Moore MAS and Metcalf D. Ontogeny of the haemopoietic system; yolk sac origin of *in vivo* and *in vitro* colony forming cell in the developing mouse embryo. *Br J Haematol* 1970; 18: 279.
2. Muller AM, Medvinsky A, Strouboulis J, Grosveld F and Dzierzak E. Development of hematopoietic stem cell activity in the mouse embryo. *Immunity* 1994; 1: 291-301.
3. Witte ON. Steel locus defines new multipotent growth factor. *Cell* 1990; 63: 5-6.
4. Williams DE, de Vries P, Namen AE, Widmer MB and Lyman SD. The Steel factor. *Dev Biol* 1992; 151: 368-376.
5. Geissler EN, McFarland EC and Russell ES. Analysis of pleiotropism at the dominant white-spotting (W) locus of the house mouse: A description of ten new W alleles. *Genetics* 1981; 97: 337-361.
6. Ogawa M, Nishikawa S, Yoshinaga K, Hayashi S-I, Kunisada T, Nakao J, Kina T, Sudo T, Kodama H and Nishikawa S-I. Development and function of c-kit in fetal hemopoietic progenitor cells: transition from the early c-kit-independent to the late c-kit-dependent wave of hemopoiesis in the murine embryo. *Development* 1993; 117: 1089-1098.
7. Ogawa M, Matsuzaki Y, Nishikawa S, Hayashi S-I, Kunisada T, Sudo T, Kina T, Nakauchi H and Nishikawa SI. Expression and function of c-kit in hemopoietic progenitor cells. *J Exp Med* 1991; 174: 63-71.
8. McCulloch EA, Siminovitch L and Till JE. Spleen colony formation in anemic mice of genotype W/W^v. *Science* 1964; 144: 844-846.
9. McCulloch EA, Siminovitch L, Till JE, Russell ES and Bernstein SE. The cellular basis of the genetically determined hemopoietic defect in anaemic mice of genotype Sl^d/Sl^d. *Blood* 1965; 26: 399-410.
10. Boggs DR, Boggs SS, Saxe DS, Gress RA and Canfield DR. Hematopoietic stem cells with high proliferative potential. Assay of their concentration in marrow by the frequency and duration of cure of W/W^v mice. *J Clin Invest* 1982; 70: 242-253.
11. Harrison DE and Astle CM. Lymphoid and erythroid repopulation in B6 W-anemic mice: A new unirradiated recipient. *Exp Hematol* 1991; 19: 374-377.
12. Ikuta K and Weissman IL. Evidence that hematopoietic stem cells express mouse c-kit but do not depend on steel factor for their generation. *Proc Natl Acad Sci USA* 1992; 89: 1502-1506.

13. Miller CL, Rebel VI, Lemieux ME, Helgason CD, Lansdorp PM and Eaves CJ. Studies of W-mutant mice provide evidence for alternate mechanisms capable of activating hematopoietic stem cells. *Exp Hematol* (in press).
14. Nocka K, Tan JC, Chiu E, Chu TY, Ray P, Traktman P and Besmer P. Molecular bases of dominant negative and loss of function mutations at the murine c-kit/white spotting locus: W^{37}, W^v, W^{41} and W. *EMBO J* 1990; 9: 1805-1813.
15. Rebel VI, Dragowska W, Eaves CJ, Humphries RK and Lansdorp PM. Amplification of Sca-1$^+$ Lin$^-$ WGA$^+$ cells in serum- free cultures containing Steel factor, Interleukin-6, and erythropoietin with maintenance of cells with long-term *in vivo* reconstituting potential. *Blood* 1994; 83: 128-136.
16. Szilvassy SJ, Humphries RK, Lansdorp PM, Eaves AC and Eaves CJ. Quantitative assay for totipotent reconstituting hematopoietic stem cells by a competitive repopulation strategy. *Proc Natl Acad Sci USA* 1990; 87: 8736-8740.
17. Lemieux ME, Rebel VI, Lansdorp PM and Eaves CJ. Characterization and purification of a primitive hematopoietic cell type in adult mouse marrow capable of lympho-myeloid differentiation in long-term marrow «switch» cultures. *Blood* (in press).
18. Sutherland HJ, Hogge DE, Cook D and Eaves CJ. Alternative mechanisms with and without Steel factor support primitive human hematopoiesis. *Blood* 1993; 81: 1465-1470.
19. Kodama H, Nose M, Yamaguchi Y, Tsunoda J, Suda T and Nishikawa S. *In vitro* proliferation of primitive hemopoietic stem cells supported by stromal cells: Evidence for the presence of a mechanism(s) other than that involving c-kit receptor and its ligand. *J Exp Med* 1992; 176: 351-361.

Résumé

Le *Steel factor* est une cytokine pléiotropique qui agit sur un grand nombre de types cellulaires du système hématopoïétique. Le récepteur du SF est codé par le proto-oncogène *c-kit* identifié chez la souris comme le locus *white spotting* (W). Les mutations germinales affectant, soit le SF, soit son récepteur, provoquent une anémie macrocytaire, des modifications de la couleur des poils ainsi qu'une stérilité. Des études antérieures ont également montré que ces mutations modifient l'activité *in vivo* des cellules souches hématopoïétiques. Pour étudier cet aspect, nous avons comparé le nombre et l'activité de ces cellules dans le foie fœtal et dans la moelle adulte de souris normales et W41/W41. Les résultats montrent qu'un nombre normal de cellules souches hématopoïétiques peut être produit et maintenu pendant le développement fœtal et la vie adulte en absence d'une réponse SF fonctionnelle. De plus, les cellules souches W41/W41 stimulées *in vitro* dans des conditions qui n'impliquent pas SF ont une capacité de réponse proliférative normale. Par ailleurs, l'expansion du système hématopoïétique chez la souris adulte au cours de la récupération hématopoïétique secondaire à une chimiothérapie est dépendante de la stimulation du SF, contrairement à l'expansion indépendante du SF observée pendant le développement fœtal. Cette modification du rôle du SF pendant la vie fœtale est associée à une diminution correspondante de la capacité du système hématopoïétique adulte d'être régulé par des mécanismes alternatifs importants pour le contrôle de la prolifération cellulaire au cours de la vie fœtale.

2) Ontogeny of the immune system

2) *Ontogénie du système immunitaire*

Cytokine/receptor control points in murine T cell development

James P. Di Santo

INSERM U 429, Hôpital Necker-Enfants Malades, 149, rue de Sèvres, 75015 Paris, France, fax: (33 1) 46 77 84 37

Abstract

Lymphocyte development results from the expansion and differentiation of committed precursor cells under the influence of bone marrow, thymic and gut microenvironments, and requires both stem cell-stromal cell contact and interactions between soluble cytokines and their receptors. A variety of lymphokines play a role in T-cell differentiation, acting both intrathymically during the early develomental stages or later in the peripheral effector phases of immune responses. Modifications of genes in the germline via homologous recombination represents a powerful approach to define the role of cytokines and their receptors in lymphoid development. This paper will present the results from a number of cytokine/receptor "knock-outs" which help to define control points for the various pathways of T-cell differentiation.

A review of the relationship of cytokines and their receptors to immune development would be better the subject of a book rather than a short review, and instead the focus of this paper will be the analysis of recent data linking certain cytokines and their receptors to pathways of T-cell development. T lymphocytes comprise various compartments based on anatomical location, phenotype and function. As discussed in-depth by other authors in this book, the pluripotent hematopoietic stem cell continually generates both T-lineage restricted and less restricted precursors which can seed the thymus. Further T-lineage committment occurs here. Early T-cell precursors divide and generate large numbers of immature thymocytes which express specific markers including CD3, CD4 and CD8, and a diverse repetoire of T-cell receptors (TCRs). Maturation of these cells involves the processes of positive and negative selection to yield functional, mature CD4 or CD8 lymphocytes which exit the thymus to seed the peripheral secondary lymphoid organs, primarily including the spleen and lymph nodes, the Peyers Patches in the gut wall. Natural killer (NK) cells in part arise from a common T/NK precursor which may or may not pass through the thymus, before seeding the periphery [1]. Another TCR+ cell compartment includes those developing in the absence of a thymus (similar to NK cells), which can be found primarily in the gut epithelia (intraepithelial lymphocytes, IEL), and also in the liver. These "thymo-independent" lineage differs in many respects from the classical thymus-derived

T-cells, and appear to arise from a distinct mechanism [2]. Thus T- and NK-cells comprise various compartments with respect to their developmental pathway and their distribution in the periphery. These different T/NK populations also differ in their cytokine requirements as well.

Cytokines and T-cell development

The role of cytokines and their receptors in T-cell development has been demonstrated by various technical approaches. Clearly, most cytokines were biochemically purified and subsequently cloned based on *in vitro* cellular assays, such as colony formation, proliferation, or effector functions such as cytotoxicity or antibody production. These assays can give a general estimation of the range of cytokine activity. These assays, however, do not allow for a comparison of the relative potency or importance between cytokines which have biological activity. Further neutralization of cytokine activity by antibody neutralization or blocking of the cognate receptor *in vitro*, in *ex vivo* organ culture, or *in vivo* may help to substantiate the biological importance of a cytokine/receptor system. For example, an antibody against the interleukin-2 (IL-2) receptor alpha chain (CD25), specifically identified a subpopulation of early precursors in the thymus and blocked thymocyte development in fetal thymic organ culture (FTOC), suggesting that interactions between IL-2 and its receptor may be important for intrathymic T-cell development *in vivo*. Exogenous cytokine administration *in vivo* is another useful approach in that one begins with an intact immune system and any pertubations can be followed with time. A complementary approach using transgenic mice overexpressing a cytokine can target expression to a particular lymphoid compartment depending on the nature of the transgenic promoter. Lastly, targeted disruption of a gene using homologous recombination in embryonic stem cell provides a certain definitive approach, in that development in complete absence of any gene product can be evaluated. Still, gene knock-outs may suffer from certain peculiarities inherent to the immune system, as will be discussed.

What have cytokine/receptor gene KO mice told us about the role of these factors in T-cell development ? Specifically, do certain cytokines interactions determine lineage development, and within certain compartments, are there differential effects during intrathymic and peripheral stages ? What can be learned about cytokine redundancy ? and immune plasticity (specifically the ability of the immune system to respond through expansion of otherwise minor subpopulations) ?

IL-2 deficient mice

Since the hypothesis that IL-2 plays a role in thymic development has already been mentioned, let us summarize the IL-2 deficient mouse [3]. The most surprising feature of the IL-2 KO mouse is what initially seems like such a normal immune system can become so very abnormal. First, despite the impressive amount of data demonstrating the capacity of IL-2 to support lymphocyte proliferation *in vitro,* and the effects of CD25 antibodies in FTOC, it appears that IL-2 does not play a role in the thymus. Cell numbers, phenotype and mechanisms of positive and negative selection are completely normal in IL-2$^{-/-}$ thymi [3, 4]. Moreover, peripheral cell number, phenotype, distribution, and many *in vivo* immune responses are normal or only minimally afffected in 3-4 week-old mice: antiviral responses, T-mediated antigen-specific immunologlobulin production, and NK activity are present [5]. The generation of thymus-independent gut

IEL and liver T-cells has not yet been reported. Overall, young IL-2 deficient mice are relatively normal. However, by 6-8 weeks of age, a number of abnormalities have developed including severe anemia, and splenomegaly with polyclonal B-cell activation, causing death in 50% of mice, whereas the other 50% develop an inflammatory bowel disease [6]. These pathophysiology underlying these processes are not well understood, but they seem to involve an expansion of $CD4^+$ cells, which are presumably unregulated and upset immune homeostasis. These effects are mediated by T cells, as IL-2 deficient *nu/nu* mice do not suffer the disease. Thus, IL-2 may be viewed as a key mediator of immune regulation, specifically with respect to T-cells, in contrast with its original assumed role as a strictly proliferative agent.

IL-4 deficient mice

IL-4 was also originally identified as a growth factor for lymphoid cells, and as an important B-cell differentiation factor for immunoglobulin (Ig) isotype switch. IL-4 action is pleiotropic with additional growth and differentiation activities for hematopoietic precursors, mast cells and macrophages. However, the IL-4 deficient mice have surprisingly few hematopoietic system abnormalities [7]. $IL-4^{-/-}$ mice have no intrathymic abnormalities, nor any peripheral T-cell dysfunction. NK cells are present, but any effects on gut IEL development has not yet been reported. B-cells are present in normal numbers, however, these cells fail to produce IgE and levels of IgG1 are reduced, while other Ig isotypes appear unaffected. Infection with the nematode *Nippostrongylus brasiliensis* induces a massive production of IgE in normal mice, while similar infection of IL-4 deficient mice results in no IgE secretion [7]. Taken together, these results suggest that the major role of IL-4 lies in Ig switch regulation, specficially to that of IgE. It could be agrued that other lymphokines may be able to replace IL-4 for T-cell development, implying a redundancy at the level of IL-4 function. The alternative argument is that IL-4 has no role in T-cell development. Unlike IL-2 deficient mice, IL-4 deficient mice do not develop autoimmune manifestations with increasing age.

Mice doubly-deficient for IL-2 and IL-4 have been analyzed [8]. These mice have normal intrathymic and peripheral T-cell compartments, suggesting that these two cytokines are not redundant for eachother in mainstream T-lymphocyte development.

IL-7 deficient mice

IL-7 was initially described as a growth factor for pre-B cells and additional *in vitro* studies demonstrated the ability of IL-7 to stimulate growth of many other hematopoietic cell types, including T-cells. When administered to mice, antibodies to IL-7 or its receptor arrest B-cell development, and decrease thymic cellularity, while injection of IL-7 or constituitive IL-7 production by transgenes in mice result in increase numbers of peripheral T and B-cells. Recently, mice deficient for IL-7 and its receptor have been described [9, 10]. The $IL-7R^{-/-}$ mice have a more complicated phenotype, which may relate to interactions between the IL-7R and ligands other than IL-7 *(see below)*. Therefore, it is simpler to first discuss the $IL-7^{-/-}$ mice. Unlike IL-2 and IL-4 knock-outs, IL-7 deficient mice show a dramatic thymic phenotype with a 25-fold decrease in total thymocyte cell numbers. Interestingly the remaining cells demonstrate a normal CD4/CD8 pattern and proliferate in mitogenic assays with responses similar to wild-type thymocytes. The peripheral T-cell compartment is likewise decreased in size, but normally responsive *in vitro*. NK cells are present and functional. Gut IEL have not yet been analyzed, and there is no evidence of regulatory dysfunction or autoimmune disease in older IL-7$^{-/-}$ mice. Thus, IL-7 plays a major role in intrathymic T-cell development (and early B-cell development, although space limits the discussion here), probably during the immature (CD4-CD8-) stage. It is known that IL-7R are present on early thymocytes and that IL-7 can stimulate their proliferation *in vitro*. Therefore it is likely that IL-7 interacting with its receptor plays a major role in the expansion of intrathymic precursors. Since this block is not complete, other factor(s) can poorly compensate resulting in partial thymocyte development and small numbers of peripheral splenic T-cells. Moreover, the fact that residual lymphocytes in IL-7$^{-/-}$ mice do not expand in the periphery suggests that IL-7 also plays a critical role in peripheral lymphoid homeostasis. Although severely lymphopenic, IL-7 deficient mice are not immunodeficient. Thus IL-7$^{-/-}$ mice demonstrate the tremendous plasticity of the immune system, where compensatory mechanisms can recover some level of immune development in an animal otherwise missing a critical cytokine.

IL-2Rγ deficient mice

Recently, the IL-2Rγ chain has attracted a great deal of interest because mutations in this molecule are associated with an X-linked severe combined immune deficiency in humans (SCIDX1) characterized by a complete block in T-cell development. Although this receptor chain was first described as a functional component of the IL-2R, the absence of any T-cell deficiency in IL-2 deficient states in mice or man [3, 11] strongly suggested the IL-2Rγ chain participated in other cytokine receptor systems. Over the past year it has be shown that IL-2Rγ participates in the receptors for multiple cytokines, including IL-2, IL-4, IL-7, IL-9 and IL-15 [12]. The IL-2Rγ chain appears obligatory for IL-2 and IL-15 binding and function. While IL-4R and IL-7R can bind their resepctive ligands, transfection experiments have shown that the IL-2Rγ chain augments the affinity of IL-4 and IL-7 receptors. Still it remained unclear whether these receptors could function in the absence of IL-2Rγ. More importantly, the stage at which IL-2Rγ deficiency blocked the development and function of lymphoid cells was unclear. To address these questions and to generate an animal model for SCIDX1, we disrupted the IL-2Rγ chain by a modified gene targeting approach.

The LoxP/Cre bacteriophage recombinase system was used to create a defined deletion of the IL-2Rγ chain gene. LoxP sites are small (34 bp) sequences which are specifically recognized by the enzyme Cre [13]. The Cre enzyme mediates a recombination event at these sites, resulting in the specific deletion of DNA sequences between two in-phase LoxP sites. This process functions in many cell types, and has been used to create site-specific deletions in the mammalian genome. In our experiment, the targeting vector contained a single LoxP site into the first intron and a LoxP-flanked neomycin resistance cassette into the sixth intron of the IL-2Rγ gene [14]. Following homologous recombination in ES cells, the endogenous gene was replaced with the LoxP-modified version. The Cre enzyme was then expressed by transient transfection in the ES clones. Different deletion events between the LoxP sites were anticipated. Deletion between upstream LoxP1 and LoxP3 removed the neo gene and exons 2 through 6 of the IL-2Rγ gene. As these exons encode the entire extracellular and transmembrane domains of the molecule, this would result in a locus unable to produce any IL-2Rγ protein (γ-). A deletion between LoxP2 and LoxP3 removes only the neo cassette, and results in a IL-2Rγ locus with LoxP sites remaining in the first and sixth introns. These sites should not in principle disrupt the ability of the gene to produce a functional IL-2Rγ protein, and this locus is referred to as "flanked by Lox P" or "floxed" (g^{flox}). Mice carrying either of these two modified IL-2Rγ loci in the germline were generated. Results of the initial analysis of these mice have been recently reported [15].

As expected, T-cell development in IL-2Rγ-deficient male mice is abnormal. The thymus of IL-2Rγ⁻ mice is small with a 30 fold reduction in cell number (roughly 5-10 x 10^6 cells/thymus). Interestingly, no single stage of T-cell differentiation is uniquely affected as thymocytes show near normal patterns of expression for CD4 and CD8 molecules. Spleens of IL-2Rγ-deficient mice have a 8-fold reduction in lymphoid cell numbers, and a small number mature T- and B-cells are present. Strikingly, NK-cells and gut IELs are not found in IL-2Rγ⁻ mice, and Peyer's patches are not detected.

Functionally, thymocytes and splenocytes from IL-2Rγ-deficient mice are poorly responsive to mitogens *in vitro* with or without added cytokines (IL-2, IL-4, IL-7, IL-9). PMA with IL-4 is a strong stimulus for normal thymocytes, but fails to activate thymocytes from IL-2Rγ⁻ animals. Consistent with the absence of phenotypically defined NK-cells, IL-2Rγ-deficient mice lack NK activity against the YAC target cell line. Splenic B-cells also fail to undergo IL-4 mediated Ig isotype switch. Taken together, these results strongly suggest that in the absence of the IL-2Rγ chain, the function of multiple cytokines, including IL-2, IL-4, IL-7 and IL-9 is impaired. Mice carrying "floxed" IL-2Rγ loci were immunologically normal, as were female mice who were heterozygous carriers of the IL-2Rγ⁻ mutation.

IL-2Rγ⁻ mice, which can be considered IL-2, -4, -7, -9, -15 deficient mice, also develop some autoimmune features similar to IL-2 mice, such as splenomegaly with secondary hematopoiesis and decrease in B cell numbers with age. The mice also are extremely susceptible to infection, and manifest a global immune deficiency with early death (within 12 weeks in conventional facilities). A puzzle remains to determine which cytokines are responsible for the development of the residual lymphoid cells seen in these mice. Recently, a new factor called thymic stromal lymphopoeitin, TSLP, has been identified [10]. This factor binds the IL-7Rα chain and a new receptor chain called IL-7Rβ, and thus may be able to function in the absence of IL-2Rγ chain. The identification of TSLP may also help to explain the more severe thymic phenotype seen in the IL-7R(α)-deficient mice, which would logically be unresponsive to either IL-7 or TSLP.

Conclusions

T-cell development may be viewed a passing through a number of cytokine checkpoints. IL-7 plays an important role both intrathymically and peripherally. The strong effect of IL-7 deficiency in the thymus mirrors that of IL-2Rγ, and suggests that most of the thymic phenotype in IL-2Rγ-deficient mice is likely due to the lack of IL-7 function. The dependence of certain cell populations on IL-2Rγ expression, such as NK or gut IEL, for example, which are spared by all single cytokine deficient mice, suggest that these populations likely depend on a combination of cytokines (likely to be IL-2 plus IL-15) for their initial production and/or maintenance. This hypothesis may soon be supported with the IL-2Rβ-deficient mice, which should share this phenotype. Interestingly, the cytokines once thought to be the major mediators of T-cell proliferation (such as IL-2 and IL-4), seem to be important in peripheral immune regulation rather than in the establishment of the lymphoid system. It is clear that future cytokine/receptor deficient mice will allow us to build on this model.

The technique of homologous recombination to target genes in ES provides a powerful approach to discern the function of cytokines and their receptors in immune function. The analysis of various mouse strains deficient in cytokines and their receptors has demonstrated a their roles in the development of certain T and NK lineages, and in discerning function in primary, secondary and regulatory aspects of immune development. The caution in this approach, however, remains in the immune response to the KO gene. Compensatory mechanisms may allow for unexpected degrees of immune reconstitution (for example the development of mature T cells in IL-2Rγ^- mice). An alternative approach may lie in the analysis of chimeric animals, in which gene targeted cells could be marked and easily followed. In this scenario, the competition and interaction between normal and deficient cells might also give some insight into the importance of a particular gene in the function of the immune system.

References

1. Rodewald H.-R. Pathways from hematopoietic stems cells to thymocytes. *Curr Opin Immunol* 1995; 7: in press.
2. Rocha B, Guy-Grand D, Vassalli P. Extrathymic T cell differentiation. *Curr Opin Immunol* 1995; 7: in press.
3. Schorle H, Holtschke T, Hünig T, Schimpl A, Horak I. Development and function of T cells in mice rendered interleukin-2 deficient by gene targeting. *Nature* 1991; 352: 621-24.
4. Krämer S, Mamalaki C, Horak I, Schimpl A, Kioussis D, Hünig T. Thymic selection and peptide-induced activation of T cell receptor-transgenic CD8 T cells in interleukin-2-deficient mice. *Eur J Immunol* 1994; 24: 2317-22.
5. Kündig, TM, Schorle H, Bachmann MF, Hengartner H, Zinkernagel RM, Horak I. Immune responses in interleukin-2-deficient mice. *Science* 1993; 262: 1059-61.
6. Sadlack B, Merz H, Schorle H, Schimpl A, Feller A, Horak I. Ulcerative colitis-like disease in mice with a disrupted interleukin-2 gene. *Cell* 1993; 75: 253-61.
7. Kühn R, Rajewsky K, Müller W. Generation and analysis of interleukin-4 deficient mice. *Science* 1991; 254: 707-10.
8. Sadlack B, Kühn R, Schorle H, Rajewsky K, Müller W, Horak I. Development and proliferation of lymphocytes in mice deficient for both interleukins-2 and 4. *Eur J Immunol* 1994; 24: 281-84.
9. von Freeden-Jeffry U, Vieira P, Lucian LA, McNeil T, Burdach SEG, Murray R. Lymphopenia in interleukin-7 gene-deleted mice identifies IL-7 as a nonredundant cytokine. *J Exp Med* 1995; 181: 1519-26.
10. Peschon JJ, Morrissey PJ, Grabstein KH, Ramsdell FJ, Maraskovsky E, Gliniak BC, Park LS, Ziegler SF, Williams DE, Ware CB, Meyer JD, Davison BL. Early lymphocyte expansion is severely impaired in interleukin 7 receptor deficient mice. *J Exp Med* 1994; 180: 1955-60.
11. DiSanto JP, Keever CA, Small TN, Nichols GL, O'Reilley RJ, Flomenberg N. Absence of interleukin-2 production in a severe combined immunodeficiency disease syndrome with T cells. *J Exp Med* 1990; 171: 1697-1704.
12. Taniguchi T. Cytokine signaling through nonreceptor protein tyrosine kinases. *Science* 1995; 268: 251-5.
13. Sternberg N, Hamilton D. Bacteriophage P1 site-specific recombination I: recombination between LoxP sites. *J Mol Biol* 1981; 150: 467-86.
14. DiSanto JP, Certain S, Wilson A, MacDonald HR, Avner P, Fischer A, de Saint Basile G. The murine interleukin-2 receptor g chain gene: organization, chromosomal localization aand expression in the adult thymus. *Eur J Immunol* 1994; 24: 3014-18.
15. DiSanto JP, Müller W, Guy-Grand D, Fischer A, Rajewsky K. Lymphoid development in mice with a targeted deletion of the interleukin-2 receptor gamma chain. *Proc Natl Acad Sci USA* 1995; 92: 377-81.

Résumé

Le développement lymphocytaire résulte de l'expansion et de la différenciation de cellules précurseurs « engagées », sous l'influence de la moelle osseuse, des microenvironnements thymiques et digestifs, et nécessite à la fois un contact entre les cellules souches et les cellules stromales et des interactions entre des cytokines solubles et leurs récepteurs. De nombreuses lymphokines interviennent au cours de la différenciation lymphocytaire T, et agissent à la fois au niveau intrathymique au cours des stages précoces du développement ou plus tard au cours des phases effectrices de la réponse immunitaire. La modification de gènes dans la lignée germinale par recombinaison homologue permet dorénavant de définir le rôle de ces cytokines et de leurs récepteurs au cours du développement lymphocytaire. Dans cette revue, nous présenterons les résultats de plusieurs expériences d'inactivation de gènes de cytokines/récepteurs qui permettent de définir les points de contrôle des différentes voies de différenciation des cellules T.

Materno foetal relationship

Gérard Chaouat

INSERM CJF 92-09 et Hôpital Antoine-Béclère, Bâtiment de Gynécologie obstétrique, avenue de la Porte-de-Trivaux, 92140 Clamart, France, tel. and fax: (33 1) 45 37 44 50

Abstract

We first recall briefly the status of inflammatory cytokines in early implantation period. We then describe the status of LIF production in an vitro relatively short term human decidual explant culture system. We then review the status of local immunosuppression in established pregnancy, and describe the molecules involved. We finish this brief review by giving some hints about the involvement of inflammatory cytokines in the onset of parturition.

Many of the concepts presented in this paper owe a lot to the tremendous impetus that was impulsed by the enunciation by the late Tom Wegmann of the original immunotrophic hypothesis [1], deduced from common work on a murine abortion model [2]. Much of my work would not have been possible without him, and indeed he was also quick to realise the interest of cytokine in early implantation [3]. I want specifically in the introduction to pay this tribute to his memory.

Pregnancy is often viewed from Medawar enunciation of the problems that were associated from the view point of a transplantation immunologist for the survival of the conceptus as a semiallogeneic allograft [4]. Whereas this is a concept that has allowed Reproductive Immunology to thrive and evolve, it must now be replaced by the concept of the use of immuologically defined molecules in a continuous crosstalk between the maternal decidua and the placenta, of which mastering rejection of the foetus is only a part.

Those steps begin to be very well known at Molecular level, and our knowledge of the feto maternal relationship is now far from the pseudo science status that serious immunologist still attribute to the Field, in ignorance of the clear cut demonstration of the role of cytokines in parturition, and ... the aforementioned demise of by gone theories and concepts such as "blocking factors" of undetermined origin, the role of antibodies in establishing tolerance, the TLX theory, etc. The involvement of immunologic mechanism is demonstrated unambiguously by gene knock out animals, isolation and /or cloning of suppressor molecules, precise quantitative PCRs as well as RNAse protection assays, etc.

The cytokine crosstalk is programmed, and in fact "inflammatory like" mechanisms, triggered by the reaction of the mother reproductive tract to the foreign bodies that are spermatozoa, and later on blastocyst(s), are at first absolutely mandatory for implantation to occur in the proper hormonal context which also triggers local growth factor production (EGF, IGF, CSF-1, etc). Nature has even opened his News and views section by the provocative "could there be life without LIF?" which replace the field in its exact perspective.

After the process occurs (and it is far from this review, but it must also be said, the immunologic like dialogue is involved in inducing the expression of adhesion molecules and integrins on the placenta and decidua), its persistence could lead to high local expression of TNF and gamma IFN which are embryo toxic /embryo cytostatic. Therefore, the process is very quickly down regulated by the shift towards a local and systemic "Th2" cytokine profiles, whereas the embryo also makes use of its own cytostatic molecules, the placental interferons (tau ones in most species), to prevent local NK activation expansion that would be detrimental to itself. The beauty of the process is that those molecules… are of prime endocrine function in most species since they maintain the corpus luteum.

In the early post implantation period, and in the established pregnancy, a very important local immunosuppression is observed, exerted both by decidual and placental suppressor molecules, and a progesterone dependent suppressor circuit. This is when the conceptus is the most akin in mice and rats where the placenta is MHC H-2 K and D positive on the external layers of the placenta to the semiallogenic allograft status, protected by local immunosuppression, that most of you still think about when dealing with mother foetus relationship.

Finally, at the end of pregnancy, and I will briefly review it in this paper, there is now very solid evidence for the involvement of inflammatory mediators in the very process of delivery.

Let us first discuss implantation.

In mice and rats, leukocyte like cells migrate and accumulate on Day 1 very close to the uterine lumen [5-7]. This is a seminal fluid dependent migration, no such cell trafficking being seen following mating with vasectomised males are used [7]. "Immunologically" speaking, this is very akin to an inflammatory reaction, and one can indeed detect a marked secretion by both lymphocytes and cells from the uterine tract itself, *e.g.* decidual epithelial or glandular cells of IL-1,TNF,IL-6, G-CSF, CSF-1, M-CSF and IL 3 [7,8]. Most of those lymphokines will come back to normal by days 3, and still be expressed at low levels after implantation [9] except for CSF [10]. The important role of IL-1 is exquisitely shown by C. Simon [11] who showed that IL-1 receptor antagonist prevents successful implantation in mice. The role of CSF-1 is shown by elegant work of J Pollard who have shown that CSF-1 regulated placental development and that op/op mutant mice who have no CSF-1 are of low fertility and almost completely sterile ([10] and personal communications, and in press).

The most important cytokine at this stage is HILDA-LIF (Human Interleukin for Leukocyte Differentiation Antigen, Leukaemia Inhibiting Factor). In mice, by gene knock out technology, Stewart *et al* [12], confirmed by a French group with the same technology [13] have shown that LIF- / LIF- homozygous mutants are sterile albeit they are fertile) because embryos (be them LIF-/LIF- or LIF+/LIF+) do not implant in such mice, except if these are supplemented by recombinant LIF is given via an osmotic pump.

We have recently shown that when we compared samples from fertile women and a group of women suffering from sterility of unknown aetiology, despite successful IVF since implantation repeatedly fails the later have a very low LIF production *in vitro*. Our data strongly suggest that, in some well defined cases, repeated implantation failures after successful IVF could be due to a LIF deficiency. Since recombinant LIF is available, such a diagnosis could pave the way to further substitutive therapeutics analogue to what was performed in the mutant mice.

As I said, it is then necessary to down regulate the inflammatory reaction, and indeed the last prediction of Tom Wegmann was that "successful allopregnancy is a TH2 phenomenon" [14].

Indeed, a TH2 profile can be observed in normal pregnancy whereas similar results are obtained using quantitative PCR [15, 16]. Conversely, the immunological profile of mice undergoing early pregnancy loss is biased towards an excess TH1 profile [17,18], and indeed TH1 cytokines are abortifacient in normal mice [19-22].

Conversely, exacerbation and or prolongation of the local inflammatory component by DS RNA ([6, 23] and Kachkache et al, submitted for publication) leads to malimplantation.

It was tempting to speculate that TH2 secretion is required to down regulate the local post coital inflammatory response, and then all along pregnancy, with a peak as deduced from kinetics studies at the perimplantation period [15,16].

When we tested by sensitive specific ELISA, decidual and placental IL 10, IL 3, and IL 4, almost no production was noticed in CBA x DBA/2 (abortion prone murine mating) compared to CBA x BALB/c [24]. Recombinant IL-10 prevents foetal wastage in CBA x DBA/2 mice in a very very effective fashion, much more than did in previous series of experiments, or in recent parallel ones, IL 3 or GM-CSF [22]. This effect is not observed in non abortion prone mating. The obvious explanation is that these have no tendency as CBA to produce high titres of placental and decidual TNF and gamma INF (the latter fact is certainly the reason for the extreme difficulty to perform embryo transfers in the CBA foster mothers, compared to the ease of use of C57BL/6 recipients, for example [25].

In contrast, *in vivo* neutralisation of gamma interferon reduces the CBA x DBA/2 foetal wastage as well as sensitivity of various strains of mice to TNF, LPS, or Ds RNA promoted increases in resorbtion rate. Most important, alloimmunisation of CBA/J against BALB/c corrects local IL10 production in the CBA x DBA/2 combination.

What could be the signal for TH2 cytokine production? Let us recall that placenta secrets in a variety of species high levels of interferons, which also perform endocrine functions of prime importance: in ovine, bovine, etc *e.g.* species devoid of chorionic gonadotrophin, they insure corpus luteum maintenance [26-30]. Similar material might also exist in human [31, 32]. Such materials are immunosuppressive *in vitro* and *in vivo,* which make them ideal candidates for early pregnancy associated local immunosuppression [33, 34]. In addition, we had observed that CBA x DBA/2 foetal wastage could be prevented by *in vivo* injection of a single, pre or peri implantation tau interferon [35-37].We predicted that this could be due to induction by R.oTP of TH2 secretion profile characteristic of successful pregnancy more than its local cytostatic effects. Indeed, such an injection induces high levels of decidual suppressor activity, and part of it is mediated by an increase in decidual and placental IL 10 as well as IL 3 and IL 4.

The increase is in general more marked in placentae than deciduae.

Those data show a key role for immune endocrine interactions mediated by placental interferons. These would not only act as a local cytostatic agent and maintain the corpus luteum in a variety of species, devoid of CG, but a single molecule (tau INF) could thus exert the functions of both endocrine signalisation of early pregnancy maternal recognition of pregnancy and install the isotypic regulation and down play of cellular immune responses characteristic of pregnancy before maternal allorecognition of the foeto placental unit occurs via IL 10 regulation of the production of the otherwise abortifacient cytokines, TNF and gamma INF. It is relatively simple to imagine how placental interferons could exert their effect on TH2 like (like because this secretion is very unlikely to be mainly due to lymphocytes). As in other situations, TH2 secretion s would act as feed back to the (quite enormous) constitutional secretion of interferon by placenta, perceived as an "abnormal" interferon response which immediately calls for down regulation signals. Another possibility would be an interferon action on IL 10 receptors. Such a role could be the logical explanation for conservation of tau interferon structure across species.

The establishment of the Th2 profile is, as stated, a characteristic of the then ongoing established pregnancy. At that stage, placental and decidual IL-10 are part of an important local immunosuppresive gradient.

Other immune endocrine pathways need mentioning. Szekeres Bartho on one hand, Beaman and colleagues on the other hand have described progesterone dependent secretion of suppressive factors [40-43] and indeed monoclonal antibody to one of such factor which is cloned in both mice and human (TJ6) is indeed abortifacient [43] without affecting placenta l and embryo development *per se* [42].

The existence and involvement of lymphocytic progesterone receptors is now demonstrated by FACS analysis, ELISA, as well as Molecular Biology on activated lymphocytes [44-46].

The factor(s) we have here quoted suppress an MLR, an NK assay directed against human embryonic fibroblast, and in an MLR/CML boost cells of the suppressor induced phenotype and down regulate inside the CD8 pool expansion differentiation of cells of the cytotoxic subset [47].

In mice and human, similar properties have been ascribed to placental secreted immunosuppressive materials. The material has now been identified in the supernatants of human short term culture of human term placental cells or explants as a low MW (< 1 Kd) suppressor molecule which acts as an "anti IL2". In fact, the material is acting by preventing lymphokine or TCR or CD3 initiated lymphocyte replication, and block the cells very early in the replication cycle, leading to a state of functional anergy, with hyper expression of alpha beta TCR. *In vivo*, the material blocks a local GVH reaction as well as a general one provided the host is repopulated with adult, mature T cells and dose not involve bone marrow stem cells in the early steps of the repopulation [48-55], and De Smedt and Chaouat, submitted and in press).

In this respect, cord blood lymphocytes are sensitive to the action of the material, but when stem cells are injected into a lethally irradiated host, the half life of the product is too short for it to act long enough, *e.g.;* to be still present when/ before these cells engage in an alloantigen induced expansion after in a first step their differentiation into mature T cells.

On the other hand, adult T cells (splenocytes) are anergised only if they have a TCR specificity making them react with the allogenic component of the host. Otherwise they expand normally and do repopulate the host, giving it a normal immunocompetence when they encounter an antigen much later on, by then in absence of the suppressor product.

Another component which is of importance in the establishment of the local immunosuppression is decidual associated suppression. This is exerted by small non T non B cells, of the natural suppressor phenotype, which are recruited/migrate from bone marrow under trophoblast influence, and which act by secreting a soluble suppressor which is convincingly demonstrated to be a TGF beta 2 homologue material [56-59]. Lack of production of this factor is associated with abortion in mice [60].

Other local immunosuppressive agents are the expression by the placenta of complement regulatory molecules (which locally transform cytotoxic antibodies in non complement "actionable" ones, *eg* give them locally an enhancing function [61-64].

Indeed, enhancing antibodies and suppressor cells are demonstrable at systemic level during allopregnancy [65, 68-73]. But it must be stated with force that they are not mandatory for successful allopregnancy [74, 75].

Other important regulatory events/proteins are in the human selective expression on extravillous trophoblast of a monomorphic MHC class I molecule, whose expression is restricted to the placenta, HLA-G. HLA-G is the SOLE MHC molecule expressed in situ by human trophoblasts, and transfection experiments strongly suggest that it is a molecule whose expression confers hyposensitivity to NK mediated lysis [76-79].

Finally, at term, lymphokine do play an important role in delivery.

Let us mention here without detailing that LPS and TNF can induce labour in mice. This was first observed by Parand and Chedid, and confirmed by ourselves, and studied in great detail by Romero and colleagues in mice, and subsequently Chwalicsz in guinea pigs [80-83].

We have, using a classical PHA assay, as well as a miniaturised one that we have developed specially for that purpose, and a miniaturised NK assay, studied the capacity of lymphocytes from women in different state of parturition to produce Progesterone Induced Blocking Factor. We have also confirmed that the production of such a factor is abrogated during normal labour. We have then studied ocytocin induced labour and successful induced delivery. We have observed that the production of PIBF remains normal in such conditions.

Using a sensitive and specific ELISA as well as the L 929 bioassay, we have made a longitudinal study of TNF seric values from the very start of pregnancy (using IVF ET individuals with early positive HCG values). TNF (seric values) rise progressively in the second and third term of pregnancy, It is impossible at present to assess whether the lack of increase in seric TNF values observed in the first term reflects merely a dilution effect of low doses produced at that stage at the feto maternal interface, or whether there is a low (or lack of) production at the interface at that stage. Serious technical, financial, and ethical constraints limits studies of the first term at the feto maternal interface in primates and, indeed!, humans!

If one turns then to normal labour, seric TNF levels rise sharply during the early parturition onset (up to 5 cm cervical dilatation) (not shown). We have then been able to survey RU 486 induced labour. TNF values are enhanced again after one or two days of RU 486 ingestion (whichever the dose).They peak when the contraction start up to 5 cm dilatation. The increase of TNF during pregnancy is accompanied by an increase in seric soluble TNF receptors, be them the 55 Kd or 80 Kd form.

When ones studies normal or, interestingly, RU 486 induced parturition, not only is TNF production further enhanced (be it measured by ELISA or L 929 bioassay) compared to pregnancy, but seric soluble TNF receptors levels do rapidly decrease, thus causing an amplification of the bioactive TNF. Seric IL 1 also increases during labour [84].

Having reviewed materno foetal relationship, the main conclusion for this meeting is that at the materno foetal interface there exists a profound gradient of immunosuppression that would render any lymphocyte trafficking from mother to foetus, or vice versa, functionally inert, if not in fact anergised.

For this meeting, it means that it is very unlikely that cord blood lymphocytes would be populated with maternally derived functional lymphocytes, thus rendering very theoretical the threat of a cord blood derived GVH threat.

References

1. Wegmann TG. Foetal protection against abortion: is it immunosuppression or immunostimulation? 1984. *Ann immunol* Inst Pasteur 135 D. 309.
2. Chaouat G, Kiger N et Wegmann TG, 1983. Vaccination against spontaneous abortion in mice. *J Reprod Immunol* 389-392.
3. Wegmann TG, 1991. The role of lymphohaemopoietic cytokines in signalling between the immune and reproductive system. In Strauss II JF, Little CR (Eds). In uterine and embryonic factors in early pregnancy. *Plenum Press.* New York. P 87 96.
4. Medawar PB. Some immunological and endocrinological problems raised by the evolution of viviparity in vertebrates. Symp. *Soc Exp biol* 1953. 7. 320-338.
5. Noun A, Acker G, Chaouat G, Antoine JC and Garabedian M, 1989. Macrophages and T lymphocyte bearing antigens bearing cells in the uterus before and during ovum implantation in the rat. *Clin Exp Immunol* 78.434-438.

6. Kachkache M, Acker GM, Chaouat G, Noun A and Garabedian M, 1991. Hormonal and local factors control the immunohistochemical distribution of immunocytes in the rat uterus before conceptus implantation: Effects of ovariectomy, fallopian tube section and RU 486 injection. *Biology of Reproduction.* 45. 860-868.
7. Mac Master MT, Newton RC, Sudhanski K Dey and Andrews GK, 1992. Activation and distribution of inflammatory cells in the mouse uterus during the preimplantation period. *J Immunol* 148. 1699-1705.
8. Sanford TR, De M and Wood G, 1992. Expression of colony stimulating factors and inflammatory cytokines in the uterus if CD1 mice during days 1 to days 3 of pregnancy. *J Reprod Fert* 94.1. 213-220
9. De M, Sanford TR and Wood G, 1993. Expression of IL1 , IL 6 and TNF alpha in mouse uterus during preimplantationperiod of pregnancy. 97. *J Reprod Fert* 63-69
10. Arceci B, Shanahan F, Stanley ER and Pollard JW, 1989. The temporal expression and localisation of colony stimulating factor (CSF-1) and its receptor in the femal reproductive tract are consistent with CSF-1 regulated placental development. *Proc Nat Acad Sci* 86.8811-8818.
11. Simon C, Frances A, Piquette GN, Danasouri IE, Zurawski G, Dang W and Polan ML, 1994. IL-1 receptor antagonist prevents successful implantation in mice. *Endocrinology* 134.2. 521.
12. Stewart C, Kaspar P, Brunet LJ, Bhatt H, Gadi I, Köntgen F and Abbondanzo S, 1992. Blastocyst implantation depends on maternal expression of leukemia inhibitory factor. *Nature.* 359, 76-79.
13. Escary JL, Perreau J, Dumenil D, Ezine S and Brulet P, 1993. Leukaemia inhibitory factor is necessary for maintenance of haematopoietic stem cells and thymocyte stimulation. *Nature.* 363, 361-364.
14. Wegmann TG, Lin H, Guilbert L and Mossman TH, 1993. Bidirectional cytokines interactions in the materno fetal relationship: successful allopregnancy is a Th2 phenomenon. *Immunol Today.* 14. 353-355.
15. Lin H, Mossman TR, Guilbert L, Tuntipopipat S and Wegmann TG, 1993. Synthesis of T Helper -2 cytokines at the maternal fetal interface. *J Immunol* 151.9.4562.
16. Delassus S, Countinho GS, Saucier S, Darche S and Kourilky P, 1994. Differential cytokine expression inmaternal blood and placenta during murine gestation. *J Immuno*l 152, 2411-2420
17. Tangri S and Raghupathy R, 1993. Expression of cytokines in placenta of mice -undergoing immunologically mediated fetal resorption. *Biol Reprod* 49.4.840-850
18. Tangri S, Wegmann TG, Lin H, Raghupathy R, 1994. Maternal anti placental reactivity in natural, immunologically mediated fetal resorption. *J Immunol* 152: 4903.
19. Parand M, L Chedid, 1964. Protective effects of chlorpromazine against endotoxin induced abortion. *Proc Soc Exp Biol Med* 116: 906
20. Mattsson, R., R. Holmdahl, A. Scheynius, F. Bernadotte, L. Mattsson. 1991. Placental MHC class I antigen expressionis induced in mice following in vivo treatment with recombinant interferon gamma. J. Reprod. Immunol. 19. 2: 115.
21. Tezabwala, B. U., P. M. Jonhson, R. C. Rees. 1989.Inhibition of pregnancy viability in mice following IL-2 administration. Immunology. 67: 115.
22. Chaouat, G., E. Menu, M. Dy , M. Minkowski, D. A. Clark, T. G. Wegmann. 1990. Control of fetal survival in CBA x DBA/2 mice by lymphokine therapy. J. Fert. Steril. 89 : 447.
23. Kinsky, R., G. Dealge G., N. Rosin, M. N. Thang, M. Hoffman, G. Chaouat. 1990. A murine model of NK cell mediated resorption. Am.J.Reprod.Immunol. 23 : 73.
24. Chaouatg., Assal Meliani A., Martal J., Raghupathy R., Elliot J.E. , Mossmann T.R. , And Wegmann T.G. . Il-10 prevents inflammatory cytokine-mediated fetal death and is inducible by tau interferon.J Immunol. In press.
25. Paldi A : Genomic imprinting and feto maternal relationship. In Biologie cellulaire et moléculaire de la relation materno fetale. Colloque INSERM 254.Editions INSERM John Libbey.1991 : 61-66.
26. Charlier, M., D. Hue, J. Martal , P. Gaye. 1989. Cloning and expression of cDNA encoding ovine trophoblastin : its identity with a class-II alpha interferon. Gene. 77 : 341.
27. Charpigny, G., P. Reinaud, J. Huet, M. Guillomot, M. Charlier, J. C. Pernollet, J. Martal. 1988. High homology between a trophoblastic protein (trophoblastin) isolated from ovine embryo and interferons. FEBS Letters. 228 : 16.

28. Martal, J., E. Degryse, G. Charpigny, N. Assal, P. Reinaud, M. Charlier, P. Gaye, J. C. Lecocq. 1990. Evidence for extended maintenance of the corpus luteum by uterine infusion of a recombinant alpha interferon (Trophoblastin) in sheep. J. Endocrinol 127: R5-R8.
29. Pontzer CH, Torres BA, Valette JL, Bazer FW, Johnson H, 1988. Antiviral activity of the pregnancy recognition hormone ovine trophoblast rotein (oTP) 1. *Biochem Biophys Research Commun* 152: 801.
30. Martal J, Chene N. Functions of embryonic interferons and the main serum proteins specific for pregnancy. Trophoblast. *Research,* 6, 1992. 73-122.
31. Whaley E, Caroll RS, Imakawa K, 1991b. Cloning and analysis of a gene encoding ovine interferon a-II. *Gene,* 106, 281-282.
32. Whaley AE, Caroll RS, Nephew KP, Imakawa K, 1991a. Molecular cloning of unique interferons from human placenta. In workshop of annual meeting of the International Society for Interferon Research. Nice (France). J; IFN *Res* 11. Suppl. Abstr. 69.
33. Fillion C, Chaouat G, Reinaud P, Charpigny JC and Martal J, 1991. Immunoregulatory effects of trophoblastin (oTP): all 5 isoforms are immuno suppressive of PHA driven lymphocyte proliferation. J.Reprod. *Immunol.* 19.237-249.
34. Assal-Meliani A, Charpigny G, Reinaud P, Martal J and Chaouat G, 1993. Recombinant ovine trophoblastin (r.otp) inhibits ovine,murine and human lymphocyte proliferation. *J Reprod Immunol* 25 148-165
35. Chaouat G, Menu E, David F, Djian V, Kinsky R. Reproductive Immunology 1989-1992: some important recent advances about feto maternal relationship. Progress in immunology VIII. 8th international congress in immunology, Springer Verlag, 1992. p 825.
36. Chaouat G, Menu E, David F, Djian V, Kinsky R. Lymphokines, cytokines,MHC allorecognition and pregnancy success or failure. *Reproductive Immunology,* Elsevier Serono, 1992, p 107.
37. Assal Meliani A, Kinsky R, Martal J and Chaouat G, 1995. *In vivo* effects of recombinant otp trophoblastin: r.otp prevents local gvh reaction in mice (pln assay), prevents resorptions and favours implantation in the CBA/J x DBA/2 mating combination. *Amer J Reprod Immunol* 33.
38. Fiorentiono DF, Bond MW, Mossman TR, 1989. Two types of mouse (T helper cells IV) TH2 clones secret a factor that inhibit cytokine production by TH1 cloes. *J Exp Med* 170: 2081.
39. Fiorentino DF, Zlotnik A, Vieira P, Mossman TR, Howard M, 1991. IL-10 acts on the antigen presenting cell to inhibit cytokine production by TH1 cells. *J Immunol* 146: 344.
40. Szekeres-Bartho J, Kilar F, Falkay G, Csernu V, Torok A and Pacsa AS, 1985. Progesterone treated lymphocytes release a substance inhibiting cytotoxicity and prostaglandin synthesis. *Amer J Reprod Immunol* 1985. 9.15-.
41. Lee CK, Ghoshal K, Beaman KD, 1990. Cloning of a cDNA coding for a T cell molecule with putative immunoregulatory role. *Mol Immunol* 1990.27.1137-1134.
42. Hoversland R.C. And Beaman K.D.1991. The lack of effect of a monoclonal antibody against murine T cell suppressor factor on murine embryo development in vitro. Am. J. Reprod. Immunol. 26:84-88.
43. Beaman K.D., Hoversland R.C. 1988. Induction of «spontaneous» abortion by blocking antigen specific suppression. J. Reprod. Fert. 1998.82. 135-139.
44. Szekeres Bartho J, Szekeres G, Debre P, Autran B, Chaouat G. Reactivity of lymphocytes to a progesterone receptor specific monoclonal antibody. *Cell Immunol* 1990.125.273.
45. Paldi A, D'auriol L, Misrahi M, Bakos A, Chaouat G and Szekeres Bartho J. Expression of the gene coding for the progesterone receptor in activated human lymphocytes. Endocrine journal.2.317 319
46. Szekeres Bartho J., Reznikoff Etievant M., Varga P., Pichon M.F., Varga Z. And Chaouat G. . Lymphocytic progesterone receptors in human pregnancy. J.Reprod. Immunol.1989.1989.16.239.
47. Szekeres Bartho J, Autran B., Debre P., Andreu G., Denver L., Blot P. And Chaouat G. Immunoregulatory effects of a suppressor factor from healthy pregnant women's lymphocytes after progesterone induction. Cell. immunol.1989.122.281.
48. Chaouat G and Kolb JP. Immunoactive products of murine placenta. II) Afferent suppression of maternal cell mediated immunity by supernatants from short term enriched cultures of murine trophoblast enriched maternal cell populations. *Ann Immunol.* Institut Pasteur. 1984. 135C.205.
49. Kolb JP, Chaouat G and Chassoux DJ. Immunoactive products of placenta. III) Suppression of Natural Killing activity. *J Immunol* 1984.132. 23O5-2312.
50. Chaouat G and Kolb JP. Immunoactive products of placenta.IV) Impairment by placental cells and their products of CTL function at effector stage. *J Immunol* 1985. 135. 215-221.

51. Menu E, Kaplan L, Andreu G, Denver L, Chaouat G. Immunoactive products of human placenta. I - An immunoregulatory factor obtained from explant cultures of human placenta inhibits CTL generation and cytotoxic effector activity. *Cell Immunol* 1989; 119:341.
52. Menu E, David V, Bensussan A, Chaouat G. Immunoactive products of human placenta. II -Direct inhibition of non-MHC specific, non-MHC restricted cytolytic activity of human alpha beta, but not gamma delta positive T cell clones. *J Reprod Immunol* 1988; 16:137.
53. Menu E, Jankovic Dl, Theses J, David V, Chaouat G. Immunoactive products of human placenta. III - Characterization of an inhibitor affecting lymphocyte proliferation. *Regional Immunology* 1991; 3:254.
54. Menu E, Kinsky R, Hoffman M, Chaouat G. Immunoactive products of human placenta. IV - Immunoregulatory factors obtained from cultures of human placenta inhibit local and general murine graft versus host reactions (GVHR). *J Reprod Immunol* 1991; p.195.
55. Khrishnan L, Menu E, Chaouat G, Talwar Gp, Raghupathy R. *In vitro* and *in vivo* immunosuppressive effects of supernatants from the human choricarcinoma cell line. *Cell Immunol* 1991; 138:313.
56. Clark DA, Mc Dermott M and Sczewzuk MR, 1980. Impairment of host versus graft reaction in pregnant mice: II) Selective suppresion of Cytotoxic cell generation correlates with soluble suppressor activity and successful allogeneic pregnancy. *Cell Immunol* 1980. 52.106-118.
57. Clark DA. Maternal Immune response to the fetus. EOS-Revista di Immunologia et Immunofarmacolagia. 1985.2:114-117.
58. Clark DA, Flanders KC, Banwatt D, Millar-Book W, Manuel J, Stedronska-Clark, Rowley B, 1990. Murine pregnancy decidua produces a unique immunosuppressive molecule related to transforming growth factor beta-2. *J Immunol* 144-12.3008-3004.
59. Clark DA, Richard G, Lea, Judith Denburg, Daljeet Barwatt, Justin Manuel, Najim Daari, Jenny Underwood, Magdy Michel, James Mowbray, Salim Daya et/and Gerard Chaouat. Transforming growth factor beta related factor in mammalian pregnancy decidua : homologies between the mouse and human in successful pregnancy and in recurrent unexplained abortion. Biologie cellulaire et moléculaire de la relation materno fetale. Editions INSERM John Libbey. 131-141
60. Clark DA, Chaput A, Tutton B. Active suppression of host versus graft reaction in pregnant mice. VII. Spontaneous abortion of CBA x DBA/2 fetuses in the uterus of CBA/J mice correlates with deficient non-T suppressor cell activity. *J Immunol* 1986. 136.1668-1771.
61. Hsi BL, Fenichel P and Cervoni F, 1991. Expression of complement regulatory proteins on human gametes and trophoblast.Biologie cellulaire et moléculaire de la relation materno fetale. Editions INSERM John Libbey Pages 3-13
62. Holmes CH, Simpson KL, Wainwright SD, Tate CG, Houlihan JM, Sawyer JH, Roger IP, Spring FA, Amstee DJ and Tanner MJ, 1990. Preferantail expression of the comlement regulatory protein Decay Aceelerating Factor at the fetomaternal interface during human pregnancy. *J Immunol* 144.3099-3115.
63. Jonhnson PM, Risk JM, Mwenda JM, Hart CA, Purcell DFJ and Dacon NJ, 1986. Human trophoblast expression of retroviral like activity and CD 46 (membrane cofactor protein, Hu Ly-m5and H316 TLX antigen). In Reproductive Immunology 1989. L Mettler and W D Billington Eds. Amsterdam. 1990.
64. Purcel DFJ, Brown MA, Russel SM, Clark CJ, Mc Kenzie IFC and Deacon NJ, 1989. The cDNA cloning of human CD 46, an antigen system incorporating TLX and MCP. Existence of multiple alternative splice variants. *J Reprod Immunol* Supp. 207.
65. Voisin G and Chaouat GA, 1974. Demonstration, nature and properties of antibobies eluted from the placenta and directed against paternal antigens. Journal of Reproduction and Fertility. Suppl. 21, p. 89.
66. Bell SC and Billington WD, 1980. Major antipaternal allo antibody induced by pregnancy is non complement fixing IgG1. *Nature* (London) 1980.288-387-388.
67. Bell SC and Billington WD, 1983. Anti fetal alloantibody inthe pregnant female. *Immunological Rewiew*. 75. 5-30.
68. Chaouat G, Voisin GA, Escalier D and Robert P, 1979. Facilitation reaction (enhancing antibodies and suppressor cells) and rejection reaction (sensitized cells) from the mother to the paternal antigens of the conceptus. *Clin Exp Immunol,* 35 :13-24.
69. Baines MG, Millar KG and Pross HF. Allograft enhancement during normal murine pregnancy. *J Reprod Immunol* 1980.2.141-148.

70. Smith RN and Powell AE, 1977. The transfer of pregacy induced hyporesponsivenes to male skin grafts with thymus dependent spleen cells. *J Exp Med* 156.899-911.
71. Engleman EG, Mc Michael AJ and Mc Devitt HO. Suppression of the mixed lymphocyte reaction in man by a solubleT cell factor: specificity of the factor for both the responder and the stimulator. *J Ex Med* 1978. 147. 1037-1045.
72. Chaouat G and Voisin GA, 1979. Regulatory T cell subpopulations in pregnancy. I. Evidence for suppressive activity of the early phase of MLR. *J Immunol*, 122: 1383-1388.
73. Mattson R, Mattson A and Sulila P, 1985. Allogeneic pregnancy in B cell depleted CBA/Ca mice. Effects on fetal survival and maternal lymphoid organs. *Dev Comp Immunol* 1985. 9. 709-713.
74. Monnot P, Chaouat G, 1984. Systemic active suppression is not necessary for successful allopregnancy. *American J Reprod Immunol,* 1984, 6, 5-8.
75. Mattson R and Holmdal R, 1987. Maintained allopregnancy in rats depleted of T cytotoxic/suppressor cells by OX8 monoclonalantibody treatment. *J Reprod Immunol* 1987.
76. Ellis SA, Sargent IL, Redman CWG, Mcmichael AJ, 1986. Evidence for a novel HLA antigen found on human extravillous trophoblast and choriocarcinoma cell line. *Immunology,* 59, 595-601.
77. Kovatts S, Main EK, Libbrach C, Stublebline M, Fischer SJ, De Mars R, 1990. A class I antigen, HLA-G, expressed in human trophoblasts. *Science.* 248 :220-223.
78. Ellis SA, 1990. HLA-G: at the interface. *Am J Reprod Immunol* 23: 84-86.
79. Kovatts S, Librach C, Fisch P, Main EK, Sondel PM, Fischer SJ and De Mars R, 1991. The role of non classical MHC class I on human trophoblast. In Biologie cellulaire et moléculaire de la relation materno fetale. G Chaouat and J Mowbray Eds. Editions INSERM John Libbey. Paris. 1991. Pages 41-51. Pages 13-21.
80. Romero R, Mazor M, Tartakowsky B, 1991. Systemic administration of interleukin 1 induces preterm parturition in mice. *Am J Obst Gyn* 165.969-971.
81. Branch DW, Dudlay DJ, Mitchel MD, 1992. Prostaglandin E2 production by murine dcidua is increased in response to abortifacient doses of LPS. Annual meeting of the American Society for Immunology of Reproduction. Charleston. SC. Abstract * 325.
82. Chwalisz C, Scholz P, Hegele-Hartung CH, Roth G and Bukowski R, 1993. Cervical ripening with interleukin 1 Beta,interleukin 8, and tumor necrosis factor alpha in pregnant guinea pigs. Submitted for publication.
83. Bukowski R, Scolz P, Hasan SH and Chwalisz C, 1993. Induction of preterm parturition with the interleukin 1 beta, Tumor necrosis factor alpha, and with LPS guinea pigs. In press.
84. Chaouat G, Delage G, Christophe Lelaidier, Catherine Bertrand et Frydman R, 1994. Bases immunologiques de la mise en route du travail. In IXème JTA. JTA ARETEM editions. M Azoulay, A Ioian, R Mezin Editeurs. Tome 1. Pages 57-79.

Résumé

Après avoir passé en revue le rôle des cytokines et plus particulièrement des cytokines inflammatoires dans l'implantation, nous décrivons la gestation établie et les événements immunosuppresseurs locaux rattachés, et, finalement, le rôle des lymphokines dans la parturition.

Hematopoietic cell commitment during embryonic development

Ana Cumano[1], Françoise Dieterlen-Lièvre[2], Christopher J. Paige[3] and Isabelle Godin[2]

[1] INSERM U. 277, Unité de Biologie Moléculaire du Gène, Institut Pasteur, Paris, France, tel.: (33 1) 40 61 30 56, fax: (33 1) 45 68 85 48; [2] Institut d'Embryologie du CNRS et du Collège de France, Nogent-sur-Marne, France; [3] The Wellesley Hospital Research Institute, Toronto, Canada

Abstract

Long-term reconstitution of irradiated recipients has been the only available assay to detect multipotent hematopoietic stem cells. We developed a clonal in vitro system that allows the differentiation of myeloid cells, and of T and B lymphocytes and therefore, the detection of multipotent cells. Using this assay we established that the first B-cell precursors detected in embryonic development, in the mouse, are located in the yolk sac and in the para-aortic splanchnopleura, at the stage of 8-10 somites. All precursors analyzed were multipotent hematopoietic cells capable of generating multiple lineages of myeloid cells, B cells and TcR α/β and γ/δ expressing T cells.

The same type of analysis done with precursors isolated from day 12 fetal liver revealed that in addition to multipotent precursors, intermediate hematopoietic cells could be detected that had retained T-cell and myeloid potential, or macrophage and B-cell potential. A model of commitment in the developing embryonic hematopoietic system is discussed.

All hematopoietic cells derive from a multipotent precursor, present in the bone marrow of adult mice and in the fetal liver, during embryonic life. This cell type is rare and is defined by two main characteristics, multipotentiality and self-renewability.

Hematopoietic stem cells have been identified by the capacity to reconstitute all hematopoietic cell lineages for a period longer than 5 to 6 months, when transferred to a lethally irradiated host. A combination of surface markers has been defined that, although not exclusively, is present in all long term reconstituting cells from bone marrow of adult mice [1] or fetal liver, in embryos [2], and allow the enrichment of this cell type. Long term reconstitution of irradiated hosts has thus been the only available assay to identify hematopoietic stem cells.

Hematopoietic lineage commitment is a complex process in which a multipotent cell becomes restricted to a single lineage developmental pathway. The mechanisms leading to lineage commitment in hematopoietic cells are not understood. However, the myeloid pathway of differentiation has been extensively characterized when *in vitro* systems allowing the differentiation of myeloid precursors were established. These clonal assays allowed to define intermediate myeloid precursors and growth factors required for the progression in the differentiation pathway. In contrast to myeloid cells little is known in the lymphoid pathway of differentiation.

In the last years we established an *in vitro* culture system that allows multipotent hematopoietic precursors to differentiate in all blood cell types. Although this test does not assay for self-renewability, it allowed us to identify the first sites where hematopoietic cells can be detected in embryonic development. We determined their differentiation potential and detected intermediate precursors in the lymphoid pathway of differentiation, in fetal liver, allowing a better understanding of the process of hematopoietic commitment.

B-cell precursors can be detected in two different locations in 10 somite mouse embryos

Fetal liver is the main hematopoietic organ during embryonic life, in the mouse. The first precursors can be detected at day 10 of gestation in the liver rudiment. Before that stage, however, lymphoid precursors were identified in the yolk sac and in the body of the embryo [3]. Taking the avian hematopoietic development as a model, Godin and collegues established that the para-aortic splanchnopleura (P-Sp) in a mouse embryo at day 8.5 of gestation harboured cells that can differentiate into B lymphocytes, when grafted under the kidney capsule of an immunodeficient (SCID) mouse [4].

We used a modification of an *in vitro* assay system that allows uncommitted precursors [5] to differentiate into mature B cells, to define the number and differentiation potential of the first B-cell precursors detected in the embryo *(Figure 1)*. Yolk sac and para-aortic splanchnopleural cells were isolated together with the remaining embryo proper. Cell suspensions from these three different origins were cultured under limiting dilution conditions, in an assay system allowing lymphocyte as well as myeloid cell differentiation. *Figure 2* shows the number of B-cell precursors detected per isolated organ at different stages of embryonic development. The first precursors can be detected both in the yolk sac and in the P-Sp at the stage of ten somites. Absolute numbers of precursors increase thereafter and in 25 somite embryos more than ten precursors were detected in both locations. The body of the embryo deprived of the P-Sp does not contain detectable B-cell precursors [6].

All detected B-cell precursors in pre-liver embryos are multipotent hematopoietic cells

The experiments described above indicate that before fetal liver repopulation, hematopoietic precursors can be found in the para-aortic splanchnopleura and in the yolk sac. These precursors arise apparently at the same time in both locations.

Using micromanipulation of single cells into culture conditions that allow multilineage hematopoietic cell differentiation we established that all lymphoid precursors detected at the stage of 22 somites in the P-Sp are multipotent cells *(Figure 1)*. Erythroid and myeloid cells are detected using a combination of *c-kit ligand*, granulocyte-macrophage colony stimulating factor (GM-CSF), macrophage-colony stimulating factor (M-CSF) and erythropoietin (Epo), as growth factors. B lymphocyte precursors can be expanded in the presence of stromal cells and interleukin 7 (IL-7), furthermore they can differentiate into plasma cells when they are stimulated by lipopolyssacharide (LPS). T lymphocytes were detected when embryonic thymic lobes were repopulated by cells originated *in vitro* from these precursors. The T-cell precursors detected in these

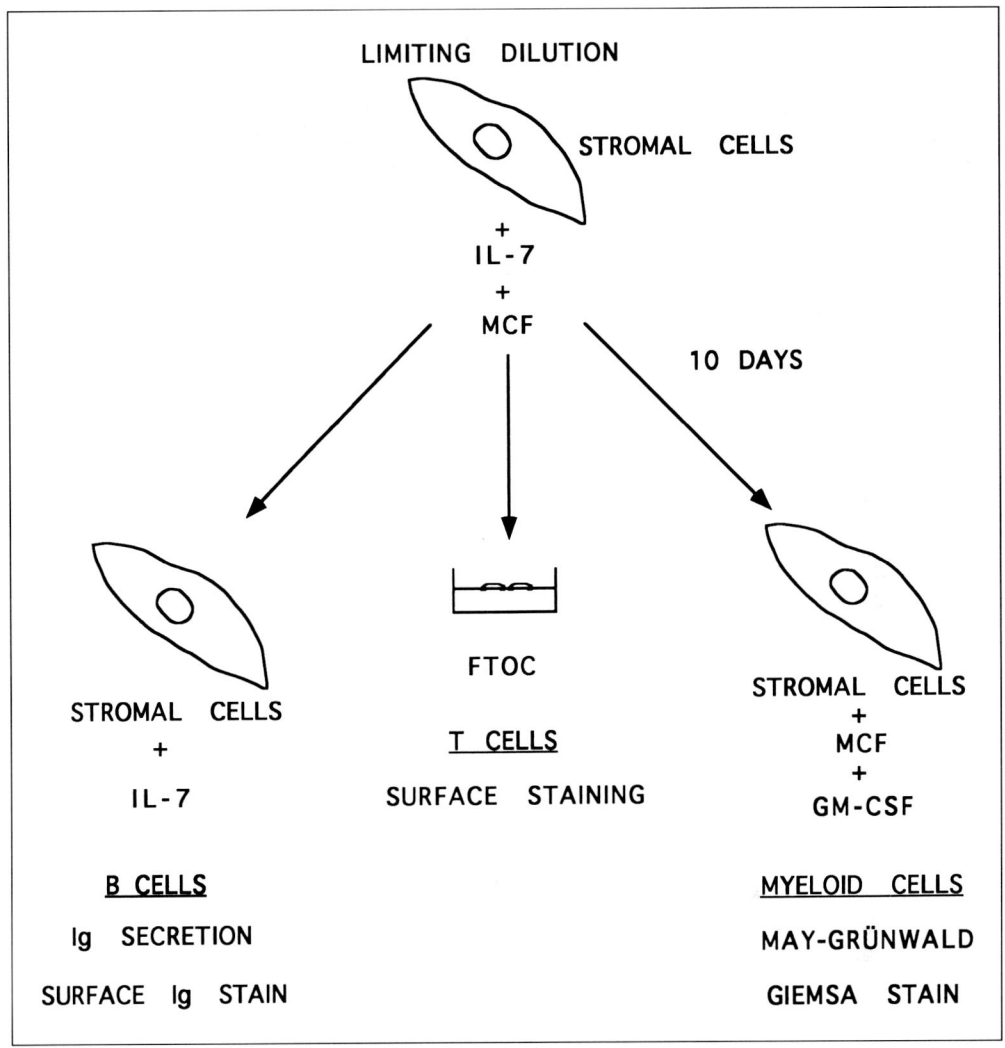

Figure 1. Schematic representation of the culture conditions used to detect myeloid, B- and T-lymphoid potentialities, from single cells.

cultures can generate α/β as well as γ/δ bearing T-cells from which Vg 5 expressing cells are a majority. The nature of the precursors generated *in vitro*, capable of repopulating embryonic thymic lobes is unknown. It is conceivable that commitment to the T-cell pathway of differentiation occurs in culture; alternatively, multipotent precursors could be kept quiescent or could proliferate without commitment, in this assay system.

It is worth mentioning that circulation between the yolk sac and the embryo proper is established around the stage of 9 somites. All multipotent precursors characterized in this study are isolated after circulation was established and therefore we cannot rule out that they recirculated from the yolk sac to the P-Sp.

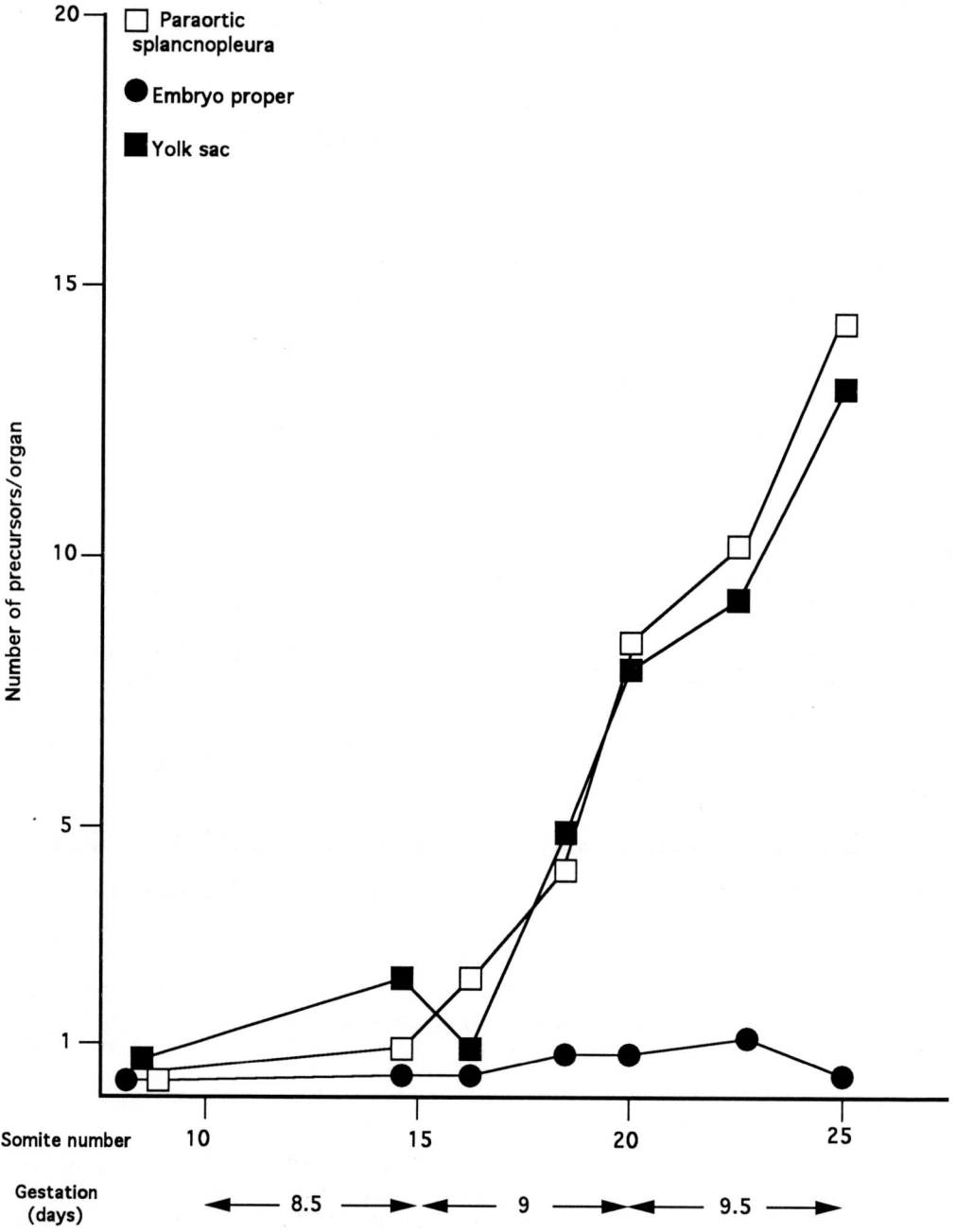

Figure 2. Quantification of B-cell precursors found in the yolk sac, The P-Sp and the remaining embryo body at different times of development. Each cell suspension was prepared from 20-30 pooled embryos.

Intermediate lymphoid precursors in fetal liver, at day 12 of gestation

The fetal liver is seeded by hematopoietic precursors at day 10 of gestation. In day 12 fetal liver, most B-cell precursors do not express the B220 marker and are uncommitted for the B-lineage pathway of differentiation. At this stage of gestation we have identified an intermediate bipotent cell, capable of differentiating into B cells and macrophages, but into no other myeloid cell type [5]. This experiment suggested that few lymphoid committed cells are present and that most B-cell precursors detected *in vitro* are intermediate hematopoietic precursors with lymphoid potential. We analyzed the differentiation potential of hematopoietic clones derived from day 12 fetal liver in the same experimental scheme used to detect multipotent cells, in day 9 embryos.

Four different types of clones were detected: 1. Multipotent precursors that could generate myeloid cells as well as T and B lymphocytes. 2. Intermediate precursors that could generate myeloid and T cells but no B-cells. 3. Intermediate precursors that could generate B cells and macrophages but no T-cells and no other myeloid cells. 4. Myeloid restricted precursors that could neither generate B nor T lymphocytes. From this result, a scheme of hematopoietic commitment in embryonic development emerges. Multipotent precursors would first loose the capacity to differentiate into B cells. Then myeloid committed cells would be generated by the loss of T cell potential. The bipotent macrophage/B-cell precursor would constitute a B-cell precursor that maintain the capacity to become macrophage, for a short period of time since both differentiation programs are closely related. The observation that many pre-B cell lines can differentiate into macrophages *in vitro* supports this hypothesis.

Commitment in the hematopoietic system could be seen as a gradual, stepwise process in which a decreased probability to become B then T cells would accompany a loss of self-renewability. This scheme implies the existence of T and B lymphocyte committed precursors.

References

1. Spangrude GJ, Heimfeld S and Weissman IL, 1988. Purification and characterization of mouse hematopoietic stem cells. *Science,* 241:58-62.
2. Jordan CT, McKearn JT and Lemischka IR, 1990. Cellular and developmental properties of fetal hematopoietic stem cells. *Cell,* 61:953-963.
3. Tyan M and Herzenberg LA, 1968. Studies on the ontogeny of the mouse immune system. II. Immunoglobulin-producing cells. *J Immunol* 101:446-452.
4. Godin I, Garcia-Porrero JA, Coutinho A, Dieterlen-Lèvre F and Marcos MAR, 1993. Para-aortic splanchnopleura from early mouse embryos contains B1a cell progenitors. *Nature,* 364:67-70.
5. Cumano A, Paige CJ, Iscove NN and Brady G, 1992. Bipotent precursors of B cells and macrophages in murine fetal liver. *Nature,* 356:612-615.
6. Godin I, Dieterlen-Lièvre F and Cumano A, 1995. Emergence of multipotent hematopoietic cells in the yolk sac and para-aortic splanchnopleura of 8.5 dpc mouse embryos. *Proc Natl Acad Scien U.S.A.* 92:773-777.

Résumé

Les cellules hématopoïétiques souches sont couramment détectées par leur capacité de reconstituer tout le système hématopoïétique d'un animal receveur irradié. Nous avons établi un système de culture qui nous permet de détecter *in vitro* des cellules hématopoïétiques multipotentes. Grâce à ce système, nous avons étudié la capacité de différenciation des premiers précurseurs hématopoïétiques détectés dans l'embryon de souris. Il s'agit de cellules multipotentes localisées à la fois dans le sac vitellin et dans la splanchnopleure para-aortique d'embryons à partir de 10 somites. Ces cellules ont la capacité de générer différents types de cellules myéloïdes ainsi que des lymphocytes B et des lymphocytes T exprimant soit le TcRα/β, soit le TcRγ/δ.

Une telle analyse appliquée aux précurseurs du foie fœtal isolés à jour 12 de gestation suggère l'existence de précurseurs lymphoïdes intermédiaires qui ont gardé un potentiel de différenciation en cellules T et myéloïdes, et d'autres en macrophages et cellules B. Un modèle de détermination de lignée en hématopoïèse embryonnaire est proposé.

3) Animal models

3) *Modèles animaux*

Human stem cell engraftment in sheep

Graca Almeida–Porada[1], Alan W. Flake[2], Christopher Porada[1], James Ruthven[1], Jujuan Ruthven[1], Esmail D. Zanjani[1]

[1] Department of Veterans Affairs Medical Center, University of Nevada School of Medicine, Reno, NV 89520, USA, tel.: (702) 786 7200, fax: (702) 786 7200; [2] Children's Hospital of Michigan, Detroit, MI 48201, USA

Abstract

We have created a model that offers an ideal assay system to study the biology of human hematopoiesis. In this system, we took advantage of the permissive environment of the early gestational sheep fetus to engraft human hematopoietic stem cells (HSC) and achieve long-term multilineage expression of human cells in an immunologically normal recipient. Because of the unresponsiveness of the human cells to sheep growth factors, we are also able to assess in vivo *the role of human regulatory factors in normal and abnormal hematopoiesis. The small size of the fetus permits us to investigate the engraftment ability of small numbers of human stem cells from different sources, while the relatively large size of the chimeric sheep allows long-term evaluation and assessment of the long-term repopulating ability of the human HSC.*

Human hematopoiesis is maintained throughout life by a highly specialized population of primitive hematopoietic progenitor cells known as the hematopoietic stem cells (HSC) [1]. Unlike other cells, HSC are thought to be capable of both multilineage differentiation and of giving rise to progeny cells with functional characteristics similar to their own [2]. The pluripotential differentiation capacity of HSC is the process by which these cells generate the various blood cell lineages, whereas their ability to produce additional stem cells, a process known as self-renewal, is a cardinal function that prevents stem cell extinction. The existence of the HSC and its long-term repopulating ability have been well established in animal and man [3]. In mice, the use of lethally irradiated recipients as an *in vivo* assay has permitted the study of not only the repopulating ability of HSC but also its self-renewal capacity [3, 4]. Much of what we know about human HSC has been provided by data derived from *in vitro* studies. *In vitro* studies have shown that immature HSC isolated from adult marrow, cord blood, and fetal liver differ in their ability to produce hematopoietic progenitors in cytokine supplemented suspension cultures *in vitro*, and that the proliferative capacity of these HSC decrease markedly with age [5]. These studies indicate the existence of significant ontogeny related functional differences between HSC [5]. These types of information, if confirmed by *in vivo* evaluations can be used to considerable advantage in clinical transplant settings. It is understood, however, that the *in vivo* long-term multilineage and self-renewal potential of the human HSC is generally not fully addressed by *in vitro* assays. The practical and ethical limitations of *in vivo* analyses of HSC in human patients prevent the direct *in vivo* evaluation of the biological functions of the candidate human HSC.

To overcome the lack of appropriate *in vivo* assays for human HSC, a number of investigators have developed systems utilizing several strains of immunodeficient mice by which to test the *in vivo* behavior of these cells [6-9]. These murine models have been extremely valuable for the study of human HSC activity from a variety of sources and have been applied to the study of human infectious disease, neoplasia, and autoimmune disease [10-12].

We have taken advantage of the permissive environment of the early gestational age fetus and developed a large animal model of human hematopoiesis in sheep. The permissive environment of the developing fetus characterized by its immunological naivete and available hematopoietic sites [13-15] has permitted the long-term engraftment and multilineage expression of human HSC in sheep [16-19].

Materials and methods

Transplantation procedure and donor cell preparation

Using the amniotic bubble procedure, as previously described, [20] the recipients, in all cases preimmune 54-65 day gestation sheep fetus, were transplanted with donor (human) cells. Human cells of postnatal origin were derived from adult bone marrow, peripheral blood and cord blood. In most cases, highly purified preparations of adult human cells were employed. The methods for preparation of post-natal HSC (whole or purified) and human fetal liver HSC have been previously reported [17,18]. Briefly, a single cell suspension of human fetal liver was obtained by gentle homogenization of the tissue in a hand-operated glass homogenizer after being thoroughly rinsed in heparinized media. Removal of hepatocytes was performed by sedimentation at room temperature, after which the cells were pelleted by centrifugation and resuspended in the appropriate media before injection.

Monitoring engraftment

Bone marrow mononuclear cells (BMNC) and peripheral blood cells (PBC) were analyzed for the presence of donor (human) cells by flow cytometry on a FACScan flow cytometer as previously described [18]. The samples were also examined for the presence of donor cells by karyotyping of marrow and peripheral blood cells (after PHA stimulation) and of progenitor cell derived hematopoietic colonies as previously reported [17]. Bone marrow mononuclear cells were cultured in methylcellulose with IMDM and erythropoietin at a concentration of 2 IU/ml. For optimal growth of either human or sheep colonies, human or sheep PHA-LCM was used respectively. Colonies were enumerated by type, removed from the plates individually, and processed for karyotyping on day 9 (sheep) or 19 (human) of incubation.

Results

Human fetal liver-derived hematopoietic cells were transplanted into preimmune fetal lambs at 48-54 days of gestation. The results which have previously been reported, [15-18, 21-22] are presented in *Table I*. Donor (human) cell engraftment was obtained in some of the animals, and all of the animals found to be chimeric have maintained expression of human cells for over five years. The persistence of expression of human cells for this long period of time without graft loss suggests that the engraftment of long-term repopulating human stem cells may have occurred.

This was also demonstrated by the fact that transplantation of $CD45^+$ cells isolated 3.5 years after transplant from the bone marrow of the chimeric sheep into new preimmune recipient sheep resulted in engraftment and multilineage expression of donor (human) cells in these secondary recipients *(Table II)*.

Other sources of human HSC were also tested in this model, these included purified stem cells from cord blood, adult bone marrow and adult peripheral blood. Results in *Table III* show the percentages of engraftment and expression of human cells in sheep transplanted with unpurified human HSC from different sources. As is shown, the results were similar between the different groups with regard to both incidence and efficiency of engraftment. However chimeric lambs that received crude preparations of cells from post-natal human sources developed GVHD and

Table I. Average distribution of donor (human) cells/progenitors in bone marrow of 4 different sheep at 1 year after transplantation with human fetal liver–derived hematopoietic cells[1] *in utero*.

Phenotypical analysis		Donor (human) colonies[2]	
	% positive cells		% of total colonies
CD45	6.9 ± 2.3	CFU–Mix	3.4 ± 1.2
CD34	0.4 ± 0.2	CFU–GM	7.8 ± 2.6
CD3	1.9 ± 0.5	BFU–E	3.9 ± 1.1
CD14	0.9 ± 0.3		
CD22	2.1 ± 0.7		

1. Each value represents mean ± 1 SEM of results from four chimeric lambs. Determinations were made using buffy coat cells.
2. CFU–Mix, mixed colony-forming units; CFU-GM, granulocyte–macrophage colony–forming units; BFU-E, erythroid blast–forming units.

Table II. Relative distribution of human donor $CD45^+$ cells in secondary recipients, at different time points after transplant[1].

	% Donor ($CD45^+$) Cells	
Weeks Post–Transplant	Blood	Bone Marrow
3	6.2	3
24	2.2	7
46	1.0	5
68	1.8	7

1. Each value represents mean of results from two separate secondary recipients.

Table III. Relative efficiency of engraftment of human HSC from different sources and comparative GVHD development.[1]

Source of HSC	(%) Chimeric	(%) Donor cells	(%) With GVHD
Fetal Liver	47	2 – 8	0
Cord Blood	50	4 – 11	85
Peripheral Blood	38	2 – 9	85
Adult Marrow	47	1 – 13	88

1. Each Fetus received 5×10^8 cells/Kg estimated fetal body weight. The values (range) for donor cells reflect the relative percentages of CD45$^+$ cells present in the marrow at birth.

Table IV. Comparison of human cell engraftment and the development of GVHD in human/sheep chimeras.[1]

Cells transplanted	FLVR	Crude preparations			Enriched/purified preparations		
		ABM	APB	CB	ABM	CB	APB
Engraftment	Yes	Yes	Yes	Yes	Yes	Yes	Yes
GVHD	No	Yes	Yes	Yes	No	No	No

FLVR: fetal liver; ABM: adult bone marrow; APB: adult peripheral blood; Enriched/purified preparations included CD34$^+$, Lin$^-$ cells, further characterized for the expression of either HLA$^-$DR or CD38 (see ref. 11).

Table V. Numbers of CD45$^+$ cells obtained in the primary recipient sheep.

Months after transplant	Number of CD45$^+$ Cells	% of Total	Number of CD45$^+$ cells obtained after panning
22	19×10^6	2.1	5×10^6
27	7×10^6	1.8	1.2×10^6

Table VI. Relative distribution of donor (human) cells in secondary recipient sheep.[1]

Months post-transplant	% CD45$^+$ cells		% cells with human karyotype	
	Marrow	Blood	Marrow	Blood
3	6.2	0	4.7	0
9	3.1	0	ND*	0
12	4.1	0	5.3	0
15	5.2	0	6.5	0

1. Each of the secondary recipients received 0.6×10^6 cells/fetus. Four sheep were injected, one died in utero and 3 survived. The results presented in this table are from one of the sheep that showed human cell chimerism. ND*, not determined.

died *(Tables III and IV)*. The development of GVHD in these animals is likely associated with the presence of donor mature T-cells in the graft [23]. In this regard, the transplantation of CD34$^+$- enriched/purified cells from post-natal human sources resulted in significant donor cell engraftment without GVHD *(Table IV)*.

It is of interest to note that as with whole cell preparations, lambs chimeric with purified human HSC exhibited long-term donor cell engraftment and multilineage expression. That these purified cell preparations contained long-term repopulating cells was demonstrated by the transplantation of CD45$^+$ cells isolated from bone marrow of these lambs into secondary recipients. In *Table V* numbers of CD45$^+$ cells found in the bone marrow of a chimeric sheep transplanted with adult human CD34$^+$,HLA-DR$^-$ bone marrow cells at 22 and 27 month after transplant are shown.

These cells were injected into new recipients and the phenotype of human cell subpopulations found in these secondary transplanted sheep is shown in *Table VI*. In addition, the presence of human chimerism was also confirmed by quantitating the number of cells in peripheral blood and bone marrow which exhibit a human karyotype, *(Table VI)*.

In these as well as in primary recipients, and regardless of the source of human cells/progenitors, bone marrow exhibits higher levels of human cell expression than the peripheral blood. This could be due to the fact that sheep stroma is able to maintain human progenitor cells but only minimally supports terminal differentiation [24]. In agreement with this data, we have shown that the levels of human cell expression in peripheral blood can be increased by infusion of human specific cytokines such as IL-3, GM-CSF and SCF [17] or by cotransplantation of autologous human stroma [25].

Discussion

The results presented here and previously reported make evident the successful engraftment and expression of HSC from fetal and postnatal human donors in this model [15-18,21]. The engrafted cells in our model are not only retained, but are capable of multilineage differentiation into cells bearing human surface markers, human karyotype, and *in vivo* responses to human-specific growth factors. The engraftment, now more than five years post-transplant, has been long-term and associated with multilineage expression involving donor (human) erythroid, lymphoid and myeloid cells [16]. This, and the ability to transfer such a cell population to a secondary host demonstrates that the engraftment of HSC in these chimeric lambs resulted from the engraftment of HSC with long-term repopulating ability. It is obvious from the numbers of human bone marrow cells contained in these sheep that a high degree of cellular proliferation had to occur in the primary as well as the secondary recipients in order to detect human cells in the secondary recipient. Moreover, the time frame within which these studies were conducted indicates that the original graft may have contained cells with a high proliferative potential. Our studies have also demonstrated that significant donor HSC engraftment occurs only when transplantation is performed early in gestation, showing that the engraftment of human HSC in this setting occurs because the unique aspects of fetal development, such as the immuno naivity of the recipient, and the available "homing" sites in the bone marrow, create a permissive environment for the engraftment and tolerance of immunologically foreign HSC [15]. The system may also benefit from the possible "processing" of cells by the fetal thymic microenvironment, which could theoretically result in long-term cellular and humoral tolerance. Currently, there is no ideal system able to fulfill the requirements for a perfect assay to test human HSC *in vivo*. However, our findings suggest that the human/ sheep chimeras provide a biologically useful and relevant *in vivo* model for the assay and study of the human HSC. In this model, the engraftment and multilineage expression of human HSC is likely the result of engraftment of the long-term repopulating human HSC. Furthermore, the human cell compartments in these chimeric sheep are biologically responsive to human-specific cytokines, allowing for the *in vivo* assessment of the role of human regulatory factors in normal and abnormal hematopoiesis. Another observation is that the biologic phenomenon of GVHD appears to be analogous to allogeneic transplantations. Preliminary evidence indicates that GVHD in these lambs is associated with donor mature T cells. Another attractive feature of this model is that the small size of the fetus permits the assessment of engraftment of relatively few highly purified human HSC. This, combined with the fact that the large size of the chimeric animal after birth allows sampling at regular intervals for long periods, indicates the utility of this model for evaluating the *in vivo* engraftment/differentiation and GVHD potentials of human HSC.

Supported in part by National Institutes of Health Grants No. HL46556, HL40722, and HL49042, by Department of Veterans Affairs, and by the G Harold and Leila Y Mathers Charitable Foundation.

References

1. Abramson S, Miller G, Phillips RA. The identification in adult bone marrow of pluripotent and restricted stem cells of the myeloid and lymphoid systems. *J Exp Med* 1977; 145:1567-1579.
2. Ogawa M. Differentiation and proliferation of hematopoietic stem cells. *Blood* 1993; 81:2844-2853.
3. McCune JM, Namikawa R, Kaneshima H, Shultz LD, Leiberman M, Weissman IL. The SCID-hu mouse: Murine model for the analysis of human hematolymphoid differentiation and function. *Science* 1988; 241: 1632-1639.
4. Moore MAS. Does stem cell exhaustion result from combining hematopoietic growth factors with chemotherapy? How do we prevent it? *Blood* 1992; 152: 219-224.
5. Craig W, Kay R, Cutler RL, Lansdorp PM. Expression of Thy-1 on human hematopoietic progenitor cells. *J Exp Med* 1993; 177:1331.
6. Dick JE. Establishment of assays for human hematpoietic cells in immune deficient mice. *Current Topics Microbiol Immunol* 198; 152: 219-224.
7. McCune JM, Namikawa R, Kaneshima H, Shultz LD, Leiberman M, Weissman IL. The SCID-hu mouse: Murine model for the analysis of human hematolymphoid differentiation and function. *Science* 1988; 241: 1632-1639.
8. Barry TS, Jones DM, Richter CB, Haynes BF. Successful engraftment of human postnatal thymus in severe combined immune deficient (SCID) mice. Differential engraftment of thymic components with irradiation versus anti-asialo GM-1 immunosuppressive regiments. *J Exp Med* 1991; 173: 167-180.
9. Kamal-Reid S, Dick JE. Engraftment of immune-deficient mice with human hematopoietic stem cells. *Science* 1988; 242: 1706-1709.
10. Namikawa R, Kaneshima H, Lieberman M, Weissman IL, McCune JM. Infection of the SCID-hu mouse by HIV1. *Science* 1988; 242: 2684 -1686.
11. Cannon MJ, Pisa P, Fox RI, Cooper NR. Epstein Barr virus induces aggressive lymphoproliferative disorders of human B-cell origin in SCID/hu chimeric mice. *J Clin Invest* 1990; 85: 1333-1337.
12. Krams SM, Dorshkind K, Gershwin EM. Generation of fibrillary lesions after transfer of human lymphocytes into severe combined immunodeficient (SCID) mice. *J Exp Med* 1989; 170: 1919-1930.
13. Flake AW, Harrison MR, Zanjani ED. In utero stem cell transplantation. *Exp Hematol* 1991; 19: 1061-1064 .
14. Zanjani ED, Ascensao JL, Harrison MR, Tavassoli M. Ex vivo incubation with growth factors enhances the engraftment of fetal hemopoietic stem cells transplanted in sheep fetuses. *Blood* 1992; 79: 3045-3049.

15. Zanjani ED, Ascensao JL, Tavassoli M. Liver-derived fetal hemopoietic stem cells selectively and preferentially home to the fetal bone marrow. *Blood* 1993; 81: 399-404.
16. Zanjani ED, Flake AW, Rice HE, Hedrick MH, Tavassoli M. Long term repopulation ability of xenogeneic transplanted human fetal liver hematopoietic stem cells (HSC) in sheep. *J Clin Invest* 1994; 93: 1051-1055.
17. Zanjani ED, Pallavicini MG, Ascensao JL, Flake AW, Langlois RG, Reitsma M, MacKintosh FR, Stutes D, Harrison MR, Tavassoli M. Engraftment and long term expression of human fetal hematopoietic stem cells in sheep following transplantation in utero. *J Clin Invest* 1992; 89: 1178-1188.
18. Srour EF, Zanjani ED, Brandt JE, Leemhuis T, Briddell RA, Heerema NA, Hoffman R. Sustained human hematopoiesis in sheep transplanted in utero during early gestation with fractioned adult human bone marrow cells. *Blood* 1992; 79: 1410-1412.
19. Srour EF, Zanjani ED, Cornetta K, Traycoff CM, Flake AW, Hedrick M, Brandt J, Leemhuis T, Hoffman R. Persistence of human multilineage, self renewal lymphohematopoietic stem cells in chimeric sheep. *Blood* 1993; 82: 3333.
20. Flake AW, Harrison MR, Adzick NS, Zanjani ED. Transplantation of fetal hematopoietic stem cells in utero: the creation of hematopoietic chimeras. *Science* (Wash DC) 1986; 233: 776-778.
21. Zanjani ED, MacKintosh FR, Harrison MR. Hematopoietic chimerism in sheep and non-human primates by in utero transplantation of fetal hematopoietic stem cells. *Blood Cells* 1991; 17: 349-363.
22. Zanjani ED, Silva MRG, Flake AW. Retention and multilineage expression of human hematopoietic stem cells in human-sheep chimeras. *Blood Cells* 1994; 20: 331-340.
23. Crombleholme TM, Harrison MR, Zanjani ED. In utero transplantation of hematopoietic cells in sheep: the role of T cells in engraftment and graft-vs-host disease. *J Ped Surg* 1990; 25: 885-892.
24. Almeida GD, Zanjani ED, Ascensao JL. Role of sheep stroma in supporting human hematopoiesis in human/sheep chimeras. *Clin Res* 1994; 42: 235a.
25. Almeida-Porada GD, Hoffman R, Ascensao JL, Zanjani ED. Co-transplantation of autologous stromal cells with purified auldt human hematopoietic stem cells (HSC) results in increased engraftment and early donor cell expression in sheep. *Blood* 1994; 84: 253a.

Résumé

Un modèle expérimental est proposé, qui permet d'analyser la capacité de reconstitution à long terme de cellules hématopoïétiques humaines. Ces cellules sont injectées pendant la période fœtale à des moutons. Ce modèle présente plusieurs avantages : (1) à ce stade de développement (54-65 jours), il y a tolérance immunologique, ce qui assure l'acceptation de la greffe xénogénique. Cependant, lorsque les cellules du greffon proviennent d'organes adultes, il est nécessaire d'utiliser des suspensions déplétées de cellules immunologiquement compétentes ($CD34^+$) pour éviter une GVHD. (2) La reconstitution hématopoïétique se fait dans un animal immunologiquement normal. (3) La petite taille du fœtus permet de tester les capacités de reconstitution de petits nombres de cellules présélectionnées ($CD34^+$ ou sous-populations $CD34^+HLADr^-$) d'origine différente (sang de cordon, foie fœtal, moelle osseuse adulte, sang périphérique). (4) L'étude séquentielle et prolongée du chimérisme, possible dans ces animaux de grande taille, montre que dans 40-50% des animaux, la moelle contient 2-10% de cellules humaines. La greffe de cellules souches humaines très primitives est suggérée par la persistence d'un état chimérique 5 années après la greffe et par la possibilité de transplantations secondaires.

Human hematopoiesis in SCID mice

John E. Dick, Tsvee Lapidot, Josef Vormoor, André Larochelle, Dominique Bonnet, Jean Wang

Department of Genetics, Hospital for Sick Children and Department of Molecular and Medical Genetics, University of Toronto, Toronto, Ontario, Canada, M5G1X8, tel.: (416) 813 6354, fax: (416) 813 4931

Summary

The ability to transplant human hematopoietic cells into mice provides a powerful system to characterize primitive human stem cells and to create animal models for human hematopoietic diseases such as hemoglobinopathies and leukemia. These models can be used to learn something about the basic mechanisms that underlie these diseases and to develop new treatment strategies providing better pre-clinical information. In particular we are using this system to evaluate current gene therapy procedures and vectors. This review will briefly summarize our recent work to characterize the engrafting cells from normal and leukemic patients using a variety of techniques including gene transfer.

The hematopoietic system is organized as a hierarchy that originates from stem cells that have extensive proliferative and differentiation capacity and give rise to all myeloid and lymphoid lineages [1]. Insight into the biology of these stem cells is fundamental to our understanding of the regulation of normal and abnormal hematopoiesis. Because stem cells can only be assayed by their ability to reconstitute the entire hematopoietic system, they have only been studied in the mouse where repopulation assays are readily available [2]. By contrast, our understanding of human stem cells is not well developed because of the obvious limitations in developing similar transplantation assays. Similarly, few models that replicate human hematopoietic diseases are available.

Over the last five years, several different approaches have been developed to establish *in vivo* models for human hematopoiesis by transplanting human hematopoietic cells into immune-deficient mice [3, 4]. Our group developed an approach based on conventional bone marrow transplantation protocols [5, 6]. Human hematopoietic cells from several different sources are injected via the tail vein into sublethally irradiated immune-deficient mice. Our past and present studies strongly suggest that primitive cells (probably more immature than progenitors) engraft the murine microenvironment. These immature cells proliferate and differentiate into multiple myeloid, erythroid, and B cell lineages resulting in extensive repopulation of the murine bone marrow [7]. Despite this progress, SCID mice have some limitations as hosts for human cells.

We have little success in transplanting these mice with limiting cell numbers or with purified $CD34^+$ cells. More recently, we have examined other immune-deficient mice and found NOD/SCID mice to be superior to SCID mice. These mice have multiple defects in innate immunity including defects in NK cells, complement, and macrophage killing [8]. All of our recent experiments on characterizing SRC have come from using these recipients. This review will briefly summarize our recent work to characterize the engrafting cells from normal and leukemic patients using a variety of techniques including gene transfer.

Characterization of SCID-repopulating cells (SRC)

Over the last several years we have accumulated several lines of evidence that suggest primitive cells engraft immune-deficient mice and are responsible for establishing the graft of human cells. 1) Our initial experiments showed that the transplantion of human bone marrow cells into SCID mice resulted in the engraftment of human cells in the murine bone marrow [9]. Mature cells in the peripheral blood did not engraft. 2) Mice transplanted with bone marrow or cord blood remained engrafted for at least 3 months [9, 10]. The levels of human cells could be greatly stimulated if the mice were regularly treated with human cytokines such as stem cell factor (SCF, MGF, kit-ligand), PIXY321 (IL-3/GM-CSF fusion protein, and EPO [7]. Cytokine treated mice contained high levels of human myeloid, erythroid, and B cell lineages. There was no difference in the stimulation of human hematopoiesis if cytokines were given directly after the transplant or after a delay of 3 months. These data indicate that primitive human cells homed to the murine microenvironment, survived there for at least several months, and remained responsive to cytokine stimulation. 3) Flow cytometry analysis of engrafted mice detected immature $CD34^+CD38^-$ cells [11] and $CD34^+thy^+$ cells (in preparation) in the marrow of engrafted mice. These cell surface markers detect a small population of very immature cells in human bone marrow [12]. Clinical human transplants have shown that CD34 is expressed on stem cells (as well as more committed cells). 4) Only $CD34^+$ cells and not $CD34^-$ cells engraft immune-deficient mice (in preparation). 5) Committed progenitors for all myeloid and erythroid lineages, as well as the ealiest known multipotential progenitors (CFU-blast, CFU-GEMM) were found in engrafted mice [7]. In addition, human long-term culture intiating cells (LTC-IC) were detected 1-2 months after the transplant (in preparation). 6) Our initial kinetic studies suggested that there was an increase in the number of CFU-GM during the first month after the transplant [13]. Recently we have carried out a much more extensive kinetic study that indicated there was a rapid and large expansion of progenitors, LTC-IC, and $CD34^+thy^+$ cells over the first 28 days of engraftment (in preparation). These studies suggest that the expansion is derived from the proliferation and differentiation of the engrafting cell. 7) As outlined in more detail below, gene marking experiments have found that the vast majority of progenitors that are assayed in colony assays, as well as a proportion of LTC-IC are not responsible for maintaining the graft of human cells. Taken togther, these data argue that the engrafting cell is very primitive. We have termed this cell the SCID-Repopulating Cell (SRC). Only additional gene marking studies will prove whether SRC is pluripotential and capable of self-renewal. Using similar approaches, we have also identified and characterized a new class of primitive leukemic stem cells based on their ability to initiate leukemia after transplantation [14]. These AML stem cells are in the $CD34^+CD38^-$ fraction for at least some patients.

Models for gene therapy

The ability to introduce new genes into hematopoietic cells provides a novel approach to correct human genetic diseases [15]. To achieve permanent correction, the target for gene transfer must be the pluripotent stem cell because mature cells and committed progenitors do not have the proliferative capacity to reconstitute the entire hematopoietic system. Most studies, over the past 10 years, have used highly infectious retrovirus vectors to introduce genes into stem cells [16]. Methods for retrovirus-mediated gene transfer were first developed using mouse bone marrow because of the availability of repopulation assays for pluripotent stem cells. These studies showed that retroviruses could efficiently transduce pluripotent stem cells that completely reconstituted the entire hematopoietic system of the mouse [17]. Surprisingly, the same methods of retrovirus infection were much less efficient for canine [18, 19] or primate [20, 21] stem cells where the level of genetically marked cells after reconstitution were generally lower than 1%. The early experience in human clinical trials [22] also suggests that gene transfer into normal human stem cells is inefficient. Therefore, significant species differences exist in the efficiency of retrovirus infection, pointing out the importance of extensive pre-clinical evaluation of vectors and conditions specific for human stem cell gene transfer.
We have made two advances to develop pre-clinical models for gene therapy. The first is to determine the efficiency of retrovirus-mediated gene transfer into SRC and the second is to create animal models for human genetic diseases.

Gene transfer into SRC

The SCID transplant system provides the means of assessing the efficiency of gene transfer into SRC. We [23] and Nolta *et al* [24] have previously reported that low numbers of genetically manipulated cells could be detected in transplanted immune-deficient mice. However, these mice were engrafted with low levels of human cells and few mature cells developed in the mice, hence it difficult to determine the nature of the engrafting cell. We have now used the improved transplant system, with NOD/SCID mice and cytokine treatment to assay the efficiency of gene transfer into progenitors and SRC from human bone marrow or cord blood (in preparation). Human cells were stimulated with cytokines for one day and then co-cultuvated with virus-producing cell lines for two days before plating in colony assays and transplantation into mice. Our preliminary data using these standard gene transfer methods indicate that while progenitors are efficiently infected (>50%), gene transfer into SRC is much lower (<0.1%), highlighting the need to use appropriate assays for pre-clinical studies (Vormoor *et al*, unpublished). This data is consistent with the low stem cell gene transfer observed in earlier canine [18, 19], primate [20, 21] studies, and recent human clinical trials [22]. Clearly new vectors and approaches need to be developed for efficiently transducing human stem cells. There are at least two possibilities of why SRC can not be infected. Either they do not express the retrovirus receptor or they can not be induced to enter the cell cycle during the 3 days in culture. These results also confirm our hypothesis that SRC are more primitive than progenitors since few marked cells were detected in the mice 1 month post-transplant.

Animal models for human genetic diseases

Until recently, the most significant difficulty in developing and evaluating gene transfer protocols for human cells was the lack of a relevant *in vivo* re-population assay that detects genetically deficient human hematopoietic stem cells and their diseased differentiated progeny. β-thalassemia and sickle cell anemia (SCA) are two common human genetic disorders of the β-globin gene that present special problems for gene therapy [25]. The newly introduced globin genes must be introduced into stem cells, expressed only in erythroid cells and be precisely regulated in order to produce a functional hemoglobin molecule. An animal model was created by transplanting bone marrow cells from human β-thalassemia and SCA patients into immune-deficient mice [11]. Primitive bone marrow cells from β-thalassemia major and sickle cell anemia patients engraft immune-deficient mice, giving rise to high levels of human erythroid and myeloid cells in response to treatment with human cytokines. The bone marrow of transplanted mice contained the entire erythroid lineage from BFU-E to mature erythrocytes expressing human γ, β or β^s-globin. Moreover, human erythroid cells from mice transplanted with sickle cell anemia bone marrow showed characteristic sickling under reducing conditions in an *in vitro* assay. This model provides a powerful *in vivo* system that can be used to evaluate the efficiency of globin gene transfer into primitive human hematopoietic cells, lineage-specfic expression in mature erythrocytes, and ultimately correction of the cellular defect found in the erythroid lineage. Although we have focussed on hemoglobinopathies, this approach should be applicable to create animal models for any genetic defect involving the human hematopoietic system.

References

1. Till JE, McCulloch EA. Hematopoietic stem cell differentiation. *Biochim Biophys Acta* 1980; 605: 431-459.
2. Phillips R. Hematopoietic stem cells: concepts, assays, and controversies. *Sem Immunol* 1991; 3: 337-347.
3. McCune J, Kaneshima H, Krowka J, Namikawa R, Outzen H, Peault B, Rabin L, Shih C, Yee E, Lieberman M, Weissman I, Schultz L. The scid-hu mouse: A small animal model for HIV infection and pathogenesis. *Annu Rev Immunol* 1991; 9: 399-429.
4. Torbett B, Picchio G, Mosier D. Hu-PBL-SCID mice: a model for human immune function, AIDS, and lymphomagenesis. *Immunol Rev* 1991; 124: 139-164.
5. Dick J, Lapidot T, Pflumio F. Transplantation of normal and leukemic human bone marrow into immune-deficient mice: Development of animal models for human hematopoiesis. *Immunol Rev* 1991; 124: 25-43.
6. Dick J, Sirard C, Pflumio F, Lapidot T. Murine models of normal and neoplastic human hematopoiesis. *Cancer Surveys* 1992; 15: 161-181.
7. Lapidot T, Pflumio F, Doedens M, Murdoch B, Williams DE, Dick JE. Cytokine stimulation of multilineage human hematopoiesis from immature cells transplanted into SCID mice. *Science* 1992; 255: 1137-1141.
8. Shultz L, Schweitzer P, Christianson S, Gott B, Birdsall-Maller I, Tennent B, McKenna S, Mobraaten L, Rajan T, Greiner D, Leiter E. Multiple defects in innate and adaptive immunological function in NOD/LtSz-*scid* mice. *J Immunol* 1994; in press.
9. Lapidot T, Pflumio F, Doedens M, Murdoch B, Williams D, Dick J. Cytokine stimulation of multilineage human hematopoiesis from immature cells transplanted into scid mice. *Science* 1992; 255: 1137-1141.
10. Vormoor J, Lapidot T, Pflumio F, Risdon G, Patterson B, Broxmeyer HE, Dick JE. Immature human cord blood progenitors engraft and proliferate to high levels in severe combined immunodeficient mice. *Blood* 1994; 83: 2489-97.
11. Larochelle A, Vormoor J, Lapidot T, Sher G, Furukawa T, Li Q, Shultz L, Oliveri NF, Stamatoyannopoulos G, Dick JE. Engraftment of immune-deficient mice with primitive hematopoietic cells from β-thalassemia and sickle cell anemia patients: implications for evaluating human gene therapy protocols. *Human Molecular Genetics* 1995; 4: 163-172.
12. Terstappen L, Huang S, Safford M, Lansdorp P, Loken M. Sequential generations of hematopoietic colonies derived from single non-lineage-committed CD34$^+$CD38$^-$ progenitor cells. *Blood* 1991; 77: 1218-1227.

13. Kamel-Reid S, Dick JE. Engraftment of immune-deficient mice with human hematopoietic stem cells. *Science* 1988; 242: 1706-1709.
14. Lapidot T, Sirard C, Vormoor J, Murdoch B, Hoang T, Caceres-Cortes J, Minden M, Paterson B, Caliguri MA, Dick JE. A cell initiating human acute myeloid leukaemia after transplantation into SCID mice. *Nature* 1994; 367: 645-648.
15. Morgan RA, Anderson WF. Human gene therapy. *Ann Rev Biochem* 1993; 62: 191-217.
16. Mulligan RC. The basic science of gene therapy. *Science* 1993; 260: 926-932.
17. Dick JE, Magli MC, Huszar D, Phillips RA, Bernstein A. Introduction of a selectable gene into primitive stem cells capable of long-term reconstitution of the hemopoietic system of W/Wv mice. *Cell* 1985; 42: 71-79.
18. Schuening F, Kawahara K, Miller A, To R, Goehle S, Stewart D, Mullally K, Fisher L, Graham T, Applebaum F, Hackman R, Osborne W, Storb R. Retrovirus-mediated gene transduction into long-term repopulating marrow cells of the dog. *Blood* 1991; 78: 2568-2576.
19. Carter RF, Abrams-Ogg AC, Dick JE, Kruth SA, Valli VE, Kamel-Reid S, Dube ID. Autologous transplantation of canine long-term marrow culture cells genetically marked by retroviral vectors. *Blood* 1992; 79: 356-364.
20. van Beusechem V, Kukler A, Heidt P, Valerio D. Long-term expression of human adenosine deaminase in rhesus monkeys transplanted with retrovirus-infected bone marrow cells. *Proc Natl Acad Sci USA* 1992; 89: 7640-7644.
21. Bodine DM, Moritz T, Donahue RE, Luskey BD, Kessler SW, Martin DI, Orkin SH, Nienhuis AW, Williams DA. Long-term *in vivo* expression of a murine adenosine deaminase gene in rhesus monkey hematopoietic cells of multiple lineages after retroviral mediated gene transfer into CD34[+] bone marrow cells. *Blood* 1993; 82: 1975-1980.
22. Kohn D, Weinberg K, Parkman R, Lenarsky C, Crooks G, Shaw K, Hanley M, Lawrence K, Annett G, Brooks J, Wara D, Elder M, Bowen T, Hershfeld M, Berenson R, Moen R, Mullen C, Blaese R. Gene therapy for neonates with ADA-deficient SCID by retroviral-mediated transfer of the human ADA cDNA into umbilical cord CD34[+] cells. *Journal of Cellular Biochemistry* 1994; Supple 18A: 238.
23. Dick JE, Kamel-Reid S, Murdoch B, Doedens M. Gene transfer into normal human hematopoietic cells using *in vitro* and *in vivo* assays. *Blood* 1991; 78: 624-634.
24. Nolta JA, Hanley MB, Kohn DB. Sustained human hematopoiesis in immunodeficient mice by cotransplantation of marrow stroma expressing human interleukin-3: Analysis of gene transduction of long-lived progenitors. *Blood* 1994; 83: 3041-3051.
25. Weatherall DJ, Clegg JB, 1982. The Thalassemia Syndromes. Blackwell.

Résumé

La possibilité de transplanter des cellules hématopoïétiques humaines dans des souris offre un outil très performant pour caractériser des cellules souches humaines primitives. Ce système peut aussi être exploité pour créer des modèles animaux de pathologies humaines comme certaines hémoglobinopathies ou hémopathies malignes. En particulier, de tels modèles seraient utiles pour appréhender les mécanismes physiopathologiques à l'origine de ces pathologies et pourraient aussi conduire à la mise au point de nouvelles stratégies thérapeutiques qui pourraient être testées avant leur application en clinique. Nous utilisons actuellement ces modèles pour la mise au point de stratégies de transfert de gènes. Dans ce chapitre, nous passerons en revue nos travaux récents sur la caractérisation des progéniteurs responsables de la prise de greffe après transplantation à ces souris de cellules humaines normales ou provenant de patients atteints d'hémopathies malignes.

Characteristics of human clonogenic and primitive cells engrafted into SCID mice

Françoise Pflumio, Brigitte Izac, André Katz, William Vainchenker and Laure Coulombel

INSERM U 362, Laboratoire Hématopoïèse et Cellules Souches, Institut Gustave-Roussy, 39, avenue Camille-Desmoulins, 94805 Villejuif, France, tel.: (33 1) 45 59 42 33, fax: (33 1) 45 26 92 74

The hematopoietic system is constituted by a hierarchy of cells starting from pluripotent and long term reconstituting stem cells which differentiate into lineage specific progenitors after multiple steps of divisions and differentiation. The availability of *in vivo* mouse models has greatly contributed to the present knowledge of murine hematopoiesis. On the contrary, the human hematopoietic system has been mainly studied in *in vitro* tests because of the lack of reproducible *in vivo* assays for normal human hematopoietic cells. The recent development of animal models for human hematopoiesis has opened novel areas of investigation [1-3]. The main results emerging from these studies are that immature human hematopoietic cells from fetal liver, adult and fetal bone marrow and cord blood engraft and are maintained for months in immune-deficient SCID mice or in sheep, reproducing human hematopoiesis *in vivo*. In SCID mice, the engrafted human cells remain responsive *in vivo* to human growth factors (stem cell factor, PIXY-321, EPO) and give rise to human multilineage (erythroid, granulo-monocytic, megakaryocytic) colonies when plated in methyl cellulose assays under human specific conditions. Human lymphoid B cells can also be identified among the engrafted human cells [3-5]. Although the SCID Repopulating Cell [6] is thought to be a very immature cell, nothing is known yet about its position in the hierarchy of the human hematopoietic system. In the course of developing models to understand the development and regulation of the human hematopoietic system, we have developed an animal model for human hematopoiesis using immune-deficient SCID mice transplanted with human cord blood (CB) mononuclear cells according to Vormoor [5]. The goal of this work was to characterize the engrafted human hematopoietic cells in terms of their phenotype and functionality.

Methods

The protocole was as described in Vormoor [5]. Briefly, SCID mice were sublethally irradiated (3.5Gy), intraveinously injected with human mononuclear CB cells (10-20x10^6 light-density mononuclear cells/mouse) and their bone marrow cells analysed by flow cytometry using human specific antibodies 3 to 4 weeks after the transplantation. In order to detect human progenitors, marrow cells cells from transplanted mice were plated in methyl cellulose assays in the presence of human specific growth factors (SCF, IL-3, GM-CSF and EPO).

In some experiments, human CD34$^+$ cells were sorted by flow cytometry before and after transplantation in the mice. Human clonogenic progenitors and LTC-IC were assessed respectively either by plating in methyl-cellulose containing human SCF, IL-3, EPO and G-CSF or by culture on the murine stromal cell line MS5 during 5 weeks in long term culture (LTC) medium as described in [7].

Results

When 20x10^6 human mononuclear CB cells were transplanted, human HLA-class I$^+$ cells were consistently detected in the murine bone marrow (9/11 experiments). The engraftment level varied from 0.3 to 13x10^5 human cells per 4 long bones from one experimental group to the other but was homogenous between mice transplanted with the same cord blood cells.

Phenotyping the engrafted human cells revealed the presence of mature CD19$^+$ B cells, CD15$^+$, CD33$^+$, or CD11b$^+$ granulo-monocytic cells, and glycophorin A$^+$ erythroid cells. The proportion of engrafted human immature CD34$^+$ cells was higher than in the starting sample and represented between 10 to 67% of the engrafted human HLA class I$^+$ cells. This last result could be explained by an inefficient terminal differenciation in the chimeras probably accounted for by the lack of cross-reactivity between cytokins.

On a functional point of view, the cloning efficiency of the recovered human cells was 1.4±1.1 % (n=17 mice) and 37±14 % of the clonogenic progenitors belonged to the erythroid lineage (n=23 mice) compared to 60±12 % in the original CB samples (n=6). Because the proportion of human CD34$^+$ cells among human HLA-class 1$^+$ cells engrafting SCID mice was higher than in the original CBC (1% CD34$^+$ cells), it was important to compare the functional potential of the input and the output CD34$^+$ populations as well as to test a potential enrichment in early progenitors. Thus human CD34$^+$ cells were sorted before (input) and after (output) the transplantation in SCID mice and their functionality was compared. When human CD34$^+$ cells were sorted previous to transplantation in SCID mice, the cloning efficiency was 26±7 % (n=4) compared to 4.6±2 % in output human CD34$^+$ cells. Moreover, measurement of LTC-IC frequency in human CD34$^+$ cells before and after the transplantation suggested also a loss in the LTC-IC compartment in the mice. The frequency of long term culture-initiating cells among the output human CD34$^+$ was found to be 1/275 (n=3 experiments) whereas the frequency was 1/20 in the input CD34$^+$ cells.

We have shown that human CD34$^+$ cells had different *in vitro* capabilities when tested either before or after transplantation in SCID mice in clonogenic and LTC-IC assays. In order to understand this discrepancy, immature human CD34$^+$ cells were further phenotyped by flow cytometry. Double staining with antibodies directed against human CD34 and CD38 indicated that the output CD34$^+$ population has a more mature phenotype compared to the input population, which is compatible with the results obtained in the functional assays. Experiments are in progress to clarify this point.

Conclusion

Transplantation of high numbers of CB mononuclear cells into SCID mice resulted reproducibly in the engraftment of multilineage human hematopoietic cells and progenitors during 3 to 4 weeks. Immature LTC-IC were also detected in the chimeras. However, comparison of purified human CD34$^+$ cells before and after transplantation in SCID mice revealed differences in the functionality between the 2 populations with lower cloning efficiency and LTC-IC frequencies in human CD34$^+$ cells recovered after transplantation. Whether or not these differences will be minimised by supplementation of mice with human cytokines has to be investigated. Although the results seem to indicate that human CD34$^+$ cells recovered from SCID mice are more mature than in the original sample, we could speculate that actually the engrafted human immature cells (i.e the SCID Repopulating Cell) are more immature than LTC-IC and that we do not have effective *in vitro* assays to reveal its potential.

References

1. Dick JE, Pflumio F and Lapidot T, 1991. Mouse models for human hematopoiesis. *Seminars in Immunol* **3**: 367-378.
2. Zanjani ED, Flake AW, Rice H, Hedrick M and Tavassoli M, 1994. Long-term repopulating ability of xenogeneic transplanted human fetal liver hematopoietic stem cells in sheep. *J Clin Inv* **93**: 1051-1055.
3. Kollmann TR, Kim A, Zhuang X, Hachamovitch M and Goldstein H, 1994. Reconstitution of SCID mice with human lymphoid and myeloid cells after transplantation with human fetal bone marrow without the requirement for exogenous human cytokines. *Proc Nat Acad Sci USA* **91**: 8032-8036.
4. Lapidot T, Pflumio F, Doedens M, Murdoch B, Williams DE and Dick JE, 1992. Cytokine stimulation of multilineage hematopoiesis from immature human cells engrafted in SCID mice. *Science.* **255**: 1137-1141.
5. Vormoor J, Lapidot T, Pflumio F, Risdon G, Patterson B, Broxmeyer HE and Dick JE, 1994. Immature human Cord Blood progenitors engraft and proliferate to high levels in immune-deficient SCID mice. *Blood.* **83** (9), 2489-2497.
6. Dick JE, 1994. Future prospects for animal models created by transplanting human haematopoietic cells into immune-deficient mice. *Res Immunol* **145**: 380.
7. Issaad C, Croisille L, Katz A, Vainchenker W and Coulombel L, 1993. A murine stromal cell line allows the proliferation of very primitive human CD34^{++}/CD38$^-$ progenitor cells in long-term cultures and semi-solid assays. *Blood.* **81**: 2916-2924.

Résumé

Afin de disposer de modèles d'étude du développement et des mécanismes régulant le système hématopoïétique humain, nous avons mis au point un modèle *in vivo* d'hématopoïèse humaine en transplantant des cellules mononucléées de sang fœtal humain dans des souris immunodéficientes SCID.

Les résultats obtenus indiquent une prise de greffe de plusieurs lignées du système hématopoïétique humain dans les 3 à 4 semaines suivant la transplantation. Des cellules des lignées lymphoïde B, myéloïde et érythroïde sont détectées de façon reproductible parmi les cellules de la moelle osseuse des souris de même que des cellules humaines plus immatures $CD34^+$. Du point de vue fonctionnel, l'utilisation de tests *in vitro* (test clonogénique et test de LTC-IC) a mis en évidence la présence de progéniteurs myéloïdes et érythroïdes et de LTC-IC parmi les cellules humaines ayant greffé les souris SCID. Toutefois, la comparaison entre le potentiel fonctionnel des cellules $CD34^+$ humaines obtenues avant et après la greffe aux souris a indiqué des différences importantes entre les deux populations. En effet, l'efficacité de clonage et la fréquence en LTC-IC des cellules $CD34^+$ humaines obtenues après transplantation sont plus faibles que dans la population de cellules $CD34^+$ de départ. La question de savoir si les cellules obtenues après transplantation ont perdu leur potentiel en maturant dans l'environnement murin ou si, au contraire, elles représentent une population de cellules très immatures que l'on ne peut caractériser à l'heure actuelle faute de test adéquats, reste posée.

4) Gene transfer in cord blood hematopoietic stem cells

4) *Transfert de gènes dans les cellules souches de sang de cordon*

Cord blood hematopoietic stem/progenitor cell growth and gene transduction using adeno-associated and retroviral vectors

Hal E. Broxmeyer[1-3], Scoot Cooper[1,3], Maryse Etienne-Julan[1,3], Stephen Braun[1,3], Li Lu[1,3], Stewart D. Lyman[4] and Arun Srivastava[1-3]

The Departments of [1] Medicine (Hematology/Oncology); [2] Microbiology and Immunology; the [3] Walther Oncology Center, Indiana University School of Medicine, Indianapolis, IN, USA, tel.: (317) 274 7510, fax: (317) 274 7592; [4] the Immunex Research and Development Corporation, Seattle, WA, USA

Summary

Umbilical cord blood hematopoietic stem and progenitor cells, while slowly cycling, have extensive proliferative and self-renewal capacity upon stimulation with cytokines. Clinical results using cryopreserved sibling and unrelated cord blood for transplantation are encouraging. Situations can be envisioned where there would be a need to expand the numbers of stem/progenitor cells from cord blood. Although there is not yet a quantitative assay for the human long term marrow repopulating cell, at least subsets of stem and progenitor cells can be greatly expanded ex vivo and these cells, at least prior to expansion, have been efficiently transduced with new genetic material using recombinant adeno-associated and retroviral vectors. This review briefly outlines the possibility of using viral vectors containing genes for cytokines or cytokine receptors for expansion of selected populations of immature or more mature lineage committed cells.

Hematopoietic stem and progenitor cells from human cord blood have extensive proliferative and replating capacity *in vitro* [1-3]. These cryopreserved cells have been used clinically in a sibling setting in over sixty cases and also in an unrelated setting with cells from cord blood banks in over twenty-five cases for engraftment and repopulation of the hematopoietic system of children with a variety of malignant and non-malignant disorders [1-3]. The field itself has come a long way in the short time since the initial suggestion that cord blood could serve as a source of transplantable hematopoietic stem and progenitor cells [4] and since the first successful HLA-matched sibling cord blood transplant that cured the hematological manifestations of Fanconi anemia in the affected recipient [5]. The results thus far have been encouraging. For example, Graft vs. host disease has been relatively low in recipients of sibling and unrelated cord blood, perhaps due to the lessened immunological reactivity of immune cells in cord blood [6-9]. However, there are a number of questions remaining to be answered regarding umbilical cord blood hematopoietic stem and progenitor cells, immune cells, and their use and place in transplantation [10]. Two areas needing further evaluation include the *ex vivo* expansion of hematopoietic stem and progenitor cells from cord blood and the use of stem and progenitor cells as cellular vehicles to introduce new genetic material to either cure a genetic defect or to change the proliferation/differentiation characteristics of the cells. These areas of future investigation need not be mutually exclusive and are discussed below.

Characteristics of cord blood stem/progenitor cells and attempts at their *ex vivo* expansion

Primitive progenitors in cord blood have been phenotypically characterized as being $CD34^{+++}$, $CD34^+CD45RA^{lo}CD71^{lo}$, $CD34^+CD38^-$, $CD34^+thy1^+$, and $CD34^+HLA-DR^+$. These cells are in a slow or non-cycling state usually, but they response rapidly to external stimuli to induce their proliferation [1-3]. Reasons to expand stem/progenitor cells include the collection of samples too small to be used or the need to use a sample for multiple recipients. Numerous groups have reported the extensive capacity to expand at least the more mature subsets of stem cells and the immature and mature subsets of progenitor cells from human cord blood *ex vivo* [1-3]. The read-out systems for such cells have included assays for long term culture-initiating cells (LTC-IC), high proliferative potential-colony forming cells (HPP-CFC), and multipotential (CFU-GEMM), erythroid (BFU-E) and granulocyte-macrophage (CFU-GM), granulocyte (CFU-G) and macrophage (CFU-M) progenitor cells [1-3]. However, it is not yet clear that any of these assays detect the long-term marrow repopulating stem cell (LTMRSC) [11]. It is the LTMRSC that one would want in the donor inoculum to assure the possibility for long term engraftment and it is these cells that would seem to be the best vehicle for the introduction of new genetic material in a gene therapy setting. Without a quantitative assay for the LTMRSC it is not yet possible to determine if these cells in human cord blood or any other tissue source are being increased, maintained or lost during attempts at *ex vivo* expansion. It is clear that to varying degrees LTC-IC, HPP-CFC, CFU-GEMM, BFU-E and CFU-GM are being expanded. It would seem that during *ex vivo* expansion attempts it is the mature cells that are being expanded to a greater extent and perhaps at the expense of the more immature and primitive cells [12]. A number of groups have used animals such as mice and sheep as recipients of human cells in the hope that a quantitative assay for the human LTMRSC could be developed [11,13,14]. Currently, sublethally irradiated mice with severe combined immunodeficiency (SCID) are being used in this context and cord blood has been found to engraft and repopulate the marrows of these mice to a high degree [13,14]. Whether these mice can be used as a quantitative assay for the LTMRSC or not remains to be determined, but there is variability in the capacity of different mice within a strain to be engrafted and this needs to be addressed. A number of different mouse models are being evaluated and encouraging results are apparent with transgenic SCID mice expressing the human genes for granulocyte-macrophage colony stimulating factor (GM-CSF), interleukin(IL)-3 and steel factor (SLF, also termed stem cell factor) and with mice with the non-obese diabetic (NOD) genotype in which levels of natural killer and killer cell activity is low (TA Bock, D Orlic, CE Dunbar, HE Broxmeyer, and DM Bodine, unpublished observations).

Gene transfer into cord blood stem/progenitor cells with the possibility to modify the growth characteristics of these cells

High efficiency transduction of cord blood stem/progenitor cells with new genetic material has been accomplished using recombinant retroviral [14-18] and adeno-associated viral (AVV) [19] vectors. Thus far, it appears that for high efficiency gene transduction using retroviral vectors, cells, including those from cord blood, require a pre-incubation phase of one to 3 days with growth promoting cytokines in order to place these cells into a highly cycling state [18]. In contrast, high efficiency gene transduction using AAV vectors is possible without this growth factor pre-incubation phase [19]. This latter phenomenon does not however rule out the possible need for cell division for integration of the AAV vector. It should be noted that without an assay for the human LTMRSC we do not yet have any idea of the transduction efficiency of this cell by retroviral or AAV vectors. However, with an understanding of the limitation of not knowing whether human LTMRSC are being efficiently transduced, it is possible that using viral vectors to place either genes for early acting cytokines and/or receptors for these or other cytokines into stem/progenitor cells it may be possible to enhance expansion capability *ex vivo* of these cells and their lineage committed progeny. It is within this context that we have prepared both recombinant AAV and retroviral vectors containing cDNA for human SLF and human Flt3-ligand (L), also referred to as Flk-2L. SLF and Flt3-L are potent co-stimulating cytokines for stem/progenitor cells and allow detection of early subsets of these cells [20-22]. We have previously prepared an AAV vector containing the cDNA for GM-CSF which when transduced into fibroblasts allowed expression of the transduced GM-CSF gene [23]. The AAV and retroviral vectors for SLF and Flt3-L are being prepared with and without selectable markers and schematic representations of some of these recombinant vectors are shown in *Figure 1*.

We have found that low density (<1.077 gm/cm^3) separated or sorted populations of CD34^{+++} cord blood CFU-GEMM, BFU-E and CFU-GM were efficiently transduced by AAV or retroviral vectors containing the cDNA for human SLF or Flt3-L and that these transduced cells, com-

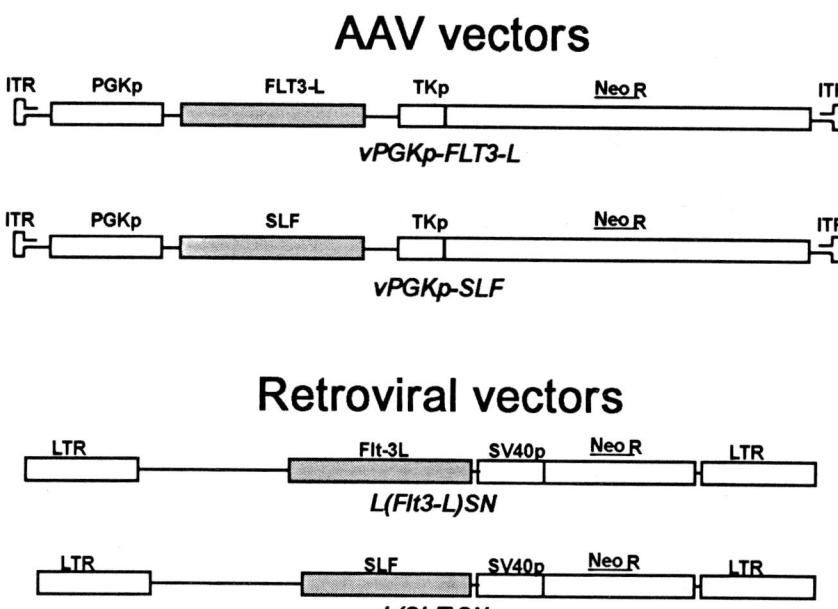

Figure 1. Schematic representation of recombinant vectors. Abbreviations: ITR, inverted terminal repeat; PGK, phosphoglycerate kinase; P, promoter; TK, thymidine kinase; *Neo*^{R}, neomycin phosphotransferase sequence; LTR, long terminal repeat.

pared to mock-infected control cells demonstrated about a doubling in cloning efficiency when the cells were plated in semi-solid medium in the presence of optimal concentrations of one or a combination of growth factors (unpublished observations). These preliminary experiments suggest the possibility that the introduction of genes for SLF and Flt-3 may allow proliferation of subsets of these cells that would not normally respond to exogenous administration of cytokines. It is possible that such maneuvers to place cytokine genes into stem/progenitor cells could in the future be used to enhance *ex vivo* expansion of cells. This might additionally be enhanced by the insertion and expression in these cells of receptors for cytokines such that cells that did not express these receptors could now express them, or that cells that did express them can now express them at higher levels, possibly making the cells more receptive to the exogenously added soluble cytokines or the endogenously produced cytokines. The introduction of new genes for cytokines and/or receptors may eventually allow for the selective expansion of early cells, perhaps through enhanced self-renewal, or of particular subsets of more committed cells.

Acknowledgement

The work cited from the authors' laboratories were supported by U.S. Public Health Service Grants RO1 HL46549, R37 CA36464, RO1 HL49202, RO1 HL54037 and a project in P01 HL53586 from the National Institutes of Health (NIH) and the National Cancer Institute to H.E.B., and by R29 AI26323, RO1 HL48342 and projects in P50 DK49218 and PO1 HL53586 from the NIH, an Established Investigator Award from the American Heart Association to AS, and by grants from the Phi Beta Psi Sorority to AS and LL. MEJ was supported in part by a grant from the Association de Recherche sur le Cancer, France, and SB was supported by NIH training program T32 DK07519 to HEB.

References

1. Broxmeyer HE. Cord blood as an alternative source for stem and progenitor cell transplantation. *Current Opinion in Pediatrics* 1995; 7: 47-55.
2. Broxmeyer HE. Clinical and biological aspects of human umblical cord blood transplantation for disease. *In* Hemopoietic Growth Factors, Oncogenes and Cytokines in Clinical Hematology. E Cacciola, AB Deisseroth & R Giustolisi, Eds. pp. 284-298. *Basel: Karger.* 1994.
3. Broxmeyer HE, Lu L, Gaddy J, Ruggieri L, Srivastava A Risdon G. Human umbilical cord blood transplantation: the immunology, expansion, and therapeutic applications of hematopoietic stem and progenitor cells. *In* Hematopoietic Stem Cells: Biology and Therapeutic Applications. DJ Levitt & R Mertelsmann, Eds. pp. 297-317. *Marcel Dekker Publishers.* New York. 1994.
4. Broxmeyer HE, Douglas GW, Hangoc G, Cooper S, Bard J, English D, Arny M, Thomas L, Boyse EA. Human umbilical cord blood as a potential source of transplantable hematopoietic stem/progenitor cells. *Proc Natl Acad Sci USA* 1989; 86: 3828-3832.
5. Gluckman E, Broxmeyer HE, Auerbach AD, Friedman HS, Douglas GW, Devergie A, Esperou H, Thierry D, Socie G, Lehn P, Cooper S, English D, Kurtzberg J, Bard J, Boyse EA. Hematopoietic reconstitution in a patient with fanconi's anemia by means of umbilical-cord blood from an HLA-identical sibling. *New Engl J Med* 1989; 321: 1174-1178.
6. Risdon G, Gaddy J, Stehman FB, Broxmeyer HE. Proliferative and Cytotoxic responses of human cord blood T lymphocytes following allogeneic stimulation. Cell Immunol 1994; 154:14-24.
7. Risdon G, Gaddy J, Horie M, Broxmeyer HE. Alloantigen priming induces a state of unresponsiveness in human cord blood T cells. *Proc Natl Acad Sci USA* 1995; in press.
8. Gaddy J, Risdon G, Broxmeyer HE. Cord blood natural killer cells are functionally and phenotypically immature but readily respond to IL-2 and IL-12. J. *Interferon and Cytokine Res* 1995; in Press.

9. Berthou C, Legros-Maida S, Soulie A, Wargnier A, Guillet J, Rabian C, Gluckman E, Sasportes M. Cord blood T lymphocytes lack constitutive perforin expression in contrast to adult peripheral blood T lymphocytes. *Blood* 1995; 85: 1540-1546.
10. Broxmeyer HE. Questions to be answered regarding umbilical cord blood hematopoietic stem and progenitor cells and their role in transplantation. *Transfusion* 1995; in press.
11. Broxmeyer HE. Consequences of human stem cells taking up residence in sheep. *J Clin Invest* 1994; 93: 919.
12. Ruggieri L, Heimfeld S, Broxmeyer HE. Cytokine-dependent *ex vivo* expansion of early subsets of CD34$^+$ cord blood myeloid progenitors is enhanced by cord blood plasma, but expansion of the more mature subsets of progenitors is favored. *Blood Cells* 1994; 20: 436-454.
13. Vormoor J, Lapidot T, Pflumio F, Risdon G, Patterson B, Broxmeyer HE, Dick JE. Immature human cord blood progenitors engraft and proliferate to high levels in severe combined immunodeficient mice. *Blood* 1994; 83: 2489-2497.
14. Orazi A, Braun SE, Broxmeyer HE. Immunohistochemistry represents a Useful Tool to Study Human Cell Engraftment in SCID Mice Transplantation Models. *Blood Cells* 1994; 20: 323-330.
15. Moritz T, Keller DC, Williams DA. Human cord blood cells as targets for gene transfer: Potential use in genetic therapies of severe combined immunodeficiency disease. *J Exp Med* 1993; 178: 529-536.
16. Lu L, Xiao M, Clapp DW, Li ZH, Broxmeyer HE. High efficiency retroviral ediated gene transduction into single isolated immature and replatable CD34^{+++} hematopoietic stem/progenitor cells from human umbilical cord blood. *J Exp Med* 1993; 178: 2089-2096.
17. Lu L, Xiao M, Clapp DW, Li ZH, Broxmeyer HE. Stable integration of retrovirally transduced genes into human umbilical cord blood high-proliferative potential colony forming cells (HPP-CFC) as assessed after multiple HPP-CFC colony replatings *in vitro*. *Blood Cells* 1994; 20: 525-530.
18. Shi YJ, Shen RN, Lu L, Broxmeyer HE. Comparative analysis of retroviral-mediated gene transduction into CD34$^+$ cord blood hematopoietic progenitors in the presence and absence of growth factors. *Blood Cells* 1994; 20: 517-524.
19. Zhou SZ, Cooper S, Kang YL, Ruggieri L, Heimfeld S, Srivastava A, Broxmeyer HE. Adeno-associated virus 2-mediated high efficiency gene transfer into immature and mature subsets of hematopoietic progenitor cells in human umbilical cord blood. *J Exp Med* 1994; 179: 1867-1875.
20. Broxmeyer HE, Maze R. Miyazawa K, Carow C, Hendrie PC, Cooper S, Hangoc G, Vadhan-Raj S, Lu L. The kit receptor and its ligand, steel factor, as regulators of hemopoiesis. *Cancer Cells* 1991; 3: 480-487.
21. Lyman SD, James L, Vanden Bos T, de Vries P, Brasel K, Gliniak B, Hollingsworth LT, Picha KS, McKenna HJ, Splett RR, Fletcher FA, Maraskovsky E, Farrah T, Foxworthe E, Williams DE, Beckmann MP. Molecular cloning of a ligand for the flt3/flk-2 tyrosine kinase receptor: a proliferative factor for primitive hematopoietic cells. *Cell* 1993; 75: 1557-1167.
22. Broxmeyer HE, Lu L, Cooper S, Ruggieri L, Li ZH, Lyman SD. Flt3-ligand stimulates/costimulates the growth of myeloid stem/progenitor cells. *Exp Hematol* 1995; in press.
23. Luo F, Zhou SZ, Cooper S, Munshi NC, Boswell HS, Broxmeyer HE, Srivastava A. Adeno-associated virus 2-mediated gene transfer and functional expression of the human granulocyte-macrophage colony-stimulating factor. *Exp Hematol* 1995; in press.

Résumé

Les progéniteurs hématopoïétiques du sang de cordon ont une capacité de prolifération et d'autorenouvellement très importante en réponse à des cytokines appropriées. Les données cliniques sur l'utilisation en transplantation de cellules de sang de cordon congelées sont encourageantes. Certaines situations cliniques en transplantation bénéficieraient de l'utilisation de populations amplifiées *in vitro*. Bien que l'on ne dispose pas encore de test permettant d'identifier et de mesurer le nombre de cellules capables de reconstituer le système hématopoïétique à long terme, il est néanmoins possible d'amplifier des sous-populations de progéniteurs *ex vivo* et ces populations peuvent être transduites avec du matériel génétique nouveau par l'intermédiaire de vecteurs de type AAV ou rétrovirus. Cet article passe en revue les possibilités d'utilisation de ces vecteurs pour transférer des gènes codant pour des cytokines ou leurs récepteurs dans le but d'amplifier des populations de progéniteurs pluripotents immatures ainsi que leur descendance plus mature.

Retroviral-mediated gene transfer into hematopoietic stem progenitor cells from fresh and cryopreserved umbilical cord blood

Li Lu[1,3], Zhi-Hua Li[1,3], Yue Ge[1,3] and Hal E. Broxmeyer[1-3]

The Departments of [1] Medicine (Hematology/Oncology); [2] Microbiology and Immunology; the [3] Walther Oncology Center, Indiana University School of Medicine, Indianapolis, IN, USA, tel.: (317) 274 7560, fax: (317) 274 7592

Summary

In consideration of the prospect for gene therapy in the future, it was considered important to know if cryopreserved umbilical cord blood (CB) cells could be enriched for hematopoietic stem (HSC)/progenitor (HPC) cells, if these cells could be transduced with foreign genes and expanded ex vivo *with stable integration and expression of the newly introduced genetic material, and if fresh cells transduced with genes could survive after the cryopreservation process. This paper briefly reviews our experience in this area using retroviral-mediated gene transfer. We found that HSC/HPC cells could be highly enriched by cell sorting after thawing the cryopreserved CB cells, the cells served as targets for high efficiency gene transduction, even at the single cell level, and the cells containing the transduced gene could be extensively expanded* ex vivo. *In addition, fresh cells transduced with new genetic material could be recovered after cryopreservation with detectable levels of the transduced gene. This information should be of use in the future considerations of CB HSC and HPC as potential transplantable source of genetically modified cells.*

Understanding of the molecular biology of some of the disorders of inherited and hematological diseases as well as the development of recombinant DNA technology has provided us with tools necessary to potentially correct defects in some of these disorders. The goal of gene therapy is to replace a defective gene with the functional genetic sequence equivalent of that gene [1]. A number of investigators have explored the use of viral vectors for transfer of new genetic material into cells as a means to develop gene-replacement therapy. The first trials have begun in this context in humans [2] but much is still to be learned with regards to the most useful target cells, the best vector systems and the most efficient transduction methods.

Umbilical CB HSC/HPC cells as targets for gene transduction

Genetic sequences can be introduced into mammalian cells. Cellular targets for gene transfer should ideally have the capacity for self-renewal and for differentiation into multiple lineages. HSC/HPC cells have been considered as ideal targets for gene transfer, since these cells are capable of self-renewal, and have the capacity to differentiate into committed mature progenitor cells for all lymphoid and myeloid cell lineages. Stable integration and expression of therapeutic genes into these primitive cells could lead to lifelong treatment of serious diseases resulting from a single efficient gene transfer event. Moreover, at least some HSC and HPC can be manipulated and expanded *ex vivo*. CB is a rich source of HSC/HPC and is easily accessible [3-6]. HSC and HPC from CB can be very highly enriched by cell sorting [7] and expanded even starting from a single isolated purified cell [8]. These cells have been used for gene transduction with high efficiency, even at the single cell level [9], with stable integration even after multiple replatings [10]. It is known that a single collection of CB contains enough HSC and HPC cells for transplantation of children [6]. Thus, we believe that CB HSC and HPC can serve as ideal targets for gene transfer and gene therapy.

Retroviral vectors

Many methods have been used for introduction of foreign genes into mammalian cells. The low frequency of HSC and HPC cells in adult bone marrow, peripheral blood or CB necessitates a very efficient method of gene transfer. In this article, we focus on retroviral-mediated gene transduction. Retroviral vectors are efficient and relatively safe tools for introduction of a non viral gene into mitotic cells *in vivo* and *in vitro*. Postmitotic cells can not be transduced, because cellular DNA synthesis/cell division seems to be a requirement for complete reverse transcription and viral integration [11]. The use of retroviruses to transfer genes into mammalian cells is possible owing to specific characteristics of the retrovirus genome and life cycle. Retroviruses have evolved to deliver their genomes efficiently into the chromosomes of the host cells that they infect. The process of virus insertion into the host DNA is a process directed by sequences in the viral long terminal repeat (LTR) and is an efficient event that preserves the integrity of the viral genome. The integrated provirus becomes a cellular gene such that it is passed on to all progeny cells in the same chromosomal location. Retroviral vector-mediated gene transfer has been currently used in gene therapy protocols for the treatment of inherited and acquired blood diseases and in gene marking and gene therapy protocols for advanced cancer.

Recently we have used a LNL6 vector containing a marker gene for neomycin resistance (Neo^R) [9, 10] and a MFG vector containing the Fanconi anemia complementation group C (FACC) gene [12] for retroviral-mediated gene transfer into HSC and HPC from fresh and cryopreserved CB cells.

Transduction protocols

Many different protocols have been used for viral-mediated gene transfer. For retroviral gene transduction, prestimulation of the cells to place them into a rapidly cycling state is required to increase transduction efficiency. The protocol we have used for gene transduction of bulk cells has been described elsewhere [9, 10]. The majority of CB HSC and HPC are in the Go/G1 phase of the cell cycle and prestimulation with cytokines is required in order to increase DNA synthesis resulting in higher transduction efficiencies [9, 10, 13, 14]. The transduction efficiency of magnetic bead separated $CD34^+$ CB cells incubated without added cytokines was low (10-20%) compared to that of the cells prestimulated with added cytokines (40-44%) [14]. In order to better study gene transfer into certain cell types, a single cell transduction protocol was developed [9]. Single $CD34^{+++}$ CB cells (those expressing the highest density of CD34 antigens) were sorted into single wells containing semi-solid culture medium in the presence of cytokines for 3 days for prestimulation of the single cells and gene transduction was performed by adding viral supernatant once a transduction efficiency of up to 80% was noted [9]. This procedure allowed us to detect an increased transduction efficiency compared to bulk-treated cells, but more importantly it allowed us to demonstrate that single cells of a known phenotype could be transduced with new genetic material. As we learn to better distinguish certain subsets of HSC/HPC it will become possible to selectively transduce these cells. Additionally, this procedure allows us to test the capacity for changing the differentiation pattern of cells by adding genes for certain cytokines and/or their receptors uncomplicated by feeder effects from other cells.

Gene transduction into cryopreserved CB cells

For gene therapy, especially where no donor cells are available for stem/progenitor cell transplantation, gene transfer and therapy using autologous cells for transplantation may in the future be a realistic possiblility. Cord blood banks are being established and if cryopreserved CB cells can be enriched for HSC and HPC, transduced with high efficiency, and expanded *ex vivo* with stable gene expression, this will have important clinical impplications. In this context, we evaluated certain characterizatics of cryopreserved CB cells.

Recovery of viable nucleated cells and HSC and HPC cells

Using a relatively unsophisticated freezing procedure which was not optimized for recovery of HSC and HPC we nevertheless found that both viable cells and hematopoietic progenitors could be recovered from non-adherent low density T-lymphocyte depleted ($NALT^-$) cryopreserved cells [15]. The immature progenitors in CB such as the multipotential colony forming cells (CFU-GEMM) were less sensitive, compared to the more mature CFU-GM, to the damage of the cryopreservation procedure [15]. More recently we found that the percent recovery of $CD34^{+++}$ cells from $NALT^-$ was similar for fresh (0.4 ± 0.07) and cryopreserved (0.4 ± 0.12) cells [12].

Gene transduction

In order to compare the capacity of gene transduction efficiency in cryopreserved cells, $NALT^-$ CB cells were transduced with a Neo^R gene prior to and after cryopreservation and similar transduction efficiencies were obtained [15]. Also, cells transduced prior to cryopreservation could be recovered which expressed the Neo^R gene [15]. Furthermore, $CD34^{+++}$ cells sorted from cryopreserved $NALT^-$ CB cells could also be transduced with new genetic material (FACC gene). Detection and expression of the transduced FACC gene in individual colonies was documented respectively by Polymerase Chain Reaction (PCR) and Reverse-transcriptase (RT)-PCR analysis [12].

Ex vivo **expansion**

Ex vivo expanded HSC and HPC may in the future be used in a clinical setting, although interpretation of such results are at present hindered by the lack of a quantitative assay for the human long-term marrow repopulating HSC. We thus evaluated the ability to *ex vivo* expand certain subsets of HSC and HPC from CB that had been treated to add new genetic material into them. Fresh and cryopreserved thawed sorted CD34^{+++} cells transduced with a FACC gene were placed into suspension culture for 7 days in the presence of cytokines prior to assay for colony formation. The efficiency of transduction and expression of FACC gene in cells from individual colonies derived from expanded cryopreserved cells transduced with this gene was similar to fresh cells by PCR and RT-PCR analysis [12].

In conclusion, cryopreserved CB cells can be enriched for HSC and HPC cells, these cells can also serve as targets for gene transduction, and be expanded *ex vivo* with stability of gene expression. Progress in the use of retroviral vector system to transduce fresh or cryopreserved HSC and HPC cells should lead to future clinical trials in patients with genetic and oncological diseases.

Acknowledgement

The studies reported from our group were supported by US. Public Health Service grants R37 CA36464. RO1 HL46549, RO1 HLS4037, RO1HL49202 and a project in PO1 HL53586 to HEB, and a research grant from the Phi Beta Sorority to LL.

References

1. Miller AD. Human gene therapy comes of age. *Nature* 1992; 357: 455-460.
2. Rosenberg SA. The immunotherapy and gene therapy of cancer. *J Clin Oncol* 1992; 10: 180-199.
3. Broxmeyer HE, Douglas GW, Hangoc G, Cooper S, Bard J, English D, Arny M, Thomas L, Boyse EA. Human umbilical cord blood as a potential source of transplantable hematopoietic stem/progenitor cells. *Proc Natl Acad Sci USA* 1989; 86: 3828-3832.
4. Broxmeyer HE, Hangoc G, Cooper S, Ribeiro RC, Graves V, Yorder M, Wagner J, Vadhan-Raj S, Benninger L, Rubinstein P, Broun ER. Growth characteristics and expansion of human umbilical cord blood and estimation of its potential for transplantation in adults. *Proc Natl Acad Sci USA.* 1992; 89: 4109-4113.
5. Hows JM, Bradley BA, Marsh JCW, Luft T, Coutinho L, Testa NG, Dexter TM. Growth of human umbilical cord blood in long term haematopoietic cultures. *Lancet* 1992; 340: 73-76.
6. Gluckman E, Broxmeyer HE, Auerbach AD, Friedman HS, Douglas GW, Devergie A, Esperou H, Thierry D, Socie G, Lehn P, Copper S, English D, Kurtzberg J, Bard J, Boyse EA. Hematopoietic reconstitution in a patient with Fanconi's anemia by means of umbilical-cord blood from an HLA-identical sibling. *N Engl J Med* 1989; 321: 1174-1178.
7. Lu L, Xiao M, Shen R-N, Grigsby S, Broxmeyer HE. Enrichment, characterization, and responsiveness of single primitive CD34^{+++} human umbilical cord blood hematopoietic progenitors with high proliferative and replating potential. *Blood.* 1993; 81: 41-48.
8. Xiao M, Broxmeyer HE, Horie M, Grigsby S, Lu L. Extensive proliferative capacity of single isolated CD34^{+++} human umbilical cord blood cells in suspension culture. *Blood Cells* 1994; 20: 455-467.
9. Lu L, Xiao M, Clapp DW, Li Z-H, Broxmeyer HE. High efficiency retroviral mediated gene transduction into single isolated immature and replatable CD34^{3+} hematopoietic stem/progenitor cells from human umbilical cord blood. *J Exp Med* 1993; 178: 2089-2096.
10. Lu L, Xiao M, Clapp DW, Li Z-H, Broxmeyer HE. Stable integration of retrovirally transduced genes into human umbilical cord blood high-proliferative potential colony forming cells (HPP-CFC) as assessed after multiple HPP-CFC colony replatings *in vitro*. *Blood Cells* 1994; 20: 525-530.

11. Miller DG, Adam MA, Miller AD. Gene transfer by retroviral vectors occurs only in cells that are actively replicating at the time of infection. *Mol Cell Biol* 1990; 10: 4239-4242.
12. Lu L, Ge Y, Li Z-H, Freie B, Clapp DW, Broxmeyer HE. CD34[+++] stem/progenitor cells purified from cryopreserved cord blood can be transduced with high efficiency by a retroviral vector and expanded *ex vivo* with stable integration and expression of Fanconi anemia complementation C gene. *Blood* 1994; 84: 355a.
13. Moritz T, Keller DC, Williams DA. Human cord blood cells as targets for gene transfer. Potential use in genetic therapies of severe combined immunodeficiency disease. *J Exp Med* 1993; 178: 529-536.
14. Shi Y-J, Shen R-N, Lu L, Broxmeyer HE. Comparative analysis of retroviral-mediated gene transduction into CD34[+] cord blood hematopoietic progenitors in the presence and absence of growth factors. *Blood Cells* 1994; 20: 517-524.
15. Li Z-H, Broxmeyer HE, Lu L. Cryopreserved cord blood myeloid progenitor cells can serve as targets for retroviral-mediated gene transduction and gene-transduced progenitors can be cryopreserved and recovered. *Leukemia* 1995; In press.

Résumé

Dans la perspective d'une utilisation thérapeutique, il semble important de déterminer les conséquences de la congélation sur les propriétés biologiques des cellules de sang de cordon, en particulier leur amplification et l'efficacité des transferts de gènes. Il était important aussi de déterminer si des cellules transduites pouvaient être congelées sans que soit perdue l'efficacité d'expression du transgène. Dans cette revue, nous détaillons notre expérience dans ce domaine. En particulier, nous montrons que des cellules de sang de cordon, après décongélation, peuvent être enrichies par tri au cytofluoromètre, puis infectées par un rétrovirus et ensuite amplifiées *ex vivo* sans perdre l'expression du transgène. A l'inverse, des cellules fraîches infectées par un rétrovirus peuvent être congelées et l'expression du rétrovirus reste détectable après décongélation. Ces observations suggèrent qu'il sera possible à l'avenir d'utiliser dans des protocoles de transplantation des cellules de sang de cordon après y avoir transféré des gènes.

5) Immunological development

5) *Développement immunologique*

Ontogeny of hematopoiesis. Aplastic anemia. Eds E. Gluckman, L. Coulombel.
Colloque INSERM/John Libbey Eurotext Ltd. © 1995, Vol. 235, pp. 123-130.

Conformation and function of MHC class II molecules on foetal B lymphocytes

F. Garban, J.-P. Truman, C. Roucard, C. Choqueux-Séébold, D. Charron and N. Mooney

INSERM U 396, Institut Biomédical des Cordeliers, 75006 Paris, France, tel.: (33 1) 42 49 90 81, fax: (33 1) 42 49 44 49

Abstract

Foetal lymphocytes are protected from antigenic encounters and are relatively anergic when compared with adult B lymphocytes. HLA class II molecules are expressed on foetal B lymphocytes, albeit at a lower level than on adult B cells. We have compared the conformation and function of class II molecules on both adult and foetal B cells. An SDS stability assay revealed that the predominant form of HLA class II molecules expressed on foetal B cells was that of aggregated dimers as opposed to the compact forms expressed on adult B cells.

These data suggested the absence of surface molecules which had been stabilized by peptide binding and the expression of 'empty' molecules which was confirmed by the binding of soluble invariant chain which is specific for empty HLA class II molecules. The generation of second messengers was estimated by the capacity to induce an intracellular calcium flux (Ca^{++}_i). Foetal lymphocytes failed to generate an Ca^{++}_i in response to stimulation via HLA-DR. Two independent outcomes of signalling via HLA-DR were examined, homotypic aggregation and apoptosis. HLA class II on foetal B lymphocytes did not induce either to the same degree as on adult lymphocytes. However, B lymphocytes from both origins were equally capable of stimulating an allogeneic response. The relationship between expression and function of HLA class II on foetal versus adult lymphocytes is discussed.

Human foetal B lymphocytes are essentially protected from foreign antigens by virtue of their privileged environment. While it can be assumed that foetal lymphocytes have been in contact with maternal alloantigens, there is little reason to believe that they have encountered exogenous antigens. Conversely, adult B lymphocytes sequestered in secondary lymphoid organs have already encountered exogenous antigen and have either undergone a primary immune response or have differentiated to become memory cells in anticipation of further stimulation by the same antigen. Adult B lymphocytes are efficient antigen presenting cells [1] and express HLA class II molecules organized as heterodimers composed of a 34kD α and a 28kD β chain. These transmembrane glycoproteins are responsable for the presentation of processed antigen to helper T lymphocytes. HLA class II molecules acquire peptide intracellularly after the dissociation of an associated protein named the invariant chain (Ii) [2], and as a result the majority of class II molecules arrive at the cell surface containing peptide. The binding of peptide increases the stability of the class II molecules in SDS detergent at room temperature and they are therefore referred to as 'compact' forms which migrate on polyacrylamide gels with an apparent molecular weight of 50-60kD. The latter property can be used to determine the presence of class II molecules stabilized by peptide. A more direct approach to the determination of whether or not HLA class II heterodimers contain peptide is the binding of a soluble, recombinant fluoresceinated-Ii that only binds to HLA class II molecules which do not contain peptide [3]. These two techniques provide complementary results for the assessment of whether or not surface HLA class II has peptide bound. Apart from the role of HLA class II molecules in presenting peptides and in stimulating allogeneic immune responses, these molecules (in common with many members of the immunoglobulin superfamily) transmit signals from the exterior to the interior of the cell [4-6]. The stringency of the immune response depends on the genetic diversity of the HLA class II molecules and this diversity is also the principal handicap to successful organ transplantation between different individuals. All of the afore mentioned roles of HLA class II molecules could influence the outcome of cord blood transplantation. Foetal lymphocytes have recently been used in transplantation as they provide a rich source of progenitor cells and appear to provoke less graft versus host (GVH) disease than lymphocytes of adult origin. We have therefore compared certain properties of HLA class II molecules on foetal and on adult lymphocytes. We report that (i.) HLA class II heterodimers on the foetal B cell surface are not in a compact conformation and that they do not contain peptide, (ii.) HLA class II molecules on foetal B lymphocytes do not generate an intracellular calcium flux, (iii.) signalling via HLA class II molecules on foetal B lymphocytes generates little homotypic aggregation but can induce apoptosis. These data lead us to suggest that while foetal B lymphocytes express functional HLA class II molecules with regard to the stimulation of allogeneic responses, neither the conformation, the fixation of peptide, the generation of second messengers nor their functional outcomes are identical to those observed on adult B splenocytes. These data may be relevant to the increased success rate of foetal versus adult mononuclear cell transplantations.

Existence of empty HLA class II on cord blood B lymphocytes

The conformation of radiolabelled immunoprecipitated HLA class II molecules on the B lymphocyte surface was examined by migration in polyacrylamide gels after incubation with SDS at room temperature. The mobility of the molecules is shown before and after boiling which permits dissociation to free α, β and Ii chains. SDS stable or compact dimers are formed after peptide binding and migrate on polyacrylamide gels with an apparent molecular weight of 50-60kD. Aggregated forms of HLA class II dimers migrate with an apparent molecular weight of greater than 110kD and the free α and β chains migrate with apparent molecular weights of 34 and 28 kD respectively. Compact forms, aggregated forms and free chains were readily detected on adult B splenocytes. The predominant form of HLA class II molecules on foetal B lymphocytes was the aggregated form (120kD) *(Figure 1)*. Compact forms were not detected even after lengthy exposure of the gels. These data lead us to suggest that the majority of HLA class II molecules on the surface of foetal B lymphocytes have not been stabilized by peptide binding.

It has already been established that a soluble, recombinant Ii only binds to empty HLA class II molecules [3]. Therefore, to support the SDS stability results, we examined the binding of a fluoresceinated Ii as a probe to detect empty HLA class II molecules on foetal and on adult B lymphocytes. *Figure 2* shows that Ii bound to a substantial proportion of foetal B cells (an average of 50%) while binding to adult B cells was considerably less. These data confirm that a considerable proportion of HLA class II molecules present on foetal B lymphocytes do not contain peptide.

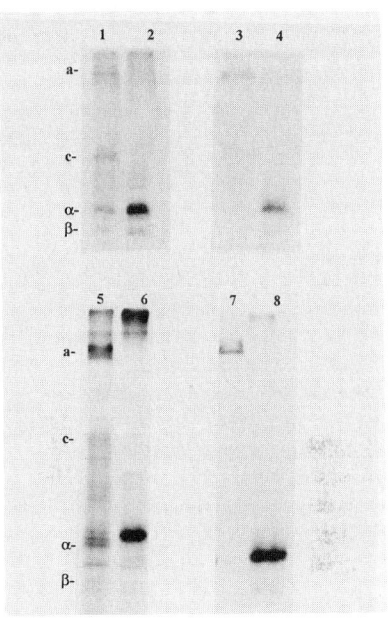

Figure 1. SDS stability of HLA class II molecules. Surface SDS stable DR complexes were detected on CA cells (lanes 1,2), B splenocytes (lanes 5,6), but not on cord blood B cells (lanes 3, 4, 7, 8). Cell surface proteins were labelled with ^{35}S methionine. DR molecules were immunoprecipitated with anti-DR antibody (D1.12). Migration was performed in a 12.5% polyacrylamide gel. For each cell type samples were boiled (lanes 2, 4, 6, 8) and not boiled (lanes 1, 3, 5, 7) in order to detect free α, β chains and stable DR complexes. The positions of aggregated forms (a), compact forms (c), and the α and β chains are shown.

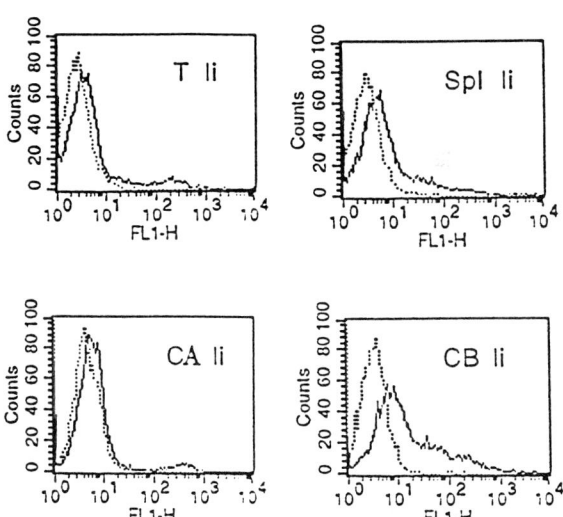

Figure 2. Detection of empty HLA class II molecules on cord blood B cells by fixation of Ii-FITC. Flow cytometry detection of empty HLA class II molecules on EBV transformed B cell line (CA), resting B splenocytes (Spl) and cord blood B cells (CB). Cord blood T cells (T) were used as a negative control. For each sample FITC-conjugated goat anti-mouse F(ab)'$_2$ was used as a negative control (....). Ii-FITC did not to fix CA cells to any greater extent than the class II negative cord blood T cells. There was minimal fixation to the splenocytes, while there was considerable fixation to the cord blood B lymphocytes.

Differences in signalling via HLA-DR on foetal B and adult B lymphocytes

The generation of an $Ca^{++}{}_i$ has been observed after cross-linking of HLA-DR molecules on adult B lymphocytes [4]. The onset of a rapid $Ca^{++}{}_i$ therefore represents one of the earliest second messengers generated by signalling via HLA-DR. An $Ca^{++}{}_i$ was not observed even after lengthy cross-linking of HLA-DR on cord blood B lymphocytes *(Figure 3)*. We also examined the capacity of surface IgM (sIgM) to generate a $Ca^{++}{}_i$ on cord blood B cells. Although the magnitude of the response was inferior to that induced via sIgM on adult B splenocytes, a significant $Ca^{++}{}_i$ was detected.

Furthermore it has been shown that homotypic or heterotypic aggregation can be readily induced after stimulation *via* HLA-DR molecules of adult splenocytes [7]. A pathway involving protein kinase C (PKC) and tyrosine protein kinases (TPK) mediates HLA class II stimulated aggregation [8]. While maximal aggregation of adult B lymphocytes was induced within one hour, we have only observed aggregation after a lengthy stimulation (>24 hours) with anti-HLA class II mAbs (data not shown). These data lead us to suggest that surface HLA-DR molecules do not generate the same second messengers on foetal versus adult B lymphocytes.

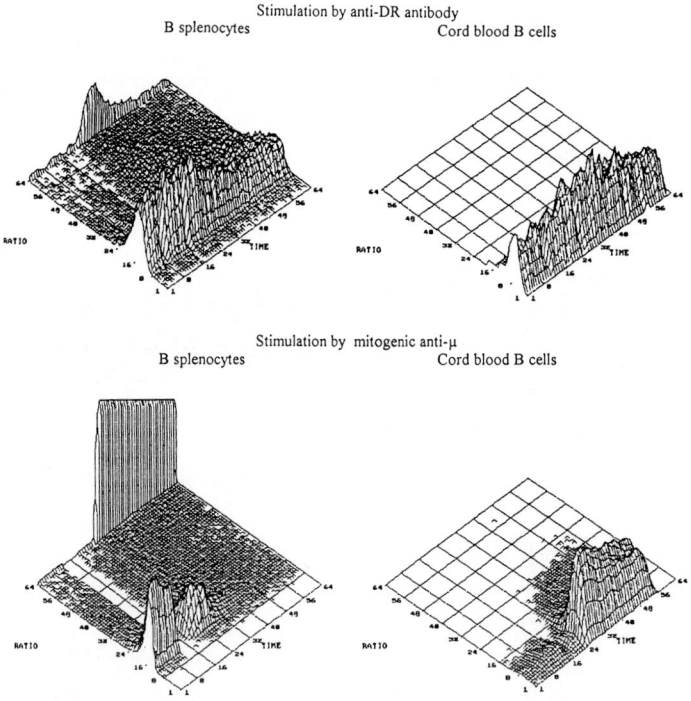

Figure 3. Variation of intracellular calcium flux on B splenocytes and cord blood B cells. The cells were first loaded with Indo-1, before reading using a flow cytometer, the diagrams represent the ratio of indo-1 complexed to calcium/ free indo-1 as a function of time. Cross-linked anti-DR antibody (D1.12) can induce a calcium flux on resting B splenocytes but not on cord blood B cells, while signalling via surface immunoglobulins (using mitogenic anti-µ mAbs) is efficient in calcium mobilization in B splenocytes as in cord blood B cells (albeit with a lower level).

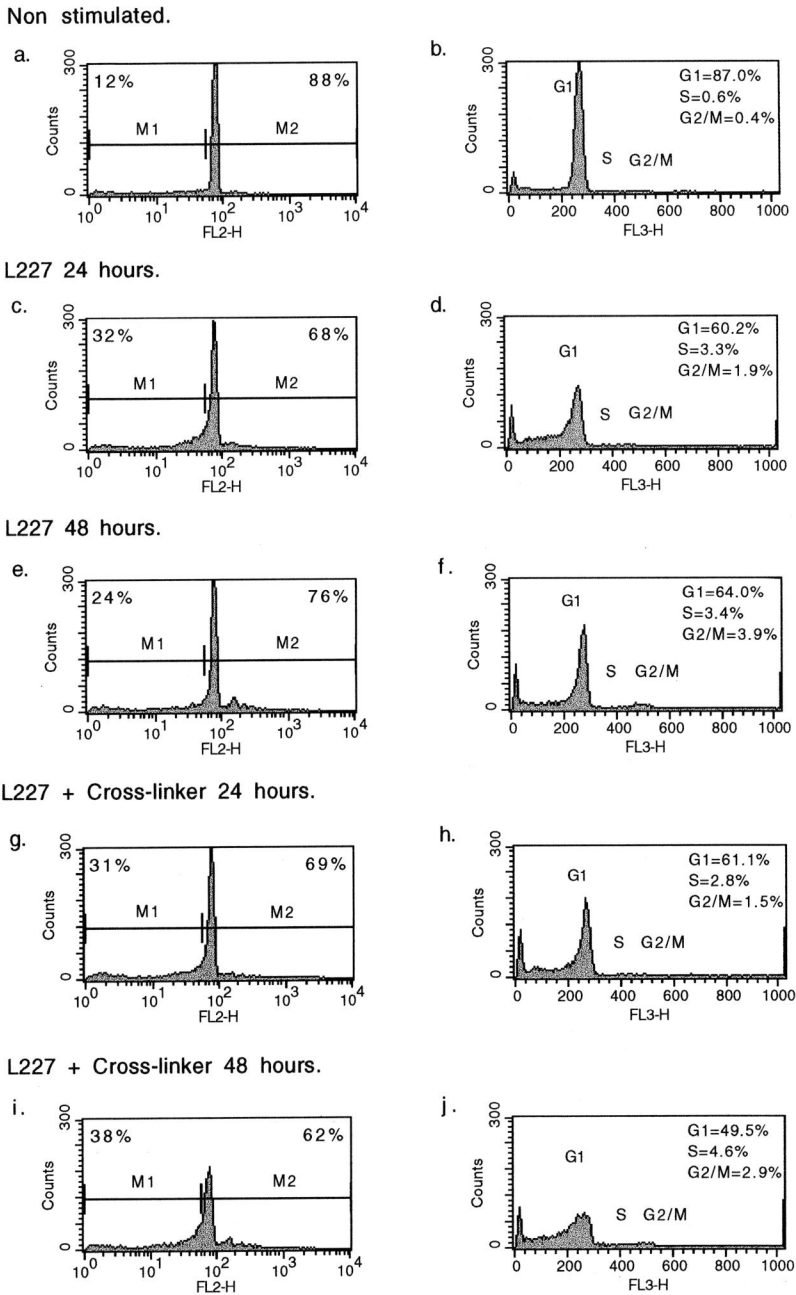

Figure 4. Anti-HLA class II antibody L227 induces apoptosis and activation in cord blood B cells. Cord blood B cells were incubated with 4 µg/ml of L227 with or without additional cross-linking with 20µg/ml of goat anti-mouse F(ab')$_2$ mAb for 24 or 48 hours (denoted as cross-linker on the figure). Afterwards, the cells were incubated overnight with a hypotonic solution containing 0.1% sodium acetate, 0.1% triton-X100, and 10 µg/ml of propidium iodide, before reading using a Becton-Dickinson FACScan with the FL2 laser for the quantification of apoptotic cells (a. c. e. g. i.), and the FL3 laser for the cell cycle data (b. d. f. h. j.), and then analysed using CellQuest V1.0 software. The M1 region contains the apoptotic nuclei, while the M2 region contains normal nuclei. The corresponding percentages are shown in their region.

Induction of apoptosis via HLA-DR on foetal versus adult B cells

We and others have previously shown that stimulation of B lymphocytes via HLA class II leads to apoptotic death demonstrated by oligonucleosomal DNA fragmentation [9] and electron microscopy [10]. Apoptotic cell death via HLA-DR was restricted to activated cells and was therefore proposed as a means of peripheral destruction of lymphocytes which have already played their role in the immune response. We have examined the capacity of HLA-DR to induce apoptosis on cord blood B cells. Stimulation via HLA-DR induced apoptosis in cord blood B cells. Furthermore, cell cycle analysis of HLA class II stimulated cord blood B cells showed that after 24 hours of stimulation, a small percentage of cells enter the cell cycle, and begin to proliferate.

Discussion

These results lead us to suggest that both the different conformation and functional properties of HLA class II molecules on foetal versus adult lymphocytes may be used as a means to distinguish these groups at a given stage in ontogeny. Low expression of MHC class II molecules has been previously reported as a major feature in B cell ontogeny in the mouse [11]. The presence of empty HLA class II molecules on antigen presenting cells is probably a consequence of the particularly privileged environment of foetal blood where little exogenous peptide is present. These molecules do however, function in stimulating an allogeneic response (data not shown) although their signal transducing capacity is limited. We cannot exclude the possibility that the low level of signalling is due to a quantitative rather than a qualitative effect. In either case, decreased signal transduction in a cognate T-B lymphocyte interaction is probably advantageous for foetal survival if only by inhibiting lymphokine production which could otherwise lead to undesirable local responses.

Since HLA class II molecules preferentially mediate death in activated human B lymphocytes, it is at first glance surprising that apoptosis is induced in foetal lymphocytes. However, these results suggest that a moderate signal first induces apoptosis in a sub-population of B cells, before activating the remaining cells. A stronger signal, in this case anti-HLA class II mAb with additional cross-linking with a goat anti-mouse F(ab')$_2$, progressively induces more apoptosis. This could be a way of destroying B cells that are aberrantly presenting antigens. It is also worth noting that a sub-population of foetal B cells express CD23, which is considered as a B lymphocyte activation marker. These cells may present an activated phenotype for HLA class II mediated cell death. Furthermore, foetal B lymphocytes express little of the Fas molecule [12] which mediates cell death in many lymphoid systems [13, 14], suggesting that these cells do not die by apoptosis as a physiological consequence. We do not yet know if Fas and the cell death induced by HLA class II signalling are related. In summary these data are important both with regard to antigen presentation and with regard to signal transduction, the study of the immunobiology of foetal HLA class II molecules may permit a more reliable prediction of the successful outcome of cord blood transplantation.

Acknowledgements

This work was supported by la Ligue contre le cancer (comité de Paris) and la Ligue National contre le cancer. J-P T. Is supported by the ARC.

References

1. Lanzavecchia A. Antigen-specific interaction between T and B cells. *Nature* 1985; 314: 537-40.
2. Roche P and Cresswell P. Invariant chain association with HLA DR molecules inhibits immunogenic peptide binding. *Nature* 1990; 345: 615-18.
3. Ericson M, Sundstrom M, Sansom D and Charron D. Mutually exclusive binding of peptide and invariant chain to major histocompatibility class II antigens. *J Biol Chem* 1994; 269: 26531-38.
4. Mooney N, Grillot-Courvalin C, Hivroz C and Charron D. A role for MHC class II antigens in B cell activation. *J Autoimmunity* 1989; 2: 215-23.
5. Mooney N, Grillot-Courvalin C, Hivroz C, Ju L and Charron D. Early biochemical events after MHC class II mediated signaling on human B lymphocytes. *J Immunol* 1990; 145: 2070-76.
6. Brick-Ghannam C, Mooney N and Charron D. Signal transduction in B lymphocytes. *Hu Immunol* 1989; 30: 202-7.
7. Mourad W, Geha R, Chatila T. Engagement of major histocompatibility complex class II molecules induces sustained, lymphocyte function-associated molecules 1-dependent cell adhesion. *J Exp Med* 1990; 172: 1513-17.
8. Ramirez R, Carracedo J, Mooney N and Charron D. HLA class II mediated homotypic aggregation: involvement of a protein tyrosine kinase and protein kinase C. *Hu Immunol* 1992; 34: 115-25.
9. Shafer P and Pierce S. Evidence for dimers of MHC molecules in B lymphocytes and their role in low affinity T cell responses. *Immunity* 1994; 1: 699-707.
10. Aramilli S, Cardoso C, Mukku P, Baichwal V and Nag B. Refolding and reconstitution of functionally active complexes of human leukocyte antigen DR2 and myelin basic protein peptide from recombinant a and b polypeptide chains. *J Biol Chem* 1995; 270: 971-77.
11. Newell K, Vanderwall J, Beard S and Freed J. Ligation of major histocompatibility complex class II molecules mediates apoptotic cell death in resting B lymphocytes. *Proc Natl Acad Sci USA* 1993; 90: 10459-63.
12. Truman J-P, Ericson M, Choqueux-Séébold C, Charron D and Mooney N. Lymphocyte programmed cell death is mediated via HLA class II DR. *Int Immunol* 1994; 6: 887-96.
13. Yonehara S, Ishii A and Yonehara M. A cell killing monoclonal antibody (anti-Fas) to a cell surface antigen co-downregulated with the receptor of tumor necrosis factor. *J Exp Med* 1989; 169: 1747-56.
14. Trauth B, Klas C, Peters A, Matzku S, Möller, Falk W, Debatin K and Kranmer P. Monoclonal antibody-mediated tumor regression by induction of apoptosis. *Science* 1989; 246: 301-4.

Résumé

Une des caractéristiques des lymphocytes fœtaux est qu'ils sont protégés de tout contact avec des antigènes extérieurs. Les molécules HLA de classe II sont exprimées à la surface des lymphocytes B fœtaux mais en moins grand nombre que sur les lymphocytes adultes. Dans ce travail, nous avons comparé la conformation moléculaire et la fonction des molécules HLA de classe II exprimées sur les lymphocytes B adultes et fœtaux. Alors que la majorité des molécules de classe II des lymphocytes B adultes est sous forme de dimères compacts, les hétérodimères agrégés de PM 120 kDa sont prédominants à la surface des lymphocytes fœtaux, suggérant qu'il n'y a pas eu stabilisation par la liaison avec le peptide. Cette hypothèse de molécules HLA « vides » a effectivement été confirmée par l'observation d'une liaison de la chaîne invariante soluble à 50% des lymphocytes B fœtaux. De plus, il n'y a pas d'induction de flux calcique dans les lymphocytes fœtaux après stimulation des lymphocytes B *via* les molécules HLA de classe II. De même, la réponse de type apoptose ou agrégation observée après stimulation *via* le HLADr est beaucoup plus faible lorsque des lymphocytes B fœtaux sont utilisés. En revanche, les lymphocytes B fœtaux sont capables d'induire une réponse allogénique aussi bien que des lymphocytes adultes. L'importance de ces observations en immunobiologie dans le cadre d'une utilisation en transplantation de cellules fœtales est discutée.

Classical and non classical HLA class I genes in the human trophoblast cells: expression, regulation and possible function(s)

Philippe Le Bouteiller and Anne-Marie Rodriguez

INSERM U 395, CHU Purpan, BP 3028, 31024 Toulouse Cedex, France, tel.: (33) 61 49 36 33, fax: (33) 61 49 97 52

Summary

Maternal acceptance of the fetal allograft is the oldest and still unsolved transplantation enigma. General absence of detectable expression of classical, polymorphic HLA-A,-B,-C and presence, at some stages, of much less polymorphic nonclassical HLA-G class I molecules at the cell surface of trophoblast cells, that constitute the materno-fetal interface during pregnancy, may be of importance. We will first present an overview of the more recent data, including ours, dealing with the constitutive, transcriptional and protein expression of each classical and non-classical MHC class I locus in the different villous and extravillous trophoblast cell subpopulations throughout the human pregnancy. Molecular regulatory mechanisms that may operate at the levels of transcription (5' CpG DNA methylation, transcription factors that bind to HLA class I cis-regulatory promoter elements, chromatin structure), translation and transport of proteins to the cell surface (availability of a pool of specific peptides and of functional β2-microglobulin, TAP1/TAP2 peptide transporters, LMP2/LMP7 proteasome subunits and calnexin molecular chaperone) will then be discussed. Functional significance of the absence of cell surface expression of classical HLA class I molecules in all trophoblast cell subpopulations, and the presence of membrane-bound HLA-G in the extravillous invasive cytotrophoblast cells will finally be questioned.

The human placental trophoblast is derived from the trophectoderm layer of the blastocyst [1] and thus possesses a fetal genome able to express both maternal and paternal antigens. Several subpopulations of trophoblast cells can be identified by their location within the placenta, morphology, state of differentiation, phenotypic markers and various endocrine properties [1, 2]. The cytotrophoblast cells are the progenitors for all subsequent trophoblast cell subpopulations. They give rise either to invasive extravillous cytotrophoblast or non invasive villous cytotrophoblast. Extravillous cytotrophoblast cells migrate from placental anchoring villi and invade the maternal decidua. They are highly proliferative during the first stages of pregnancy and then form the chorion membrane at the end of gestation. The non invasive villous cytotrophoblast constitutes the first layer of placental villi, in contact with fetal mesenchyme. The outer syncytiotrophoblast cell layer, in contact with maternal blood, is formed via fusion and differentiation of cytotrophoblast cells located beneath. Thus, both extravillous cytotrophoblast and villous syncytiotrophoblast, in contact with maternal tissues, are directly exposed to potential, cellular and humoral, maternal anti-fetal immune effectors. In normal pregnancies, these trophoblast cells must have develop defenses against these potentially harmful maternal immune agents [2]. Among the various possible mechanisms that may be involved, the lack of expression of classical, polymorphic HLA class I heavy chains and, in contrast, the presence of nonclassical, less polymorphic, HLA-G, at the cell surface of trophoblast cells, are of considerable interest [3].

The Major Histocompatibility Complex (MHC), located on the short arm of chromosome 6 in human, is compound of a set of genes that encode glycoproteins crucial for the elimination by the immune system of autologous virally infected cells, cells that have undergone oncogenic transformation or allogenic grafted cells [4]. The classical HLA-A,-B,-C class I loci encode extremely polymorphic proteins that are expressed at the cell surface of most (but not all) somatic tissues [5]. They bind intracellularly derived peptides and present them to cytotoxic T cells. In contrast to the classical HLA class I loci, the human nonclassical HLA-E,-F,-G class I loci exhibit a more limited polymorphism and their function, if any, is still unclear [5]. Although each of these nonclassical human MHC class I loci can be transcribed in a number of tissues [5], HLA-G is, to our knowledge, the only one that has been reproducibly found to be expressed as a cell surface translated product *in vivo*: HLA-G is present at the cell surface of extravillous invasive cytotrophoblast, especially at the beginning of pregnancy [2, 3, 5, 6], suggesting that it may have a specialized function.

In this chapter, after a description of the "trophoblast-specific" patterns of expression of HLA class I genes in the different human trophoblast cell subpopulations throughout pregnancy, we will examine the possible transcriptional and post-translational regulatory events that may be used by the different trophoblast cell subpopulations both to prevent expression of classical MHC class I genes and, in contrast, to favor cell surface expression of the nonclassical HLA-G class I product.

Constitutive expression of HLA class I genes in the human trophoblast cell subpopulations

We will examine both transcriptional and protein expression of the different classical and non classical HLA class I loci in the various trophoblast cell subpopulations that constitute the materno-fetal interface.

Classical HLA-A,-B,-C class I genes

It is generally admitted that none of the different human trophoblast cell subpopulations expresses detectable membrane-bound classical HLA class I molecules at either stage of pregnancy [2, 5, 6]. However, despite this lack of cell surface expression, both transcripts and translated, intracellular protein products were nevertheless detected in most trophoblast tissues. After immunoprecipitation with the anti-HLA class I W6/32 mAb, that recognizes monomorphic determinants on the a3 domain of class I heavy chains associated with β2-microglobulin (β2m), King et al [7], using S^{35} methionine metabolic labeling, identified an intracellular 45kDa heavy chain in extravillous cytotrophoblast purified from first trimester human placenta as well as in the trophoblast-derived choriocarcinoma cell line JEG-3. Using similar method and the same mAb, we recently observed the presence of a band of similar molecular weight in the cytoplasm of both villous cytotrophoblast, purified from term placenta, and, although at lower levels, of the *in vitro* differentiated syncytiotrophoblast (Rodriguez and Le Bouteiller, unpublished data). These observations confirmed the previous data obtained by immunocytochemistry on the same trophoblast cell subpopulations [8]. Although at low levels, the transcription of both HLA-A and -B class I genes was indeed demonstrated by Northern blot in these two layers of placental villi [9]. These data suggest that post-translational regulatory events are likely to prevent cell surface expression of these intracellular polymorphic MHC class I heavy chains. Although no data yet supports this hypothesis, we cannot exclude the existence of classical HLA class I soluble forms in these trophoblast cells.

Non classical HLA-E,-F,-G class I genes

We have shown that HLA-E, an ubiquitously transcribed MHC class I locus [5], also present in macaque genome [10], was the only MHC class I gene that remained transcriptionally active in the trophoblast-derived human cell line JAR [11]. Transcription of this nonclassical locus has been constantly observed in the human placenta [5, 6, 9, 12]. In our group, we have described the presence of two HLA-E messages in villous cytotrophoblast and in the *in vitro* differentiated syncytiotrophoblast isolated from term placenta [9]. However, despite such transcription, detection of intracellular and cell surface expression of HLA-E in these trophoblast cell subpopulations has never been shown. Although definitive proof of this absence will be obtained only after the use of HLA-E locus-specific mAb, these data strongly suggest that post-transcriptional regulatory mechanisms prevent its protein expression.

Very little is known about HLA-F expression in human trophoblast. Transcription of this nonclassical MHC class I locus in human placenta was demonstrated by RNase protection assay [12]. However, this study did not localize these messages in a particular trophoblast cell subpopulation.

It is now well established that the nonclassical HLA-G locus is clearly transcribed in human cytotrophoblast and, depending on the villous or extravillous subpopulation and time of gestation, sometimes translated and even expressed as a membran-bound protein [3, 5, 6, 9, 12, 13]. Five major alternatively spliced transcriptional isoforms of HLA-G have been described by Geraghty and collaborators [13, 14]. HLA-G1,-G2 and -G3 isoforms encode membrane-bound proteins containing three ($\alpha 1$, $\alpha 2$, $\alpha 3$), two ($\alpha 1$, $\alpha 3$) or one ($\alpha 1$) external domains, respectively. These three HLA-G mRNA were detected in the JEG-3 cell line, .221 HLA null lymphoblastoid cell line transfected with HLA-G, term placental tissue and extravillous membranes [14]. Using RT-PCR analysis, we confirmed their presence in the JEG-3 cell line and we also showed them in villous cytotrophoblast isolated from term placenta and, to a much lesser extent, in the *in vitro* differentiated syncytiotrophoblast [9]. However, no HLA-G mRNA was detected by Northern blot analysis in this latter trophoblast layer [9]. Intracellular protein products corresponding to these three transcriptional isoforms were detected by immunoprecipitation of .221-G transfectants, using an anti-HLA-G specific mAb [13]. Only HLA-G1 protein was immunoprecipitated with W6/32 in these human transfectants and JEG-3 [13], as well as in murine HLA-G transfectants and villous cytotrophoblast purified from term placenta (Rodriguez and Le Bouteiller, unpublished data). Extravillous cytotrophoblast was shown to express membrane-bound HLA-G proteins, especially in the early stages of gestation, whereas in villous cytotrophoblast HLA-G translated products do not reach the cell surface [5, 6, 9]. The HLA-G1 soluble form is encoded by a full length mRNA retaining intron 4, yielding a protein that lacks transmembrane and cytoplasmic domains, whereas the HLA-G2 soluble form is encoded by an HLA-G2 message retaining intron 4, yielding a protein that lacks external $\alpha 2$, as well as transmembrane and cytoplasmic domains [14]. Using transfectants containing HLA-G constructs that include the leader sequence through intron 4 and excluding or not the exons 5 through 8, it was shown that these intron containing messages encoded soluble HLA-G proteins but not membrane-bound forms [14]. Using 5' leader and 3' intron 4 primers in a PCR analysis of JEG-3, .221-G transfectants and extravillous membranes from term placenta RNA, identical messages with the coding capacity for HLA-G1 and -G2 soluble forms were detected in transfectants and tissues naturally expressing HLA-G [14]. A sixth HLA-G isoform lacking exon 4 was also detected in human first trimester placenta [15]. Although the different HLA-G transcriptional isoforms were also found in several other human tissues, including testis, keratinocytes [5], peripheral blood lymphocytes and mature lymphoid cells [15], extravillous cytotrophoblast cells in first and second trimesters of gestation appear to be, until now, the unique cell type *in vivo* that is able to express HLA-G membrane-bound proteins [5, 6]. Thus, differentiation of villous cytotrophoblast into actively proliferating, invasive extravillous cytotrophoblast is accompanied by a transport of HLA-G heavy chains to the cell surface. This strongly suggests the involvement of a highly cell-type specific post-translational regulation and a possible, specialized function in the materno-trophoblast immune relationship.

Both transcriptional and post-transcriptional regulatory mechanisms are likely to control the specific expression of each HLA class I locus in the different trophoblast cell subpopulations, depending on the stages of gestation. This is particularly obvious for the HLA-G locus, repressed in the syncytiotrophoblast, transcribed and translated in both subpopulations of villous and extravillous cytotrophoblast but expressed as a membrane-bound protein only in the extravillous cytotrophoblast. Expression of HLA-G is highest in the first trimester of pregnancy and then declines as pregnancy progresses. Generation of soluble forms of HLA-G is under the control of post-transcriptional mechanisms. As far as the classical HLA class I genes are concerned, although at low levels, it looks as if they were transcribed and translated in most trophoblast populations but the intracellular protein products are prevented from reaching the cell surface.

Transcriptional regulation

The absence of significant transcription of HLA-G in the syncytiotrophoblast and the relatively low levels of transcription of classical HLA class I genes in most trophoblast cells are in favor of some repressor molecular mechanisms of transcription in these tissues. These down-regulations can be accomplished in several ways including both *cis*- and *trans*-acting regulatory mechanisms.

Cis-acting regulatory mechanisms

Transcriptional regulation of HLA class I genes operates through an array of nuclear DNA-binding proteins that specifically bind to *cis*-regulatory elements located in the 5' untranslated promoter region [5]. Some of these elements (CCAAT and TCTAAT) are well conserved in most human class I loci, including the nonclassical. Other promoter elements (enhancer A containing a palindromic KB site, enhancer B, Interferon Consensus Sequence), present in the classical HLA-A and -B loci, are absent or deleted in the nonclassical loci, HLA-G in particular [5]. This strongly suggests that the combination of *trans*-acting factors that stimulate transcription differs between classical and nonclassical HLA class I genes and that the HLA-G specific combination of factors is likely to be present in the nuclei of cytotrophoblast cells. The use of HLA class I transgenic mice confirmed that the 5' upstream regions of these genes are largely responsible for their specific patterns of expression *in vivo*. HLA-B27 transgenic mice did not express this classical class I locus in the trophoblast cells of transgenic placenta [16]. Transgenic mice containing either a 5.7- or 6.0-kb HLA-G transgene expressed this nonclassical class I locus in both trophoblast and mesenchyme cells of the transgenic placenta [17, 18]. However, the 6.0-kb HLA-G transgene directed HLA-G expression in extraembryonic tissues far more efficiently than did the 5.7-kb transgene, suggesting that the 250-bp fragment present at the 5' end of the longer transgene should contain an important positive regulatory element [17]. The authors of this finding hypothesized that this upstream 250-bp fragment contained an important positive regulatory element that might function as a "Locus Control Region" [17]. Such *cis*-acting elements, localized outside the promoter regions, many kb upstream of linked genes, confer a high level of expression of these genes, independent of chromosomal position within the genome [19].

DNA methylation at the 5' position of the dinucleotides CpG may play a role in the repression of gene expression. CpG islands are CpG rich DNA sequences located in the 5' part of many genes, including murine and human MHC class I genes [5, 11, 20]. These regions exhibit a high frequency of methylation-sensitive restriction endonuclease sites [20]. Many studies have established an inverse relationship between the level of methylation of these "CpG islands" and the transcriptional activity of the associated coding sequences [5, 9, 11]. Alterations in DNA methylation may frequently occur in germinal cells, embryonic and extraembryonic cells, as compared with adult tissues [21]. In our group, we have demonstrated that in the HLA null, trophoblast-derived cell line JAR, the repressor mechanism that prevents significant transcriptional expression of all HLA class I genes, except HLA-E, was methylation of these CpG islands [9, 11]. This was shown first by the use of 5-azacytidine demethylating agent. After a short incubation with this drug and cell cloning, many JAR clones recovered an HLA class I expression, both at the RNA and protein levels. This was further demonstrated by double digestion of JAR genomic DNA, first with *Hind* III, and then with different methylation sensitive restriction enzymes. These studies clearly established that each HLA class I locus is heavily methylated in this cell line. The only class I locus that always appeared unmethylated and remained transcriptionally active was HLA-E [11]. Such an inverse relationship was also established in the JEG-3 cell line: HLA-A is methylated and repressed, HLA-B and -G are partially methylated but transcribed, HLA-E is unmethylated and transcriptionally active [9]. Thus, methylation of DNA is a repressor mechanism that may prevent or diminish the transcription of some HLA class I genes in trophoblast-derived cell lines. Whether this is due to the trophoblast origin of these cells, their tumoral state, or to the very long periods of culture they have been submitted to is unknown. However, the same kinds of studies performed on trophoblast cells isolated from human term placenta did not confirm that such *cis*-regulatory repressor mechanism occurs *in vivo*. Apart from HLA-E which is always unmethylated and transcribed in both villous cytotrophoblast and syncytiotrophoblast, no such relationship existed for the other class I loci [9]. Whereas HLA-A, -B and -G are undermethylated in both trophoblast layers isolated from term placenta, they are transcribed in cytotrophoblast and, although minimally, in syncytiotrophoblast [9]. Thus, the down-regulation of classical HLA class I genes and the almost total repression of HLA-G transcription in the *in vitro* differentiated syncytiotrophoblast are unlikely to be caused by DNA methylation. However, it cannot be excluded that such *cis*-acting regulatory mechanism affect the classical HLA class I gene transcription during the first steps of gestation. Possible genomic imprinting should in particular be evaluated. This transcriptional repressor mechanism that distinguishes the parental origin of genes occurs in a wide range of species including humans [22]. In the rat, the polymorphic MHC class I RT1.A and the monomorphic Pa loci are imprinted such that only the paternal antigens are expressed in the placenta, whereas the monomorphic RT1.E locus escapes this imprinting [22]. The mechanism of genomic imprinting is not known but DNA methylation could be the repressor mechanism of the imprinted loci [20]. It looks as if the genomic imprinting affecting expression of MHC class I alleles was species specific since it does not occur in murine [23] nor in equine trophoblast [24]. Whether such genomic imprinting may affect expression of classical HLA class I alleles of maternal origin in human cytotrophoblast during early gestation remains to be proven.

Trans-acting regulatory mechanisms

Transcription factors are nuclear DNA binding proteins that promote RNA transcription. They bind to *cis*-regulatory elements present in the 5' upstream region of genes (see above). Absence or very low transcription of HLA-G in the syncytiotrophoblast and relatively low expression of classical class I transcripts in cytotrophoblast may be due to lack or modifications of *trans*-acting factors that normally bind to MHC class I promoters [5]. Very little is known about the expression of such transcription factors in the different human trophoblast cell subpopulations. The ability of the class I negative trophoblast-derived human cell line JAR to express exogenous transfected HLA-A, -B [25] and -G (Le Bouteiller, unpublished data) heavy chains at their cell surface, in association with endogenous translated β2m, suggested that its nuclei contained the constitutive *trans*-acting factors necessary for the transcription of classical and nonclassical HLA class I genes to occur. Using nuclear extracts of extravillous cytotrophoblast cells isolated from first trimester human placenta, we demonstrated the presence of *trans*-acting factors that specifically bound to the palindromic KB site of enhancer A regulatory element, present in the promoter of classical HLA-A and -B class I genes [26]. The same factors were also detected in embryonic fibroblast and maternal decidual cells. In contrast, such factors were undetectable in nuclear extracts of syncytiotrophoblast isolated from the same placentas. A negative regulatory element (NRE), located 180-bp 5' to the transcription start site, has been identified in a murine MHC class I negative embryonal carcinoma cell line [27]. Sequence analysis revealed that an identical regulatory sequence is present in the human HLA-A2 gene. A recent study, using band shift assay, demonstrated that nuclear factors from JEG-3, BeWo and F9 cell lines specifically bound to this element, whereas such factors were absent in nuclear extracts from lymphocytes and other HLA class I positive cells [27]. The authors suggested that such factors may down-regulate expression of classical HLA class I genes in human trophoblast. HLA-G does not have this NRE, thus enabling its expression in these cells [27]. However, this might not be as clear, since it has been shown that JEG-3 could express a certain amount of classical HLA-B/C molecules at their cell surface [9]. The patterns of transcription of HLA-G transgene in HLA-G transgenic mice are similar to those in human [17, 18]. This implies that *trans*-acting factors that are able to bind to HLA-G *cis*-regulatory elements are also present in mice.

Despite absence of data, chromatin structure is likely to be an essential part of the transcriptional regulatory mechanisms that control expression of MHC class I genes in human trophoblast cells. One way of investigating chromatin structure is to look at DNase I hypersensitive sites within a genomic region. Such sites are the reflect of an open chromatin structure, enhancing access of *trans*-acting factors to *cis*-regulatory elements [5]. The presence of such DNase I hypersensitive sites has been demonstrated in the vicinity of enhancer A regulatory element of murine H2 genes [28].

Alternative splicings generate several alternative forms of HLA-G proteins and use of intron-retaining mRNA encodes two different soluble HLA-G proteins in human placenta and JEG-3 [14]. We hypothesize that soluble forms may also exist for the classical HLA class I transcripts in human trophoblast cells. We are currently exploring this possibility.

Post-translational regulation

Despite the presence of classical HLA class I trancripts and of intracellular translated products in villous cytotrophoblast from term placenta, no membrane-bound protein is detectable. Similarly, despite transcription and translation, HLA-G is absent at the cell surface of these trophoblast cell subpopulations, whereas this nonclassical class I molecule reaches the cell surface of extravillous cytotrophoblast, especially at the early gestation [5]. These observations suggest that post-translational regulatory mechanims are likely to operate in these trophoblast cells at the level of peptide-dependent MHC class I assembly.

Such post-translational regulation may operate through the availability of a pool of specific peptides and/or through the negative regulation of expression of a number of genes required for the MHC class I expression. Among them are the β2m, the LMP2/LMP7 proteasome subunits and TAP1/TAP2 peptide transporters that map to the class II chromosomal region in the rat, mouse and human [4], and calnexin [29].

In normal, non pathological conditions of pregnancy and in the absence of exogenous stimuli, availability of a sufficient pool of peptides able to bind to empty classical class I heavy chains in trophoblast cells is questioned. The same question can be asked regarding HLA-G: are HLA-G heavy chains able to present peptides and, if so, are these peptides present in extravillous invasive cytotrophoblast and absent in villous cytotrophoblast?

Efficient peptide binding, stabilization of the peptide/heavy chain complex, intracellular transport and cell surface expression of MHC class I molecules first depend on association with the β2m light chain [30]. In the murine placenta, the giant trophoblast cells contain MHC class I messages but not membrane-bound products in day 9.5 placentas [31]. These trophoblast cells do not express detectable levels of β2m transcripts, indicating that the noncoordinate expression of class I heavy and light chain messages might be one mechanism of control for MHC class I expression in trophoblast. β2m transcripts and moderate amounts of protein products have been detected in trophoblast-derived human choriocarcinoma cell lines [32]. We have shown that in JAR cells transfected with HLA-A, -B or -G genes, heterodimers consisting of exogenous transfected class I heavy chains linked to endogenous β2m were present at the cell surface [25]. These data demonstrated that assembly of newly synthesized MHC class I heavy chains and β2m occurred normally in this trophoblast-derived cell line, suggesting that no mutation prevented the translation of the light chain. In villous cytotrophoblast and in the *in vitro* differentiated syncytiotrophoblast from term placenta we have detected messages, but no cell surface expression, of β2m (unpublished data). Whether normal β2m translated products are present in the cytosol of these trophoblast layers remains to be determined.

Availability of other functional components of the MHC class I peptide loading machinery should also be important. Lack of expression of any of them could result in the absence of cell surface expression of MHC class I molecules in trophoblast. LMP2 and LMP7 subunits of the large proteolytic complexes, known as proteasomes, are implicated in the antigen degradation in the cytosol [4]. Peptides generated in the cytosol are transported across the endoplasmic reticulum (ER) membrane by the TAP1/TAP2 heterodimer peptide transporters [33]. They contribute to the efficient transfer of peptides to the β2m-heavy chain complex. The stable trimolecular complex can then move through the Golgi stacks and finally reach the cell surface. Cells that have defects in class I molecule assembly may have mutations in either proteasome and/or peptide transporters. The best known examples are the human B lymphoblastoid .174/T2 and mouse lymphoma mutant RMA-S cell lines that present deletions in the class II region encompassing either TAP1 alone or TAP1 and TAP2, respectively [33]. These defects result in reduced cell surface expression of MHC class I molecules [33]. In the T2 cells, most of the HLA-B5 endogenous heavy chains remain in the ER or *cis*-Golgi apparatus [33]. Mouse embryonic cells exhibiting a defect in MHC class I assembly lack TAP expression [34]. Treatment of these cells by interferon (IFN) induced appearance of peptide transporters and then cell surface expression of MHC class I molecules [34]. A recent study showed that TAP1, TAP2 and LMP7 transcripts were present in first trimester and term placentas, as well as in JEG-3 and JAR cell lines [35]. TAP1 and TAP2 messages were consistently more abundant in early than in late gestation placentas, whereas the reverse was observed for LMP7 mRNA. Although this study was performed on unpurified trophoblast cell subpopulations and did not analyze the protein products of peptide transporters and proteasome components, gestation-related differences in concentrations of specific transcripts would suggest that HLA class II associated genes may exert some control over expression of HLA class I genes in human trophoblast cells [35].

It was recently shown that the calnexin molecular chaperone, present in the ER, could associate with free empty class I heavy chains soon after their synthesis [36]. Subsequenty, an association of β2m occurs to form a transient trimolecular complex. Calnexin then dissociates from β2m/heavy chain complex. Thus, for class I molecules to bind peptides, complete their assembly and move through the *trans*-Golgi network, dissociation of class I heavy chains/β2m complex from calnexin must occur [36]. Whether such chaperone molecule plays a role in the inefficient expression of classical MHC class I molecules in human trophoblast cells is also questioned.

Thus, repression of cell surface expression of classical HLA class I genes in all human trophoblast cells and of nonclassical HLA-G in some trophoblast subpopulations can be accomplished in several ways that include transcriptional regulatory mechanisms such as DNA methylation, modifications of chromatin structure, interaction of transcription factors with promoter *cis*-regulatory elements and a variety of post-translational mechanisms.

Possible functions

Extravillous cytotrophoblast cells and syncytiotrophoblast are the two human fetal-derived, trophoblast cell subpopulations that are in direct contact with maternal tissues, decidual cells and maternal blood, respectively. Despite these locations that make them potential targets of maternal immune attack, they escape such destruction. Absence of cell surface expression of classical HLA class I molecules on both subpopulations and presence of membrane-bound HLA-G on extravillous cytotrophoblast cells are likely to be, at least a part, of the protector mechanisms developed by these extraembryonic differentiated cells. But this should not increase vulnerability to infections.

The failure of human trophoblast cells to constitutively express both the classical, polymorphic MHC class I and the MHC class II antigens, in non pathologic pregnancies, has an important consequence: any maternal anti-paternal allogenic response should be ineffective. Although no data supports this assumption yet, we cannot exclude that soluble classical MHC class I molecules secreted by trophoblast cells, would anergize potential maternal cytotoxic T cells susceptible to destroy fetal or trophoblast expressing paternal antigens. In the case of intrauterine pathogen infection, such lack of expression of classical MHC class I and class II antigens should be desastrous. We hypothesize that trophoblast cells may then develop alternative effector mechanisms of protection. Besides nonspecific responses independent of MHC [37, 38], the first mechanism of protection might be appearance of classical HLA class I molecules. It has been shown, for example, that placental cells *in vitro* and *in vivo* respond to rubella and Sendai virus challenge by upregulating IFN-γ release [37]. Up regulation of MHC can in turn occur after IFN stimulation. Such an increase of cell surface expression of MHC class I molecules, following

IFN stimulation, has been observed in murine spongiotrophoblast cells [39] and in human villous cytotrophoblast [8]. A defect in cell surface class I expression, and thus in the presentation of intracellular viral antigens, has been restored by IFN-γ in murine tumoral cell lines [40]. The second mechanism of protection could be the presentation of microbial peptides by HLA-G.

Presence of HLA-G at the cell surface of extravillous cytotrophoblast cells may also be of importance, both to the fetal allograft tolerance and to fight possible pathogen infection of the trophoblast. Although HLA-G function is currently unknown, it is likely that this nonclassical class I molecule, expressed as a membrane-bound molecule on extravillous cytotrophoblast, is able to present endogenously processed, possibly viral, peptides to maternal a/b and /or g/d T cells for the following reasons: (i) HLA-G exhibits a conserved peptide binding pocket; (ii) HLA-G can bind the CD8 molecule; (iii) β2m associates to HLA-G heavy chains [5]; (iv) once transfected in TAP1 deficient .134 cells, HLA-G expression is reduced [14]; (v) the cotton top tamarin expresses a structural homologue of HLA-G [5]; (vi) polymorphism of HLA-G appears to be more important than initially thought [41]: heterozygous fetuses may could thus present a wider variety of foreign peptides to the T cell receptors. Lysis by maternal T cells of trophoblast infected cells may thus prevent spread of infection in the placenta. Furthermore, we cannot exclude an analogy with the nonclassical murine H2-M3 molecule which can present N-formylated peptides of bacterial origin [37].

Should HLA-G be able to present paternally-derived peptides, soluble forms of HLA-G might thus anergize alloreactive T cells and prevent a maternal alloresponse, as hypothesized by Geraghty and colleagues [14].

Another possible function of the membrane-bound or soluble forms of HLA-G might also be to inactivate natural killer (NK) cells, a predominant leukocyte type, also called large granular lymphocyte, found in uterus. Although contradictory data have been obtained [5], this hypothesis is still under current investigation.

Conclusions

In this chapter, we have shown that the constitutive transcriptional and protein expression of each HLA class I locus in the human placenta appears to be trophoblast cell type and gestation-stage specific. This can be accomplished by an extraordinary diversity of transcriptional and post-translational regulatory mechanisms that are, for many of them, still to be discovered. Functional significance of the absence of classical MHC class I cell surface expression and, on the contrary, of the presence of both soluble and membrane-bound forms of the nonclassical HLA-G class I molecule in human trophoblast are also currently debated. To date, no definitive data have been provided to support or eliminate the diverse hypothesis. Among the molecular tools that would help resolving in particular the possible roles of HLA-G in the survival of the fetal allograft, we are awaiting good, HLA-G locus-specific mAbs.

Acknowledgments

We wish to thank Maryse Girr, Thierry Guillaudeux, Valérie Le Morvan and Valérie Mallet who participated to parts of the work from our laboratory presented in this chapter. We are grateful to Drs B Grandjean, P Wasmer (clinique Ambroise Paré, Toulouse) and A Berebbi (Hôpital Lagrave, Toulouse) for supplying placentas. AMR was supported by a grant from Association pour la Recherche sur le Cancer. The work in the authors' laboratory was supported by Institut National de la Santé et de la Recherche Médicale and grants to PLB from Association pour la Recherche sur le Cancer (ARC 6622) and Conseil Régional de la Région Midi Pyrénées.

References

1. Loke YW, Butterworth BH. Heterogeneity of human trophoblast populations. In: Gill TJ III, Wegmann TG, eds. *Immunoregulation and fetal survival.* New York: Oxford University Press, 1987: 197-209.
2. Hunt JS. Immunobiology of pregnancy. *Curr Opin Immunol* 1992; 4: 591-596.
3. Ellis SA. HLA-G: at the interface. *Am J Reprod Immunol* 1990; 23: 84-86.
4. Trowsdale J. "Both man and bird and beast": a comparative organization of MHC genes. *Immunogenetics* 1995; 41: 1-17.
5. Le Bouteiller P. HLA class I chromosomal region, genes and products: facts and questions. *Critical Reviews in Immunology* 1994; 14: 89-129.
6. Kovats S, Main EK, Librach C, Stubblebine M, Fisher SJ and DeMars R. A class I antigen, HLA-G, expressed in human trophoblasts. *Science* 1990; 248: 220-223.
7. King A, Chumbley G, Loke YW. In: Chaouat G, Mowbray J eds. *Cellular and Molecular Biology of the Materno-Fetal Relationship.* Paris: Colloque INSERM/ John Libbey Eurotext Ltd, 1991: 103-111.
8. Feinman MA, Kliman HJ, Main EK. HLA antigen expression and induction by γ-interferon in cultured human trophoblasts. *Am J Obstet Gynecol* 1987; 157: 1429-1434.
9. Guillaudeux T, Rodriguez AM, Girr M, Mallet V, Ellis SA, Sargent IL, Fauchet R, Alsat E, Le Bouteiller P. Methylation status and transcriptional expression of the MHC class I loci in human trophoblast cells from term placenta. *J Immunol* 1995, in press.
10. Boyson JE, McAdam SN, Gallimore A, Golos TG, Liu, X, Gotch FM, Hughes AL, Watkins DI. The MHC E locus in macaques is polymorphic and is conserved between macaques and humans. *Immunogenetics* 1995; 41: 59-68.
11. Boucraut J, Guillaudeux T, Alizadeh M, Boretto J, Chimini G, Malecaze F, Semana G, Fauchet R, Pontarotti P, Le Bouteiller P. HLA-E is the only class I gene that escapes CpG methylation and is transcriptionally active in the trophoblast- derived human cell line JAR. *Immunogenetics* 1993; 38: 117-130.
12. Wei X, Orr HT. Differential expression of HLA-E, HLA-F and HLA-G transcripts in human tissues. *Human Immunol* 1990; 29: 131-142.
13. Ishitani A, Geraghty DE. Alternative splicing of HLA-G transcripts yields proteins with primary structures resembling both class I and class II antigens. *Proc. Natl Acad Sci USA* 1992; 89: 3947-3951.
14. Fujii T, Ishitani A, Geraghty DE. A soluble form of the HLA-G antigen is encoded by a messenger ribonucleic acid containing intron 4. *J Immunol* 1994; 153: 5516-5524.
15. Kirszenbaum M, Moreau P, Gluckman E, Dausset J, Carosella E. An alternatively spliced form of HLA-G mRNA in human trophoblasts and evidence for the presence of HLA-G transcripts in adult lymphocytes. *Proc Natl Acad Sci USA* 1994; 91: 4209-4213.
16. Oudejans CBM, Krimpenfort P, Ploegh HL, Meijer LM. Lack of expression of HLA- B27 gene in transgenic mouse trophoblast. *J Exp Med* 1989; 169: 447-456.
17. Schmidt CM, Ehlenfeld RG, Athanasiou MC, Duvick LA, Heinrichs H, David CS, Orr HT. Extraembryonic expression of the human MHC class I gene HLA-G in transgenic mice. *J Immunol* 1993; 151: 2633-2645.
18. Horuzsko A, Tomlinson PD, Strachan T, Mellor AL. Transcription of HLA-G transgenes commences shortly after implantation during embryonic development in mice. *Immunology* 1994; 83: 324-328.
19. Crossley M, Orkin SH. Regulation of the beta globin locus. *Curr Opin Genet Dev* 1993; 3: 232-237.
20. Razin AC, Cedar H. DNA methylation and genomic imprinting. *Cell* 1994; 77: 473-476.
21. Guillaudeux T, d'Almeida M, Girr M, Rodriguez AM, Pontarotti P, Fauchet R, Le Bouteiller P. Differences between human sperm and somatic cell DNA in CpG methylation within the HLA class I chromosomal region. *Am J Reprod Immunol* 1993; 30: 228-238.
22. Gill TJ III. Reproductive Immunology and Immunogenetics. In: Knobil E and Neill JD, eds.*The Physiology of Reproduction.* New York: Raven Press, 1994: 783-812.
23. Drezen JM, Barra J, Babinet C, Morello D. MHC class I genes are not imprinted in the mouse placenta. *Immunogenetics* 1994; 40: 62-65.
24. Donaldson WL, Oriol JG, Pelkaus CL, Antczak DF. Paternal and maternal Major Histocompatibility class I antigens are expressed co-dominantly by equine trophoblast. *Placenta* 1994; 15: 123-135.

25. Boucraut J, Hakem R, Gauthier A, Fauchet R, Le Bouteiller R. Transfected trophoblast derived human cells can express a single HLA class I allelic product. *Tissue Antigens* 1991; 37: 84-89.
26. Boucraut J, Hawley S, Robertson K, Bernard D, Loke YW, Le Bouteiller P. Differential nuclear expression of enhancer A DNA binding proteins in human first trimester trophoblast cells. *J Immunol* 1993; 150: 3882-3894.
27. Chiang MH, Main EK. Nuclear regulation of HLA class I genes in human trophoblasts. *Am J. Reprod.Immunol* 1994; 32: 167-172.
28. Maschek U, Pulm W, Hammerling GJ. Altered regulation of MHC class I genes in different tumor cell lines is reflected by distinct set of DNase I hypersensitive sites. *EMBO J.* 1989; 8: 2297-2304.
29. Jackson MR, Cohen-Doyle MF, Peterson P, Williams DB. Regulation of MHC class I transport by the molecular chaperone, calnexin (p88, IP90). *Science* 1994; 263: 384-387.
30. Williams DB, Barber BJ, Flavell RA, Allen H. Role of β2-microglobulin in the intracellular transport and surface expression of murine class I histocompatibility molecules. *J Immunol* 1989; 142: 2796-2806.
31. Jaffe L, Jeannotte L, Bikoff E, Robertson E. Analysis of β2-microglobulin gene expression in the developing mouse embryo and placenta. *J Immunol* 1990; 145: 3474-3482.
32. Kato M, Ohashi K, Saji F, Wakimoto A, Tanizawa O. Expression of HLA class I and β2- microglobulin on human choriocarcinoma cell lines: induction of HLA class I by interferon-g. *Placenta* 1991; 12: 217-226.
33. Anderson KS, Alexander J, Wei M, Cresswell P. Intracellular transport of class I MHC molecules in antigen processing mutant cell lines. *J Immunol* 1993; 151: 3407-3419.
34. Bikoff EK, Jaffe L, Ribaudo RK, Otten GR, Germain RN, Robertson EJ. MHC class I surface expression in embryo-derived cell lines inducible with peptide or interferon. *Nature* 1991; 354: 235-238
35. Roby KF, Fei K, Yang Y, Hunt JS Expression of HLA class-II associated peptide transporter and proteasome genes in human placentas and trophoblast cell lines. *Immunology* 1994; 83: 444-448.
36. Sugita M, Brenner MB. An unstable β2-microglobulin: Major Histocompatibility Complex class I heavy chain intermediate dissociates from calnexin and then is stabilized by binding peptide. *J Exp Med* 1994; 180: 2163-2171.
37. Ojcius DM, Delarbre C, Kourilsky P, Gachelin G. Major Histocompatibility Complex class I molecules and resistance against intracellular pathogens. *Critical Reviews in Immunology* 1994; 14: 193-220.
38. Robertson SA, Seamark RF, Guilbert LJ, Wegmann TG. The role of cytokines in gestation. *Critical Reviews in Immunology* 1994; 14: 239-292.
39. Voland JR, Becker C, Hooshmand F. Overexpression of class I MHC in murine trophoblast and increased rates of spontaneous abortion. In: Hunt JS, ed. *Immunobiology of Reproduction,* Serono Symposia, New York: Springer-Verlag, 1994: 214-235.
40. Sibille C, Gould K, Hammerling G, Townsend A. A defect in the presentation of intracellular viral antigens is restored by interferon-gamma in cell lines with impaired major histocompatibility complex class I assembly. *Eur J Immunol* 1992; 22: 433-440.
41. van der Ven K, Ober C. HLA-G polymorphism in African Americans. *J Immunol* 1994; 153: 5628-5633.

Résumé

L'acceptation par la mère d'une allogreffe fœtale constitue l'énigme la plus ancienne du domaine de la transplantation. L'absence d'expression détectable des molécules polymorphiques HLA-A,-B,-C de classe I classiques et la présence, à certains stades de la gestation, de molécules HLA-G de classe I non classiques, beaucoup moins polymorphiques, à la surface des cellules trophoblastiques qui constituent l'interface fœto-maternelle pourraient avoir une implication fonctionnelle importante. Dans une première partie, nous effectuons une synthèse des résultats les plus récents concernant l'expression constitutive transcriptionnelle et protéique de chacun des loci HLA de classe I, classiques et non classiques, dans les différentes sous-populations trophoblastiques au cours de la gestation. Dans une seconde partie, nous examinons les différents mécanismes moléculaires de régulation qui pourraient contrôler la transcription de ces gènes (méthylation des îlots CpG du DNA, facteurs de transcription qui se fixent sur des éléments régulateurs en *cis* de la partie promotrice des gènes HLA de classe I, structure de la chromatine), ainsi que ceux qui pourraient contrôler la traduction et le transport des produits protéiques à la surface cellulaire (disponibilité d'un pool de peptides spécifiques, ainsi que de la β2-microglobuline, des transporteurs de peptides TAP1/TAP2, des sous-unités LMP2/LMP7 des protéasomes, et des molécules chaperones de type calnexine). Enfin, nous discutons de la signification fonctionnelle de l'absence d'expression des molécules HLA de classe I classiques à la surface de l'ensemble des sous-populations trophoblastiques, d'une part, et de la présence de HLA-G à la surface des cellules du cytotrophoblaste invasif extravilleux, d'autre part.

HLA-G expression in fetal and neonatal hematopoietic cells

M. Kirszenbaum and E. Carosella

Commissariat à l'Energie Atomique, Direction des Sciences du Vivant, Laboratoire d'Immuno-radiobiologie, Hôpital Saint-Louis, Centre Hayem, 1, avenue Claude-Vellefaux, 75010 Paris, France, tel.: (33 1) 42 49 98 24, fax: (33 1) 48 03 19 60

Abstract

HLA-G nonclassical HLA class I gene encodes the molecule that is the only MHC antigen expressed on cytotrophoblasts of placenta. This restricted expression on fetal tissue that is in contact with maternal tissue suggests that HLA-G products may play a role in materno-fetal tolerance. In these tissues HLA-G mRNA is alternatively spliced and resulting transcripts may encode molecules lacking α2 or α2 and α3 domains. We have demonstrated in the 1st trimester human trophoblast and liver a new alternatively spliced form of mRNA lacking exon 4 (HLA-G4), that may encode the α3 domain, and weak expression of the full-length mRNA copy (HLA-G1) in adult PBL. By using exon specific HLA-G primers we have demonstrated the presence of three alternatively spliced forms of HLA-G mRNA in human umbilical cord blood mononuclear cells (HLA-G2, HLA-G3 and HLA-G4). In contrast, we did not reveal any HLA-G transcripts in the $CD34^+$ fraction of cord blood cells.

The human Major Histocompatibility Complex (MHC) is located in the distal region of the short arm of chromosome 6 [6p21.3] and spans a genomic region of about 4000 kb. This region includes three subregions of MHC genes: class I, class II and class III. The class I subregion, spanning 2000 kb, is composed of more than 20 genes and pseudogenes. It comprises two groups of genes: I) classical HLA class I genes (HLA-A, HLA-B, HLA-C), which are highly polymorphic and ubiquitously expressed, encode cell surface 45-kDa glycoproteins associated with an invariant 12-kDa β2m chain that constitute the restriction elements for virus-specific and allospecific cytolytic-T-lymphocytes; II) nonclassical HLA class I genes (HLA-E, HLA-F, HLA-G) whose functions are not yet established but it is possible that each of these genes has a specific function [1]. Within nonclassical HLA class I genes, HLA-E and HLA-F are expressed in various fetal and adult tissues [2] whereas HLA-G antigen is only expressed in fetal placental tissues: in first trimester tissue high expression was detected in cytotrophoblast cells [3]; in the third trimester this expression is reduced in extravillous cytotrophoblast and increased in extravillous membrane [1]. Specific expression of HLA-G antigen restricted to fetal trophoblasts, the only fetal tissue in contact with maternal cells, which lack the classical MHC class I antigens (HLA-

A, -B, -C), may suggest a role of this gene in maternal tolerance of the placenta. The immunological mechanisms of the tolerance of semi-allogeneic fetus by the mother are still unclear [4]. Surprisingly, in fetal liver HLA-G gene is expressed in first trimester but not in the second trimester [5]. Low amounts of HLA-G transcripts were reported in fetal eye and thymus [6] but also in human adult eye tissues [7], skin [8] and germ cells [9]. HLA-G gene sequence and structure are tightly homologous to classical HLA class I genes [7] and other nonclassical HLA class I genes [2]. It is composed of 8 exons and 7 introns but encodes the protein with a shorter cytoplasmic tail. By using the PCR-SSCP technique an extensive polymorphism of HLA-G gene was recently reported in African Americans [10]. Moreover, different forms of alternatively spliced HLA-G mRNA were observed *(Figure 1)*: full-length mRNA transcript and transcripts lacking exon 3 or exons 3 and 4 [11]. Recently, by using sensitive hot-start RT-PCR technique, we have demonstrated the new alternatively spliced forms of HLA-G mRNA: HLA-G4 lacking exon 4 and HLA-G5 containing intron 4 that may encode the soluble HLA-G protein and the expression of HLA-G transcripts in various human fetal and adult cells [12,13]. We have also demonstrated that Natural Killer cells do not express HLA-G transcripts a finding which is in keeping with the proposed function of HLA-G gene products in immune-tolerance [14].

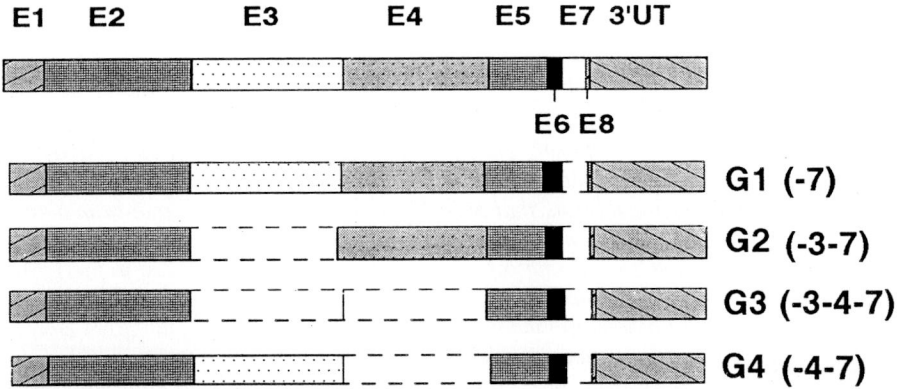

Figure 1. Structure of the alternatively spliced HLA-G transcripts. Top of the figure illustrates exon organization of HLA-G mRNA. E1: exon 1 encoding for the signal peptide; E2-E4: exons 2 to 4 encoding for a1 to α3 extracellular domains; E5: exon 5 encoding for transmembrane region; E6: exon 6 encoding for a reduced cytoplasmic region; E7 and E8: exons 7 and 8 (untranslated); 3'UT: 3'-untranslated region. G1 to G4 are alternative forms of HLA-G transcripts.

Materials and methods

Fetal liver, umbilical cord blood and adult peripheral blood cells

Human first trimester liver was obtained from voluntary terminations of pregnancy at 6 to 10 weeks of gestation. Second trimester fetal liver was obtained from therapeutic terminations of pregnancy at 16 weeks of gestation. Samples of human umbilical cord blood were obtained from full-term neonates immediately after vaginal delivery in accordance with institutional guidelines. Human peripheral blood samples were obtained from normal male volunteers. Local ethical committee approval was obtained for this study. Mononuclear cells were separated from polynuclear cells by Ficoll-Hypaque density centrifugation. The CD34+ fraction from CBMC was obtained by incubation with mouse mAb anti-CD34 (HPCA-2, Becton-Dickinson, Paris), washing then reincubation with immunomagnetic beads coated with sheep anti-mouse IgG (Dynabeads, Dynal, Paris) and separation by a magnetic device (Serva, Paris). The purity of separated CD34+ cells was approximately 89% as estimated by FACS analysis.

RNA isolation and RT-PCR amplification

Total mRNA was isolated from 2×10^7 cells or 1 g of tissue using RNA-Zol B reagent (Bioprobe Systems, France) according to the manufactor's recommendations. cDNA was prepared from 10 mg of total RNA with oligo-dT priming and M-MLV reverse transcriptase-RT (Gibco-BRL, Life Technologies). In order to reduce the number of nonspecific amplimers PCR amplification was performed using a hot-start technique. RT-PCR amplification was performed with HLA-G specific primers and 35 cycles of PCR were performed at 94°C for 1 min, 65°C for 1 min, 72°C for 1 min 30 sec. In all PCR amplifications we used as controls the RT reaction mixture without M-MLV reverse transcriptase (RT-) and PCR mixture without cDNA template (Blank).

Southern blot hybridization

The PCR products were analysed by electrophoresis in 1% agarose gel followed by alkaline blotting of the fragments in 0.4N NaOH onto a nylon membrane (Hybond N+, Amersham, France). Hybridization was performed with ^{32}P-labelled oligonucleotide HLA-G specific probes. Filters were exposed to Kodak X-OMAT AR film for 4 to 24 hours at –80°C.

Results and discussion

cDNAs from human Peripheral Blood Mononuclear Cells (PBMC) and Cord Blood Mononuclear Cells (CBMC) were amplified using HLA-G specific primers G.257 – G.1225 encompassing exons 2 to 3'-UT region of mRNA. *Figure 2* presents the Southern blot of PCR products subsequently hybridized with an exon 4 specific probe. Two bands observed in PBMC as well as in CBMC at 0.89 kb and 0.7 kb are assigned to the full length mRNA copy and to the alternatively spliced form lacking exon 3. These two bands are weak in cord blood as compared with peripheral blood cells and b-actin standard. In the aim to precise the presence alternatively spliced form of HLA-G mRNA lacking exon 4 in PBMC and CBMC, the PCR amplification was performed with G.526 forward primer specific to exon 3 and ubiquitous 3'-UT reverse primer (G.1225). Thus hybridization with the 3'-UT probe (G.1200) reveals two bands (at 0.71 kb and 0.43 kb) in PBMC assigned respectively to full-length mRNA and the alternatively spliced form lacking exon 4. In contrast in CBMC the band at 0.43 kb was not observed even if the blot was exposed for a longer time (data not shown). *Figure 3* presents the results of PCR amplification with G.526-G.1225 HLA-G specific primers on cDNA from fetal liver of 6 and 16 weeks and cord blood cells. Subsequent Southern blot hybridization with the G.1200 ^{32}P-labelled probe revealed a positive signal in 6 week fetal liver and CBMC whereas no signal was observed in 16 week fetal liver and CD34+ enriched populations (CB-CD34+). Thus the HLA-G gene seems to be expressed only in differentiated hematopoietic cells and appears to be a marker of this cells. Work is in progress to determine the type of cells from 6 week fetal liver that express HLA-G gene.

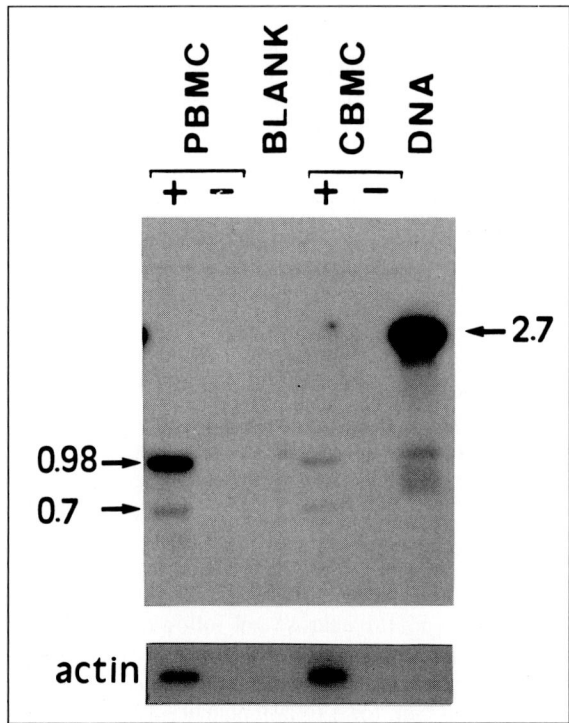

Figure 2. Strategy of detection of HLA-G alternatively spliced transcript lacking exon 3 in PBMC and CBMC cDNAs. Southern blot analysis of PCR products after amplification with primers G.257 - G.1225 and hybridization with exon 4 specific (G.647) 32P-labelled probe show the presence of 0.98 kb band of full-length mRNA and 0.7 kb band corresponding to the alternative splicing form without exon 3. Very weak intensity of hybridization signals in CBMC samples in comparison with actin control signals reveals the very weak abundance of HLA-G mRNA in CBMC.

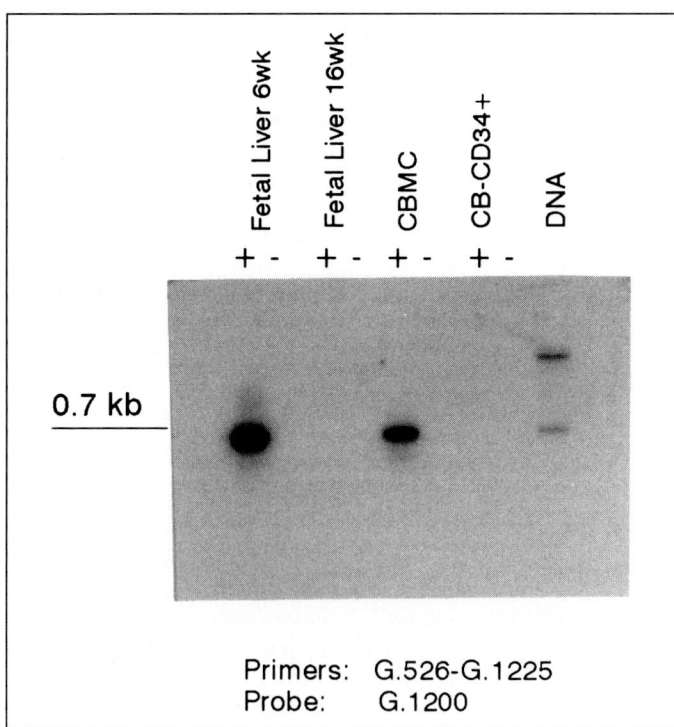

Figure 3. Expression of HLA-G gene in fetal liver and cord blood cells. After PCR amplification with G.526-G.1225 primers and subsequent Southern blot hybridization with G.1200 32P-labelled probe positive signal was observed in 6 week fetal liver and CBMC whereas no signal was observed in 16 week fetal liver and CD34+ enriched populations (CB-CD34+).

References

1. Wei XH, Orr HT. Differential expression of HLA-E, HLA-F, and HLA-G transcripts in human tissue. *Hum Immunol* 1990; 29: 131-142.
2. Geraghty DE, Wei XH, Orr HT, Koller BH. Human Leukocyte Antigen F (HLA-F). An expressed HLA gene composed of a class I coding sequence linked to a novel transcribed repetitive element. *J Exp Med* 1990; 171: 1-18.
3. Ellis SA, Palmer MS, McMichael AJ. Human trophoblast and the choriocarcinoma cell line BeWo express a truncated HLA Class I molecule. *J Immunol* 1990; 144: 731-735.
4. Herrera-Gonzalez NE, Dresser DW. Fetal-Maternal Immune Interaction – Blocking Antibody and Survival of the Fetus. *Dev Comp Immunol* 1993; 17: 1-18.
5. Houlihan JM, Biro PA, Fergar-Payne A, Simpson KL, Holmes CH. Evidence for the expression of non-HLA-A,-B,-C class I genes in the human fetal liver. *J Immunol* 1992; 149: 668-675.
6. Shukla H, Swaroop A, Srivastava R, Weissman SM. The mRNA of a human class I gene HLA G/HLA 6.0 exhibits a restricted pattern of expression. *Nucleic Acids Res* 1990; 18: 2189.
7. Geraghty DE, Koller BH, Orr HT. A human major histocompatibility complex class I gene that encodes a protein with shortened cytoplasmic segment. *Proc Natl Acad Sci USA* 1987; 84: 9145-9149.
8. Ulbrecht M, Rehberger B, Strobel I, Messer G, Kind P, Degitz K, Bieber T, Weiss EH. HLA-G – Expression in Human Keratinocytes *in Vitro* and in Human Skin *in Vivo*. *Eur J Immunol* 1994; 24: 176-180.
9. Chiang MH, Steuerwald N, Lambert H, Main EK, Steinleitner A. Detection of Human Leukocyte Antigen Class I Messenger Ribonucleic Acid Transcripts in Human Spermatozoa via Reverse Transcription Polymerase Chain Reaction. *Fertil Steril* 1994; 61: 276-280.
10. van der Ven K, Ober C. HLA-G polymorphisms in African Americans. *J Immunol* 1994; 153: 5628-5633.
11. Ishitani A, Geraghty DE. Alternative splicing of HLA-G transcripts yields proteins with primary structures resembling both class I and class II antigens. *Proc Natl Acad Sci USA* 1992; 89: 3947-3951.
12. Kirszenbaum M, Moreau P, Gluckman E, Dausset J, Carosella E. An alternatively spliced form of HLA-G mRNA in human trophoblasts and evidence for the presence of HLA-G transcript in adult lymphocytes. *Proc Natl Acad Sci USA* 1994; 91: 4209-4213.
13. Moreau P, Carosella E, Teyssier M, Prost S, Gluckman E, Dausset J, Kirszenbaum M. Soluble HLA-G molecule: an alternatively spliced HLA-G mRNA form candidate to encode it in peripheral blood mononuclear cells and human trophoblasts. *Hum Immunol* 1995; in press.
14. Teyssier M, Bensussan A, Kirszenbaum M, Moreau P, Gluckman E, Dausset J, Carosella E. HLA-G expression in human functional lymphocytes subsets. *Cell Immunol* 1995; submitted.

Résumé

Le gène *HLA-G* du complexe majeur d'histocompatibilité de classe I non classique code pour une molécule qui est le seul antigène présent sur les cytotrophoblastes placentaires. Cette expression restreinte au tissu fœtal en contact avec le tissu maternel suggère que l'antigène HLA-G peut jouer un rôle important dans la tolérance fœto-maternelle. Suite à l'épissage alternatif, dans le trophoblaste, l'ARNm du gène *HLA-G* est présent sous différentes formes qui peuvent coder pour les molécules sans domaines α2, ou α2 et α3. Précédemment nous avons démontré, dans le trophoblaste et le foie humain du premier trimestre de gestation, l'existence d'un nouveau transcrit alternatif sans exon 4 (HLA-G4) qui peut coder pour une molécule sans domaine α3, ainsi que la présence d'une faible expression d'ARNm complet dans les cellules du sang périphérique chez l'adulte. Dans ce travail, en utilisant les amorces spécifiques du gène *HLA-G,* nous avons démontré la présence de trois transcrits alternatifs (HLA-G2, HLA-G3 et HLA-G4) dans les cellules mononuclées du sang de cordon humain. En revanche, nous n'avons observé aucun transcrit du gène *HLA-G* dans la fraction DC34$^+$ du sang de cordon.

BY55 mAb delineates within human adult peripheral blood, newborn cord blood and adult bone marrow lymphocytes distinct cell subsets mediating cytotoxic activity

Valérie Schiavon[1], Edgardo Carosella[2], Indra-Gusti Mansur[1], Eliane Gluckman[2], Sana El Marsafy[2], Laurence Boumsell[1] and Armand Bensussan[1]

[1] INSERM U 93; [2] Unité de Recherche sur la Biologie des Cellules Souches, LIRB-CEA, Hôpital Saint-Louis, 1, avenue Claude-Vellefaux, 75475 Paris Cedex 10, France, tel.: (33 1) 42 39 17 63, fax: (33 1) 42 06 84 54

Abstract

We report here, with the use of BY55 monoclonal antibody, a unique cell surface protein restricted to about 20% of human circulating lymphocytes comprising most NK lymphocytes and a minor subset of $CD3^+CD8^+TCR\alpha\beta^+/CD3^+CD8^-TCR\gamma\delta^+$ lymphocytes. In contrast, only 5 to 10% of the bone marrow lymphocytes with a major proportion of $CD3^+CD8^+$ were $BY55^+$. Interestingly, within cord blood cells $BY55^+$ lymphocytes represented 20 to 35% of the lymphocytes corresponding exclusively to a $CD3^-$ cell subset. Functional studies revealed that in cord blood only NK activity was detected in association with the $BY55^+$ phenotype whereas in bone marrow and in peripheral blood the $BY55^+$ cell population contained both NK and CTL activity. Thus, BY55 mAb identifies different cytotoxic cell populations in the cord blood and in the bone marrow and therefore as they are both sources for hematopoietic stem cell transplantation these different populations might exert different consequences on the occurence of GVHD.

Natural killer cells are cytotoxic circulating lymphocytes found within the large granular lymphocyte population [1]. The characteristic surface markers expressed by circulating NK cells are CD56 [2], CD16 [3], CD11b, [4] and CD122 (IL-2R p75) [5]. Recently, several molecules including NKB1 [6], p58 molecules [7] and CD96 [8] were reported as NK cell receptors on allogeneic cloned lymphocytes. To further delineate circulating cells with cytotoxic activity, we developed a mAb obtained by repeated immunization with YT2C2, a human cell line with NK functional characteristics [9]. This monoclonal antibody, termed BY55 reacts with a novel 80 kDa protein structure expressed exclusively by YT2C2 and a subset of circulating lymphocytes [10, 11].

In peripheral blood of normal adults BY55 mAb identified CD3⁻ lymphocytes and a minor subset of CD3⁺CD8⁺ cell

In normal human peripheral blood, extensive phenotypic analysis revealed that the reactivity of BY55 mAb corresponded to 20-25% of cells including CD3 negative and CD3 positive lymphocytes. Within CD3 positive cells expressing BY55, only one third were CD8⁻CD4⁻ whereas two third were bright or dim CD8⁺ *(Table I)*. Double positive CD4/BY55 cells were never detected in circulating lymphocytes. As it is not specified on the *Table I*, it has to be noted that most of the double negative CD4/CD8 cells expressing the CD3 molecules corresponded to the TCR γδ positive T lymphocytes [10].

Table I. Frequency of BY55⁺ cells in PBL from normal individuals.

Donor No	BY55⁺ %	CD8⁺ %	CD3⁺ %	CD3⁺8⁺ %	CD3⁺8⁺ BY55⁺ %	CD3⁺8⁻ BY55⁺ %	CD3⁻8⁺ BY55⁺ %	CD3⁻8⁻ BY55⁺ %
1	11	41	87	37	4	2	3	3
2	15	19	87	18	5	5	1	9
3	30	48	61	29	6	2	9	8
4	32	37	68	19	7	3	12	10
5	22	45	70	26	3	1	9	6
6	12	29	89	25	4	1	3	4
7	26	35	75	28	5	6	5	14
8	29	29	83	42	13	2	5	8
9	19	38	89	36	9	4	2	3
10	19	41	72	27	4	2	9	7
	21.2±6.6	38.1±8.5	78.2±9.6	28.7±7.3	5.8±2.9	2.7±1.5	5.8±3.5	7.1±3.2

PBMC or blood from 10 randomly selected HIV seronegative adults were labeled for one or three color determination as described in materials and methods. Samples were analyzed by flow cytometry.
* Mean percentage ± SD

In peripheral blood of normal adults BY55 mAb identified NK and CTL activities

As most CD3⁻ lymphocytes were stained by mAb BY55, we looked at whether NK activity was exhibited by BY55⁺ cells. Thus, peripheral blood lymphocytes were labeled with BY55 and sorted into BY55⁺ and BY55⁻ cells using a FACS. The results from a representative experiment are presented in *Figure 1A*. Whole PBL and BY55 mAb-labeled PBL of this donor exhibit strong NK activity measured against the K562 cell line. As expected from the phenotypic results, the BY55⁺ cell population was greatly enriched in cells mediating NK activity, whereas the BY55⁻ population was almost deprived of cytotoxic function. It is of note that BY55 mAb did not modify NK activity. More interesting was the investigation of whether the MHC-restricted CD3⁺ CD8⁺BY55⁺ circulating cell subset also exhibited killer activity. CD3-redirected cytotoxic assays were performed with sorted CD8+BY55+ and CD8+BY55− cells: a representative cell-mediated cytotoxicity assay with unsorted and sorted effector cells is presented in *Figure 1B*. As expected, a weak but significant CD3-redirected and NK lysis against the K562 cells was observed with PBL depleted in CD4+ cells. To exclude the NK activity of CD3− CD8^{dim}BY55+ cells against K562 target cells, we separated BY55+ and BY55− cells within CD8$^{bright+}$ gated cells corresponding exclusively to TCR αβ+ cells. We found that, in contrast to CD8+BY55− cells, which never exhibited cytotoxic T-lympocyte activity (CTL), only the CD8+BY55+ cell subset mediated a strong CD3 mAb-redirected cytotoxicity. Taken together, these functional results indicate that BY55 mAb delineates in the peripheral blood of normal individuals the active cytotoxic lymphocytes including NK cells and T lymphocytes.

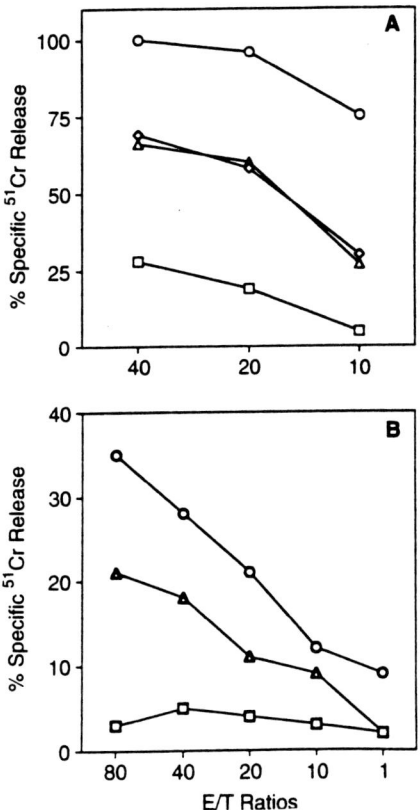

Figure 1. A. Determination of the NK activity mediated by sorted BY55+ and BY55− PBL. Freshly isolated PBL were labeled with BY55 mAb for indirect immunofluorescence. These treated cells were either used directly as effector cells (triangles), or sorted into BY55+ (circles) and BY55− (squares) effector cells by using a FACS Vantage microfluorometer (Becton Dickinson) Untreated PBL were also tested as effector cells (diamonds) against K562 target cells in a 4-h ^{51}Cr release assay. B. Determination of the CD3-redirected cytotoxicity against the Fc receptor-bearing target cell K562. Freshly isolated PBL were depleted of CD4+ cells by passage over a column and were then simultaneously labeled with FITC-conjugated BY55 mAb and PE-conjugated CD8 mAb. Cells were sorted into CD8$^{bright+}$ BY55+ (circles) and CD8$^{bright+}$ BY55− (squares) fractions. mAb-treated (triangles) and sorted cells were used as effector cells in a cytotoxic T-lymphocyte assay.

In bone marrow BY55 mAb reacted with CD3⁻ lymphocytes and T lymphocytes

Further, to determine whether the expression of BY55 molecule was restricted to any particular subset of bone marrow lymphocytes, two-color immunofluorescence staining was carried out. The results revealed that the percentage of BY55$^+$ cells was lower than in adult blood and varied from 5 to 10% of the cells gated on lymphocytes. Moreover, as shown in the representative experiments presented in *Figure 2*, half of the BY55$^+$ cells were CD3$^+$ and TCR$\alpha\beta^+$ cells. This contrasts with our results showing that the majority of BY55$^+$ cells in adult peripheral blood are CD3$^-$ lymphocytes. Furthermore half of bone marrow BY55$^+$ cells were CD8$^{bright+}$ or CD8^{dim+}, one fifth were TCR$\gamma\delta$+ cells, and half were CD16$^+$ cells.

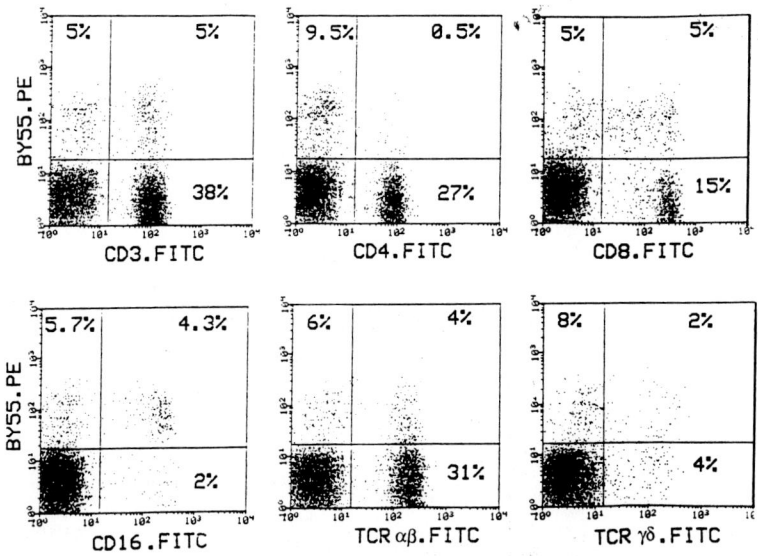

Figure 2. Two-color immunofluorescence analysis of BY55 expression in bone marrow lymphocytes. Cells from a representative donor were first labeled with CD3, CD4, CD8, CD16, TcR$\alpha\beta$ or TcR $\gamma\delta$ mAb coupled with FITC in combination with BY55 mAb, after washing, cells were incubated with a PE anti-mouse IgM. Samples were then analysed by flow cytometry. Division in quadrants was established on the basis of one-color immunofluorescence analysis of samples for each individual experiment. Number in each quadrant indicates the percent of positive cells.

In bone marrow BY55 mAb identified CTL

To study MHC-restricted killer activity of freshly isolated CD8$^+$ BY55$^+$ and CD8$^+$BY55$^-$ bone marrow lymphocytes, CD3-redirected cytotoxic assays were done with these isolated populations. A representative cell-mediated cytotoxicity assay done with unsorted and sorted effector cells is presented in *Figure 3*. We found that CD8$^+$ BY55$^+$ cell subset mediated a strong CD3 mAb- redirected cytotoxicity against the murine mastocytoma cell line P815 coated with CD3 mAb. In contrast unseparated or CD8+ BY55− cells never exhibited lytic activity *(Figure 3A)*. As expected no lysis against the P815 cells was observed with the bone marrow cells or the separated cells *(Figure 3B)*.

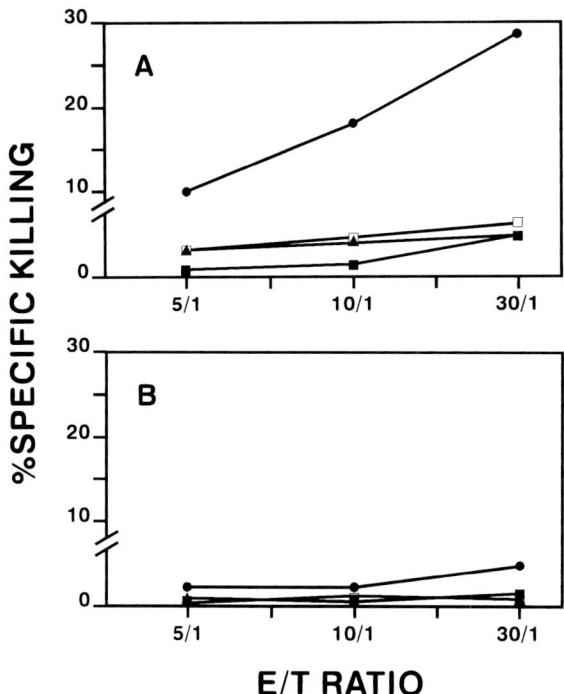

Figure 3. Determination of the CD3-redirected cytotoxicity against the Fc receptor-bearing target cells P815. Freshly isolated bone marrow mononuclear cells were simultaneously labeled with CD8 and BY55 mAb. Cells were sorted into BY55+CD8+ and BY55− CD8+ fractions. Unseparated BMC, BMC labeled with CD8 and BY55 mAb, BY55+CD8+ and BY55− CD8+ were used as effector cells against (A) P815 cells coated with CD3 mAb or (B) P815 cells alone.

In cord blood BY55 mAb identified a unique CD3− lymphocyte subset

To delineate the BY55+ lymphocyte subsets within newborn cord blood, two-color analysis was performed. Extensive phenotypic analysis performed with over twenty different samples of cord blood revealed that BY55 mAb labeled in cord blood a similar proportion as in adult blood between 22 to 35% of the cells in the lymphoid gate. The results obtained with one representative cord blood sample are shown in *Figure 4*. BY55+ lymphocytes were observed in the CD3− cell population *(Figure 4A)* and as expected from our previous studies with PBMC [10] BY55 mAb was unreactive with CD19+ cells (data not shown). Interestingly, in contrast to what was obtained with adult peripheral blood or bone marrow cells, we never found in cord blood CD3+ and/or CD8$^{bright+}$ lymphocytes reactive with BY55 mAb. In contrast, we consistently observed that half of the CD8^{dim+} cells coexpressed BY55. In addition BY55+ cells bear the NK associated structures CD56, CD16 and CD11b. The representative results from another donor with approximately one third of BY55+, CD56+, CD16+ and CD11b+ cord blood lymphocytes are

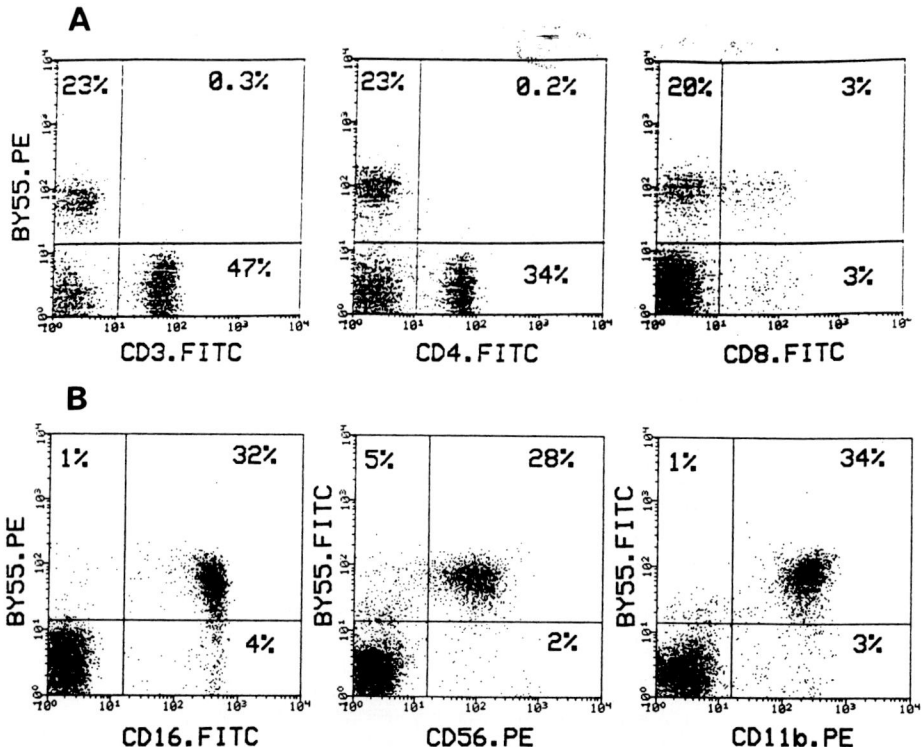

Figure 4. Two-color immunofluorescence analysis of BY55 expression in the cord blood lymphocytes. A. Cells from a representative donor were first labeled with CD3, CD4 or CD8 mAb coupled with FITC in combination with BY55 mAb. Then the cells were washed and treated with a PE-conjugated goat anti-mouse monoclonal IgM. B. Cells from a different donor were first labeled with CD56-PE, CD16-FITC or CD11b PE mAb in combination with BY55 mAb. After washing the cells were incubated either with a PE-conjugated anti-mouse IgM or with an FITC-conjugated anti-mouse IgM. Samples were then analysed by flow cytometry. Division in quadrants were established on the basis of one-color immunofluorescence analysis of samples for each individual experiment. Number in each quadrant indicates the percent of positive cells.

shown in *Figure 4B*. Among the BY55$^+$ cells most cells were CD16$^+$, CD11b$^+$ and CD56$^+$. However, a small proportion of BY55$^+$ cells did not express CD56 molecules. Furthermore 4-5% of the cells that express CD11b and CD16 molecules were unreactive with BY55 mAb. Thus, expression of BY55 surface antigen defines in cord blood a CD3$^-$ lymphocyte subset closely related but distinct from the cell subset defined by CD16, CD56 or CD11b mAb.

In cord blood BY55 mAb delineated active circulating NK lymphocytes

To determine whether BY55$^+$ lymphocytes represented the competent NK cord blood cells, CBL containing of 25% BY55$^+$ cells were separated into BY55$^+$ and BY55$^-$ cells using a FACS.

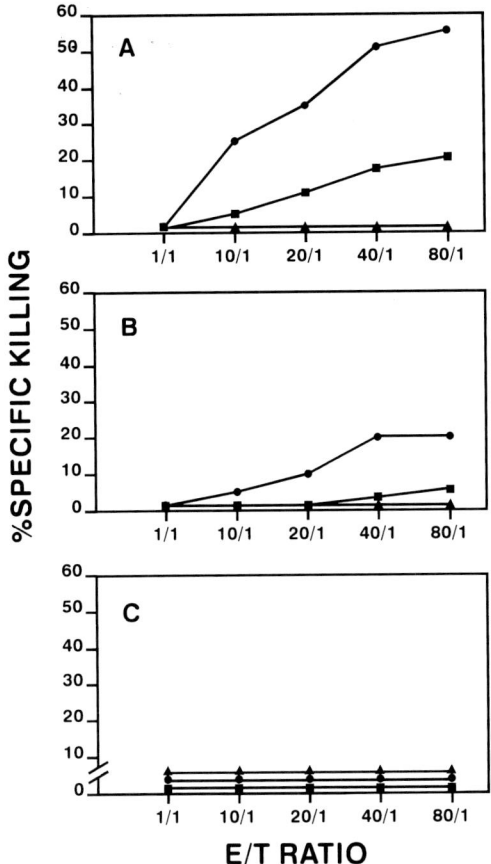

Figure 5. Determination of the NK and CTL activity mediated by sorted BY55+ and BY55− CBL. Freshly isolated CBMC were labeled with BY55 mAb for indirect immunofluorescence. These treated cells were either used directly as effector cells (squares), sorted into BY55+ (circles) or BY55− (triangles) effector cells. Effector cells were tested against (A) K562, (B) HL60 (C) P815 coated with CD3 mAb cell lines in a 4 h- ^{51}Cr release assay. Results represent mean of triplicate experiments and are expressed as percent of specific cytotoxic activity.

Reanalysis of the sorted populations revealed that less than 2% of the cells were BY55+ in the BY55− fraction whereas more than 95% of the cells were BY55+ in the BY55+ fraction (data not shown). The sorted lymphocytes and BY55 mAb labeled unseparated cells, used as control, were tested for their ability to mediate NK activity against the K562 cell line *(Figure 5A)* or against the HL60 cell line *(Figure 5B)*. The results from a representative experiment are presented. The unseparated control CBL exhibited a low but significant NK activity against the K562 target cell line whereas no killer activity was observed against HL60 cells. As expected from the phenotypic analysis, only BY55+ population was mediating NK activity and this activity was greatly enriched when compared to the control unsorted populations, as shown by a higher percentage of specific ^{51}Cr release at each E/T ratio. Interestingly, it was found that a minor but significant killer activity was also obtained against HL60 cell line in sorted BY55+ CBL. As expected from previous work done with PBMC, the BY55− cell population was totally deprived of NK killing and as expected no CTL activity was detected within the CD3+ enriched BY55− cells *(Figure 5C)*.

Expression of BY55 molecules was modified after allogeneic stimulation

One possibility to study the function of BY55 cell surface molecule is to test its expression on peripheral blood lymphocytes after stimulation with irriadiated allogeneic cells. Mixed culture lymphocyte reactions were chosen because it is well established that they induce the differentiation of cytotoxic lymphocytes with NK-like and CTL activity. The results presented in *Figure 6* revealed an almost complete disappearance of the distinct circulating BY55+ cell subset after

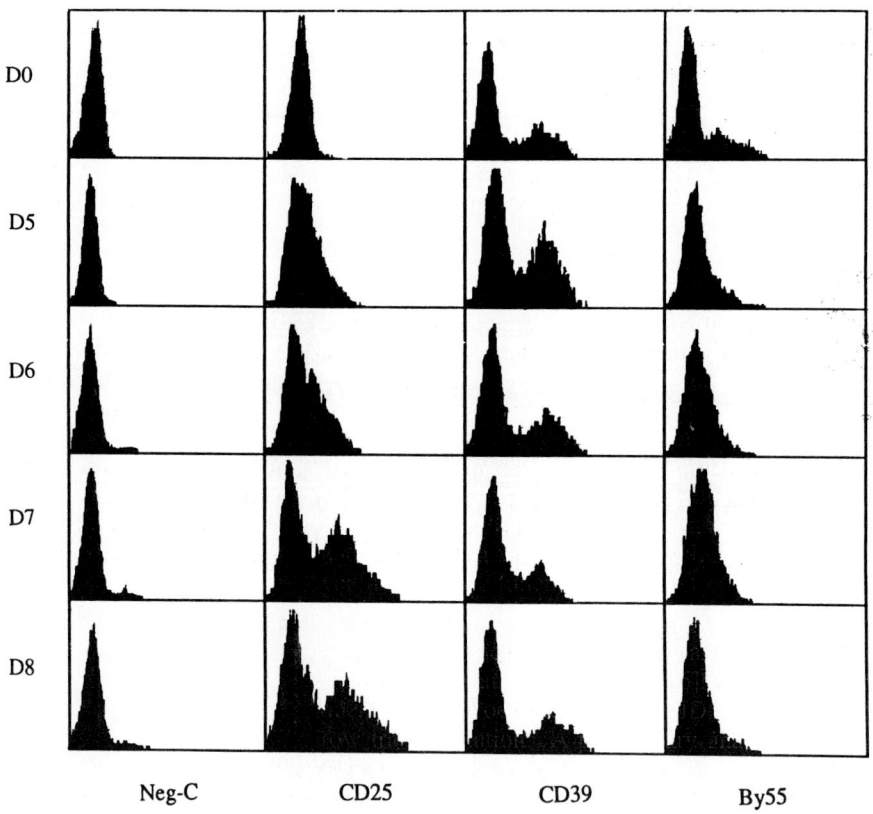

Figure 6. Kinetics of the cell-surface expression of the structure recognized by BY55 mAb after activation with irradiated allogeneic cells. PBMC were stained before (D0), and 5 days (D5), 6 days (D6), 7 days (D7) or 8 days (D8) after coculture with allogeneic irradiated PBMC for indirect immunofluorescence with an irrelevant IgM/IgG (Neg-C), CD25"BC96", CD39"BA54" or BY55 mAb. Fuorescence profiles are displayed as single parameter histograms

five to six days of co-culture with allogeneic cells. A different specific fluorescence profile was then obtained. It seemed that most alloreactive lymphocytes expressed variable low levels of BY55 molecules. In contrast, as we have already reported [12], the CD39$^+$ alloreactive T cell subset which exhibits the CTL reactivity was increased. As expected, the CD25 molecule (IL2Rα) delineated a cell subset after 5-6 days of co-culture. These results suggested that either BY55 molecules are secreted after activation as we have already demonstrated for CD106 molecules expressed on specific T cell clones [13] and/or they correspond to receptors for a soluble ligand which after ligation inhibits BY55 mAb reactivity. In addition, in both cases we postulate that BY55 molecules are probably expressed during T cell activation even though they were never identified on various IL2-dependant T lymphocyte clones tested [10].

Concluding remarks

We compared the cell surface phenotypes of cell populations defined with the BY55 mAb in peripheral blood, umbilical cord and bone marrow. Phenotypic studies of bone marrow mononuclear cells revealed that BY55$^+$ lymphocytes were less abundant than in peripheral blood from adults. However, they also consisted of an heterogeneous cell population containing CD3$^+$CD8$^+$TCR$\alpha\beta^+$, CD3$^+$CD8$^+$TCR$\gamma\delta^+$ and CD3$^-$ lymphocytes. Interestingly, the BY55$^+$CD3$^+$CD8$^{bright+}$ lymphocytes (expressing TCR$\alpha\beta^+$) sorted from adult peripheral blood and the CD8$^+$BY55$^+$ isolated from bone marrow (bearing either the TCR$\alpha\beta$ or the TCR$\gamma\delta$) were functional CTL. In cord blood BY55 mAb reacted exclusively with a cell population that corresponded to 22-35% of the lymphocytes, that lacked CD3-TCR expression and slightly differed from CD56, CD16 or CD11b-mAb defined cell subset. As expected from the phenotypic analysis, functional studies revealed that positively isolated BY55$^+$ circulating umbilical CBL exhibit highly efficient NK activity whereas no killer activity was found with the sorted BY55$^-$ population. More important was the finding that no CTL activity could be detected from the CD3 enriched BY55$^-$ cell population. Taken together these results indicate that BY55 mAb describes a unique cell surface molecule corresponding exclusively to a functional circulating lymphocyte subset which exhibits cytotoxic activity prior any in vitro stimulation. Of course, other molecules such as perforin [14] are makers of cytotoxic cells, however in contrast to the BY55 structure these molecules are intracellular and therefore they cannot be used to isolate cytotoxic cells for an *ex vivo* manipulation. In addition, the function of BY55 molecules is still unknown and, as BY55 mAb did not inhibit NK and CTL activity, they do not appear to be directly involved in cytotoxic function.

The finding that distinct cytotoxic lymphocytes are detected in the cord blood and in the bone marrow is of the utmost interest particularly because they are both sources of hematopoietic stem cell for transplantation [15,16]. These different populations might exert different consequences on the occurrence of GVHD [17] which is the most serious complication of bone marrow transplantation. A preliminary analysis of the International Cord Blood Transplantation Registry [18] has shown an absence of acute and chronic graft versus host disease in children transplanted with an HLA identical or one HLA antigen mismatched sibling cord blood transplant. The same trend has been observed in children receiving matched unrelated or two/three antigen mismatched related cord blood tranplant. This difference with patients receiving bone marrow was attributed to the immune deficiency of new born, to the young age of donor and recipient, to the presence of naive non activated T cells in cord blood and to the absence of exposure to previous CMV or other viral infections. More clinical experience is needed to confirm this finding and also to demonstrate that the diminution of GVH will not be associated with an increased incidence of rejection and leukemic relapse. Therefore, our results showing the lack of functionally active CTL in cord blood and their presence in bone marrow seems interesting. This could indicate that acute GVHD is directly attributable to CD3$^+$BY55$^+$ cells, while less severe chronic GVHD would correspond to CD3$^+$BY55$^-$ CTL precursors. Alternatively as the unique cytotoxic cell subset which was CD3$^-$BY55$^+$ in cord blood corresponded to NK cells, we cannot exclude the possibility that BY55$^+$ NK cells exert a regulatory effect [19] on the generation of effector cells responsible for GVHD. Evidence in support of this last hypothesis comes from a murine bone marrow transplantation model in which NK cells were transferred with bone marrow cells into allogeneic mice. No GVHD was noticed in these recipients [20].

This work was supported in part by grants from INSERM, Association pour la recherche sur le Cancer (ARC) and from le Comité de Paris de la Ligue contre le Cancer.

References

1. Trinchieri G. Biology of natural killer cells. *Adv Immunol* 1989; 46: 187-276.
2. Lanier LL, Chang C, Azuma M, Ruitenberg JJ, Hemperley JJ, Phillips JH. Molecular and functional analysis of human natural killer cell-associated neural cell adhesion molecule (N-CAM/CD56). *J Immunol* 1991; 146: 4421-4426.
3. Anasetti PC, Martin PJ, June CH, Hellstrom KE, Ledbetter JA, Rabinovich P S, Morishita Y, Hellstrom I, Hansen J A. Induction of calcium flux and enhancement of cytolytic activity in natural killer cells by cross-linking of the sheep erythrocyte binding protein (CD2) and the Fc-receptor (CD16). *J Immunol* 1987; 139: 1772-1779.
4. Lebow LT, Bonavida B. Purification and characterization of cytolytic and noncytolytic human natural killer cell subsets. *Proc Natl Acad Sci USA* 1990; 87: 6063-6067.
5. Tsudo M, Goldman CK, Bongiovanni KF, Chan WC, Winton EF, Yagita M, Grimm EA, Waldmann TA. The p75 peptide is the receptor for interleukin 2 expressed on large granular lymphocytes and is responsible for the interleukin 2 activation of these cells. *Proc Natl Acad Sci USA* 1987; 84: 5394-5398.
6. Litwin V, Gumperz J, Parham P, Phillips JH, Lanier L L. NKB1: A natural killer cell receptor involved in the recognition of polymorphic HLA-B molecules. *J Exp Med* 1994; 180: 537-543.
7. Bottino C, Vitale M, Olcese L, Sivori S, Morelli L, Augugliaro R, Ciccone E, Moretta L, Moretta A. The human natural killer cell receptor for major histocompatibility complex class I molecules. Surface modulation of p58 molecules and their linkage to CD3z chain, FceRIg chain and p56^{lck} kinase. *Eur J Immunol* 1994; 24: 2527-2534.
8. Moretta A, Vitale M, Olcese L, Sivori S, Bottino C, Morelli L, Augugliaro R, Babaresi M, Pende D, Ciccone E, Lopez-Botet M, Moretta L. Human natural killer cell receptors for HLA– class I molecules. Evidence that Kp43 (CD94) molecule functions as receptor for HLA-B alleles. *J Exp Med* 1994; 180: 545-555.
9. Teshigawara K, Wang H-M, Kato K, Smith, KA. Interleukin 2 high-affinity receptor expression requires two distinct binding proteins. *J Exp Med* 1987; 165: 223-238.
10. Maïza H, Leca G, Mansur I-G, Schiavon V, Boumsell L, Bensussan A. A novel 80-kD cell surface structure identifies human circulating lymphocytes with natural killer activity. *J Exp Med* 1993; 178: 1121-1126.
11. Bensussan A, Rabian C, Schiavon V, Bengoufa D, Leca G, Boumsell L. Significant enlargement of a specific subset of CD3+CD8+ peripheral blood leukocytes mediating cytotoxic T-lymphocyte activity during human immunodeficiency virus infection. *Proc Natl Acad Sci USA*. 1993; 90: 9427-9430.
12. Gouttefangeas C, Mansur I-G, Schmid M, Dastot H, Gelin C, Mahouy G, Boumsell L, Bensussan A. The CD39 molecule defines distinct cytotoxic subsets within alloactivated human CD8-positive cells. *Eur J Immunol* 1992; 22: 2681-2685.
13. Leca G, Mansur SE, Bensussan A. Expression of VCAM-1 (CD106) by a subset of TCR γδ-bearing lymphocyte clone. *J Immunol* 1995; 154: 1079-1087.

14. Tschopp J, Nabholz M. Perforin-mediated target cell lysis by cytotoxic T lymphocytes. *Annu Rev Immunol* 1990; 8: 279-285.
15. Gluckman E, Broxmeyer HE, Auerbach A, Friedman H, Douglas GW, Devergie A, Esperou H, Thierry D, Socie G, Lehn P, Cooper S, English D, Kurtzburg J, Bard J, Boyse EA. Hematopoietic reconstitution in a patient with Fanconi's anemia by means of umbilical-cord blood from an HLA-identical sibling. *N Engl J Med* 1989; 321; 1174-1178.
16. Broxmeyer HE, Douglas GW, Hangoc G, Cooper S, Bard J, English D, Arny M, Thomas L, Boyse EA. Human umbilical cord blood as a potential source of transplantable hematopoietic stem / progenitor cells. *Proc Natl Acad Sci USA* 1989; 86: 3828-3832.
17. Abruzzo LV, Mullen CA, Rowley DA. Immunoregulation by natural killer cells. *Cell Immunol* 1986; 98: 266-278.
18. Wagner JE, Kennan NA, Boxmeyer HE, Gluckman E. Allogeneic umbilical cord blood transplantation: report of results in 26 patients. *Blood* 1993; 82 (suppl 1): 86A.
19. Bensussan A, Klatzmann D, Gluckman J-C, Kalil J, Dausset J, Sasportes M. Probable role of suppressor cells and factors in kidney graft survival.*Transplant Proc* 1982; 14: 584-587.
20. Murphy WJ, Bennett M, Kumar V, Longo DL. Donor-type activated natural killer cells promote marrow engraftment and B cell development during allogeneic bone marrow transplantation. *J Immunol* 1992; 148: 2953-2960.

Résumé

Nous décrivons une nouvelle molécule membranaire à l'aide de l'anticorps monoclonal BY55 que nous avons produit contre la lignée leucémique NK, YT2C2. A l'aide de cet anticorps, nous détectons dans le sang périphérique d'un individu normal environ 20% des lymphocytes qui sont des cellules NK et une sous-population lymphocytaire T qui comprend les lymphocytes exprimant le récepteur $\gamma\delta$ et quelques lymphocytes $\alpha\beta$ qui sont essentiellement CD8. Des études fonctionnelles avec des lymphocytes séparés à l'aide d'un trieur de cellules ont démontré clairement que les cellules qui portent à la surface membranaire la glycoprotéine reconnue par BY55 ont une activité tueuse. S'agissant des lymphocytes NK, cette activité cytotoxique est mise en évidence en utilisant la cible cellulaire de référence K562 ; en revanche l'activité cytotoxique des lymphocytes T est révélée en utilisant un test « anticorps CD3-redirigé ». Ces résultats indiquent que l'anticorps BY55 reconnaît une structure membranaire dont l'expression est restreinte aux lymphocytes T cytotoxiques. Des études phénotypiques et fonctionnelles réalisées avec des cellules de la moelle osseuse et du sang de cordon de nouveau-nés indiquent que les lymphocytes cytotoxiques dans ces deux tissus correspondent à des populations lymphocytaires phénotypiquement différentes. Dans le sang de cordon, les lymphocytes cytotoxiques correspondent uniquement aux lymphocytes NK qui représentent environ 30% des lymphocytes, alors que dans la moelle osseuse les lymphocytes qui portent la molécule reconnue par l'anticorps BY55 correspondent à environ 10% des lymphocytes et contiennent à part égale à la fois des cellules NK et des lymphocytes T. Ces résultats sont discutés dans une perspective de choix du tissu pourvoyeur de cellules souches hématopoïétiques destiné à la reconstitution hématologique lors d'une greffe.

6) Clinical results of cord blood transplant

6) *Résultats cliniques des greffes de sang de cordon*

Intrauterine transplantations of foetal hematopoietic stem cells to four foetuses with haemoglobinopathies

O. Ringdén[1,2], M. Westgren[3], S. Eik-Nes[5], S. Ek[1,3], A.M. Brubakk[6], T.H. Bui[4], A. Giambona[7], C. Jakil[7], T. Kiserud[5], A. Kjaeldgaard[3], A. Maggio[7], L. Markling[1], O. Olerup[1], B.M. Svahn[2], F. Orlandi[7]

Departments of [1] Clinical Immunology; [2] Transplantation Surgery and [3] Obstetrics and Gynaecology, Huddinge Hospital, tel.: (46 8) 746 57 23, fax: (46 8) 746 68 69; Department of [4] Genetics, Karolinska Hospital, Stockholm, Sweden; Departments of [5] Obstetrics and Gynaecology and [6] Pediatrics, Trondheim, Norway; Department of [7] Obstetrics and Gynaecology, Ospedale V Cervello, Palermo, Italy

Summary

Foetal liver cell transplantations were approved by ethics committees in Sweden and Italy. Four foetuses were treated in utero *with pooled, cryopreserved foetal liver cells from five to seven donors with a cell-dose ranging from 82-270 x 10^6 and a cell viability from 86 - 93%. A foetus with α-thalassaemia underwent transplantations in the 15th and 31st gestational weeks and was also given intravascular erythrocyte transfusions prenatally. At three weeks of age, HLA-B35 was found in the peripheral blood, although it had not previously been detected in the infant, or in the parents. This child is now two years of age and depends on regular transfusions and chelation therapy. A second foetus with sickle cell anaemia underwent transplantation in the 13th gestational week and is now one year old. A third foetus with β-thalassaemia died from the procedure, which was performed in the 13th gestational week. A fourth foetus with β-thalassaemia who underwent transplantation in the 18th gestational week is now 3 months old. Engraftment was evaluated by Y-body detection, red cell phenotyping, HLA class I and class II typing and PCR for Y-chromosome specific sequence and DNA polymorphism in cord and peripheral blood. In none of these cases were we able to detect evidence of permanent allogeneic stem cell engraftment.*
In conclusion, viable foetal liver cells administered i.v. or i.p. to foetuses after the 12th gestational week failed to engraft.

Haematopoietic stem cells from bone marrow can cure a large number of severe disorders of the blood system, such as leukaemia, severe aplastic anaemia and inborn errors of metabolism [1-3]. The earlier a transplant is performed in children suffering from metabolic disorders, the more likely is the patient to benefit from enzyme replacement by bone marrow transplantation [4]. From gestational weeks 8-12, the foetal liver is the predominant haematopoietic organ in the foetus. In 1953, Billingham and co-workers reported on the induction of acquired tolerance in mice by *in utero* transplantation of allogeneic cells [5]. Subsequently, *in utero* foetal transplantation with foetal haematopoietic stem cells and tolerance induction was performed in sheep, goats, primates and humans [6-11]. In humans, Touraine and co-workers have performed three successful intrauterine transplantations, using foetal liver cells transplanted to foetuses suffering from bare lymphocyte syndrome, severe combined immunodeficiency and β-thalassaemia, respectively. These children are now alive and well at from 5 to 6 1/2 years of age (11 and this issue). Encouraged by these studies, we have created a tissue bank with cryopreserved foetal liver cells to be used for intrauterine transplantation [12,13]. We here report our experience of intrauterine transplantations in four foetuses suffering from haemoglobinopathies.

Material and methods

Ethics

The project was approved by the Regional Ethics Committee at the Karolinska Institute, Stockholm, Sweden, and Sicily, Italy. Furthermore, the project was reviewed by the Ethics Committee of the Swedish Medical Research Council, the Swedish National Council for Medical Ethics and the Norwegian Social Department. Initially, we received permission from the Regional Ethics Committee at the Karolinska Institute to perform two transplants, the results of which were reported to them. Thereafter we obtained approval to perform another 10 transplants.

Collection of foetal liver cells

Foetal liver cells were obtained from legal abortions performed with vacuum curettage in gestational weeks 5-11 [12]. After passage through a metal mesh, the cells were suspended in RPMI 1640 medium, 10% AB serum and 10% DMSO and stepwise frozen over 24 h to -190°C [14]. The women who had given their consent and donated foetal tissue were serologically screened for HIV-l, syphilis, toxoplasmosis, cytomegalovirus, hepatitis B and C, parvovirus and herpes simplex virus [13]. Sex and AB0 type were determined for selection of donors.

Intrauterine transplantation

Frozen foetal liver cells were thawed in a water bath at 37°C, diluted in RPMI with 10% AB serum and washed three times. Viability was evaluated with trypan blue. Injection of 1 ml of cells was performed with a 21-gauge spinal needle under ultrasonographic guidance.

Techniques for monitoring engraftment

Cord blood, peripheral blood or bone marrow (in case 1) were analysed to detect chimaerism, using Y-body detection (sensitivity 12-20%), red cell phenotyping (sensitivity 0.01-1%), HLA class I by serological typing and HLA class II by PCR typing (sensitivity 1-5%) [15]. Furthermore, PCR for Y, restriction fragment polymorphism and a variable number of tandem repeats were performed with a sensitivity of 0.1 to 1% [16].

Results

The first transplantation was performed in the 15th gestational week in a male foetus suffering from α-thalassaemia. The diagnosis was made in the 12th week by chorion villi biopsy. The foetus was homozygotic for α-thalassaemia with deletion of all four α-globin structured genes (Institute of Molecular Medicine, Oxford). The mother had previously given birth to a healthy boy and had lost two foetuses in the 28th week of gestation due to hydrops foetalis. About 219×10^6 cells from seven foetal livers were injected i.p. with an estimated cell dose of 2.2×10^8 cells/kg bodyweight. Cell viability was 93%. Weekly ultrasound examinations were performed during pregnancy at the National Centre for Ultrasound and Foetal Therapy in Trondheim. Due to cardiomegaly and a deteriorating condition, an erythrocyte transfusion was given to the foetus in the 29th week. No evidence of engraftment or synthesis of the α-globin chain was seen. HLA class I and HLA class II were only of the recipient type, the blood group was only 0, as previously, and only male chromosomes were detected. Therefore retransplantation was performed in the 31st week. About 270×10^6 cells from six foetal livers with a viability of 86% were injected i.v. An intravascular blood transfusion was given in the 32nd and 35th weeks. The boy was delivered by caesarean section in the 37th week due to breech presentation. Since birth, the boy has required regular blood transfusions. At three weeks of age, HLA-B35 was found. This HLA class was not found in previous samples either from the boy (HLA A1, 11; B15, 17; Cw6; DR 5,5; DQ3,3) or from his parents (mother HLA A11; B15, 16; Cw7; DR 5,5; DQ 3,3; father HLA A1, 11; B15, 17; Cw6; DR 2,5; DQ 1,3). However, chimaerism was not detected with any other technique. The boy is now two years of age and dependent on transfusions and chelation therapy. He has no signs of engraftment.

The second patient is a female with sickle cell anaemia who was given 92×10^6 cells from five foetal livers i.p. in the 13th gestational week. The cell dose was 1.3×10^8 cells/kg with a viability of 91%. Caesarean section was performed at term and the child is now eight months of age and without signs of engraftment.

The third patient was a male with β-thalassaemia, who was given 92×10^6 cells from five foetal livers from female donors. Cells were injected i.p. in the 13th gestational week. The cell dose was 1.2×10^8 cells/kg body weight. The cells were accidentally cooled on ice before injection, which was postponed due to technical difficulties. The foetus initially had normal cardiac activity, but died within 24 hrs after the procedure.

The fourth patient is a female with β-thalassaemia. In the 18th gestational week, 188×10^6 cells from five foetal livers, all male donors, were given i.v. Cell viability was 92% and the estimated cell dose was 1.7×10^8 cells/kg. The mother was delivered at term. The girl is now four months of age and shows no signs of engraftment of donor cells.

Discussion

In these foetuses, foetal liver cell transplantations were performed from the 13th to the 18th gestational week. The failure to see permanent evidence of engraftment of transplanted cells occurred most probably because the transplantations were performed too late. We believe that graft failure was due to allograft rejection in all three surviving children. After the 12th gestational week, immunocompetence starts to develop in the human foetus [17, 18].

Our experience contrasts with that of Touraine et al, whose first two transplantations were performed in the 26th and 28th weeks [10, 11]. However, both these foetuses had severe immunodeficiencies and therefore were unable to mount an immune response towards the transplanted cells, even at this late gestational age. In children with severe combined immunodeficiencies, before the transplantation, conditioning is not always needed because of immunoincompetence and an inability to reject allogeneic cells. In their third patient, a foetus suffering from thalassaemia major, transplantation was performed in the 12th gestational week, which was probably before immunological maturation had started and tolerance was therefore induced [11].

In contrast to Touraine and co-workers, we used cryopreserved cells from several donors. Touraine used non-frozen foetal liver cells from one or two donors. However, in our foetal haematopoietic cells, viability was above 86% in all cases. In our experience, *in vitro* studies have shown that cryopreservation is well tolerated by foetal liver cells [14, 19]. After the frozen cells thawed, the proportion of CD34-positive cells tended to increase [14]. Thawed cryopreserved foetal liver cells had the same capacity as non-frozen cells for colony formation of CFU-E, CFU-GM and CFU-GEMM colonies [19]. Thus, these studies demonstrated that the transplanted foetal liver cells indeed contained haematopoietic stem cells and precursor cells.

The third foetus unfortunately died after the procedure. The reason for this may have been the i.p. injection of 1 ml of cold cells, which may have caused arrhythmia and heart failure.

Three of our transplants were performed via the i.p. route and two were given i.v.. The i.p. route is less efficient than the i.v. However, it is technically more difficult to inject cells via the umbilical vein than to inject them i.p. at early gestational ages. One can perform an intracardiac injection, but this may be risky for the foetus. When we injected radiolabelled foetal liver cells 24 hrs prior to abortion, we obtained a four-fold higher radioactivity in the foetal liver after i.v. than when using i.p. injection (Westgren, in preparation). Therefore, i.v. injection is preferred whenever technically possible. However, Touraine *et al* noted engraftment after i.p. *in utero* transplantation in the 12th gestational week (Touraine *et al*, this issue).

Using various techniques to detect chimaerism, we were able to detect engraftment in foreign cells only in the first patient having a transient appearance of HLA-B35 three weeks after birth. This finding may have been due to transient engraftment of some foreign cells injected at the second transplant in the 31st gestational week.

Slavin and co-workers used T-cell-depleted bone marrow from parents or siblings of patients with metachromatic leukodystrophy and thalassaemia major [20]. They failed to achieve engraftment following *in utero* transplantation. However, this is in accordance with experiments using adult T-cell-depleted bone marrow in experimental animals in which engraftment was rarely achieved [7].

To conclude, we used viable foetal liver cells from the 5th to 11th gestational week with a high colony-forming capacity. Nevertheless, we failed to achieve engraftment *in utero* when performing transplantations in the 13th to 18th gestational week in four foetuses suffering from haemoglobinopathies. In foetuses showing metabolic disorders other than severe immunodeficiencies, intrauterine transplantations should probably be performed no later than the 12th gestational week because of the risk of allograft rejection.

Acknowledgements

This study was supported by grants from the Swedish Medical Research Council (B95-16X-05971-15B), the Swedish Cancer Society (0070-B95O9XCC), the Children's Cancer Foundation (1994/060) and the Tobias Foundation.

References

1. Thomas ED, Storb R, Clift RA, Fefer A, Johnson FL, Neiman PE, Lerner KG, Glucksberg H, Buckner CD. Bone marrow transplantation I and II. *N Engl J Med* 1975; 292: 832-843, 895-902.
2. Hobbs JR. Bone marrow transplantation for inborn errors. *Lancet* 1981; ii: 735-739.
3. Groth CG and Ringdén O. Transplantation in relation to the treatment of inherited disease. *Transplantation* 1984; 38: 319-327.
4. Hugh-Jones K, Hobbs JR, Vellodi A, Hancock M, Sheldon J, Jones S. Long-term follow-up of children with Hurler's disease treated with bone marrow transplantation. In: Hobbs JR ed. Correction of Certain Genetic Diseases by Transplantation, 1989. London: COGENT 1989; 103-111.
5. Flake AW, Harrison MR, Adzick NS, Zanjani ED. Transplantation of foetal haematopoietic chimeras. *Science* 1986; 233: 776-778.
6. Harrison MR, Slotnick NR, Crombleholme TM, Golbus MS, Tarantal AF, Zanjani ED. In-utero transplantation of foetal liver haematopoietic stem cells in monkeys. *Lancet* 1989; 2: 1425-27.
7. Pearce RD, Kiehm D, Armstrong DT, Little PB, Callahan JW, Klunder LR, Clarke JTR. Induction of haematopoietic chimerism in the caprine foetus by intraperitoneal injection of foetal liver cells. *Experientia* 1989; 45: 307-8.
8. Zanjani ED, Pallavicini MG, Ascensao JL, Flake AW, Langlois RG, Reitsma M, MacKintosh FR, Stutes D, Harrison MR, Tavassoli M. Engraftment and long-term expression of human foetal hemopoietic stem cells in sheep following transplantation *in utero*. *J Clin Invest* 1992; 89: 1178-1188.
9. Billingham RE, Brent L, Medawar PB. Actively acquired tolerance of foreign cells. *Nature* (Lond). 1953;172: 603-606.
10. Touraine JL, Raudrant D, Royo C, et al. In utero transplantation of stem cells in the bare lymphocyte syndrome. *Lancet* 1989; i: 1382.
11. Touraine JL, Raudrant D, Royo C, Rebaud A, Barbier F, Roncarolo MG, Touraine F, Laplace S, Gebuhrer L, Bétuel H, Frappaz D, Freycon F, Vullo C. *In utero* transplantation hemopoietic stem cells in humans. *Transpl Proc* 1991; 23(1): 1706-1708.
12. Westgren M, Ek S, Bui T-H, Hagenfeldt L, Markling L, Pschera H, Seiger A, Sundstrom E and Ringdén O. Establishment of a tissue bank for foetal stem cell transplantation. *Acta Obst Gynecol Scand* 1994; 73: 385-388.
13. Ek S, Westgren M, Ringdén O, et al. Infectious screening in foetal stem cell collection. *Foetal Diagn Ther* 1994; 9: 357-361.
14. Ek S, Ringdén O, Markling L, Dahlberg N, Pschera H, Seiger A, Sundstrom E and Westgren M. Effects of cryopreservation on subsets of foetal liver cells. *Bone Marrow Transplant* 1993; 11: 395-398.
15. Olerup O, Zetterquist H. HLA-DR typing by .PCR amplification with sequence-specific primers (PCR-SSP) in 2 hours: An alternative to serological DR typing in clinical practice including donor-recipient matching in cadaveric transplantation. *Tissue Antigens* 1992; 39: 225-235.
16. Bailey DM, Affara NA, Ferguson-Smith MA. The X-Y homologous gene Amelogenin maps to the short arms of both the X and Y chromosomes and is highly conserved in primates. *Genomics* 1992; 14: 203-205.
17. van Furth R, Schuit HRE, Hijmans W. The immunological development of the human foetus. *J Exp Med* 1965; 122: 1173-1187.
18. August CSA, Berkel I, Driscoll S, Merler E. Onset of lymphocyte function in the developing human foetus. *Pediatr Res* 1971; 5: 539-547.
19. Ek S, Markling L, Westgren M, Kjaeldgaard A, Ringdén O. Effects of cytokines on the formation of human foetal haematopoietic cells from the human fetal liver. Submitted for publication.
20. Slavin S, Naparstek D, Xiegler M. Intrauterine bone marrow transplantation for correlation of geneitic disorders in man. *Exp Hematol* 1990; 18: 658.

Résumé

La transplantation de cellules de foie fœtal a été approuvée par les comités d'éthique de différents pays : France, Suède et Italie. Trois fœtus ont été traités *in utero* avec un pool de cellules de foie fœtal cryopréservées provenant de 5 à 7 donneurs, le nombre de cellules injectées a été de 82 à 270×10^6 avec une viabilité de 86% à 93%. Un fœtus atteint de α-thalassémie a été transplanté entre la 15e et la 31e semaine de gestation, il a également reçu une transfusion de culot globulaire *in utero*. A l'âge de 3 semaines, HLA-B35 a été retrouvé dans le sang alors que cet antigène n'était pas présent chez l'enfant ou ses parents. Cet enfant actuellement âgé de 2 ans est thalassémique, traité par transfusions et chélation du fer. Un second fœtus, atteint de drépanocytose, a été transplanté à l'âge de 13 semaines de gestation, il est actuellement âgé de 1 an sans signe de prise de la greffe. Un troisième fœtus atteint de β-thalassémie a été transplanté à l'âge de 18 semaines de gestation, il est maintenant âgé de 3 mois. La prise de la greffe a été étudiée par détection de Y, phénotype érythrocytaire, typage HLA de classe I et II, et PCR pour les séquences spécifiques de l'Y et le polymorphisme du DNA dans le cordon et le sang. Dans aucun de ces cas, il n'a été possible de montrer un chimérisme durable. En conclusion, des cellules viables de foie fœtal administrées IV ou IP après la 12e semaine de gestation n'ont pas été capables d'être greffées.

In utero transplantation of fetal liver stem cells into human fetuses for immunodeficiency and thalassemia treatment

Jean-Louis Touraine

Département de Transplantation et Immunologie clinique, Pavillon P, Hôpital E-Herriot, place d'Arsonval, 69437 Lyon Cedex 03, France, tel.: (33) 72 11 01 51, fax: (33) 72 11 02 71

Summary

Following 19 years of experience in postnatal fetal liver transplantation (FLT), we have developed a new therapeutic method, namely the in utero *transplantation of stem cells from the human fetal liver. This early transplant takes advantage of the immunological tolerance that exists in young fetal recipients. The six fetuses that we treated were 28, 26, 17, 17, 14 and 12 weeks postfertilization. Three patients had immunodeficiencies, two others had thalassemia major and the last one had Niemann-Pick disease (type A). Donor cells were obtained from 7- to 13- week-old fetuses, with conditions approved by the National Committee for Bioethics. Donors and recipients were not matched. Under ultrasonic visualization, the fetal cells were infused through the umbilical vein of four patients and injected intraperitoneally into the 2 other ones. The first patient, born in 1988, has evidence of engraftment and reconstitution of cell-mediated immunity. This child, who had bare lymphocyte syndrome, has no clinical manifestation of the disease and lives normally at home. The second child was born in 1989; donor cell engraftment has been proven (distinct HLA phenotype) and the severe immunodeficiency has been corrected to a large degree. One fetus with chronic granulomatous disease developed fatal bradycardia after a second* in utero *FLT. One fetal patient with thalassemia major had cardiac arrest following the intravenous infusion. The fifth patient, transplanted intraperitoneally at 12 weeks of fetal age, to treat thalassemia major, has evidence of donor cell take (Y chromosome in a female patient) and a partial effect on thalassemia has been obtained (HbA increased up to 30%, one year after birth). The last patient treated by* in utero *FLT had Niemann-Pick disease. He is now in excellent condition and we are waiting for birth to know whether or not the disease can be cured. In all three patients who were born, no side-effect developed in the mother nor in the fetus. Several advantages appear to be associated with* in utero *FLT: increased probability of graft take with development of specific immunological tolerance, ideal isolation of patient (in the uterus), and optimal environment for fetal cell development (in the fetal host). Immunological tolerance, in T cells deriving from donor stem cells, after education within host thymus, was shown to involve clonal deletion for donor antigens (deletion induced by donor dendritic cells and macrophages), and clonal anergy for host antigens (anergy induced by host thymic epithelial cells). High IL-10 production persisted for many years and was likely to play a role in the stable chimerism and tolerance maintenance.*

In our Department, the transplantation of fetal liver cells, in association with syngeneic thymic cells, was used to treat patients with severe combined immunodeficiency (IDD) when there was no HLA-identical donor available for a bone marrow transplantation as well as patients with inborn errors of metabolism (IEM) or with severe aplastic anemia. Over the last 19 years, we have performed more than 230 fetal tissue transplants (FLT) to treat 63 patients. In both IDD and IEM, FLT into postnatal recipients has demonstrated beneficial effects. More precisely, 67% of the patients were either cured or improved significantly because of the treatment, and the survival curves showed a durable efficacy *(Figure 1)*. However, almost one-third of the patients did not experience significant improvement after fetal liver or thymus transplantation. In most cases, this lack of efficacy was due to either of two factors: first, an insufficient graft take in patients with rejection capabilities, and, second, late diagnosis of the initial disease and the presence of severe infection prior to transplantation. To overcome these two difficulties, we recently developed *in utero* transplantation into fetuses with conditions diagnosed during pregnancy. We reasoned that much earlier transplants (before immune development and before exposure of the host to microorganisms) would lead to an increased probability of graft take and a lower risk of infection.

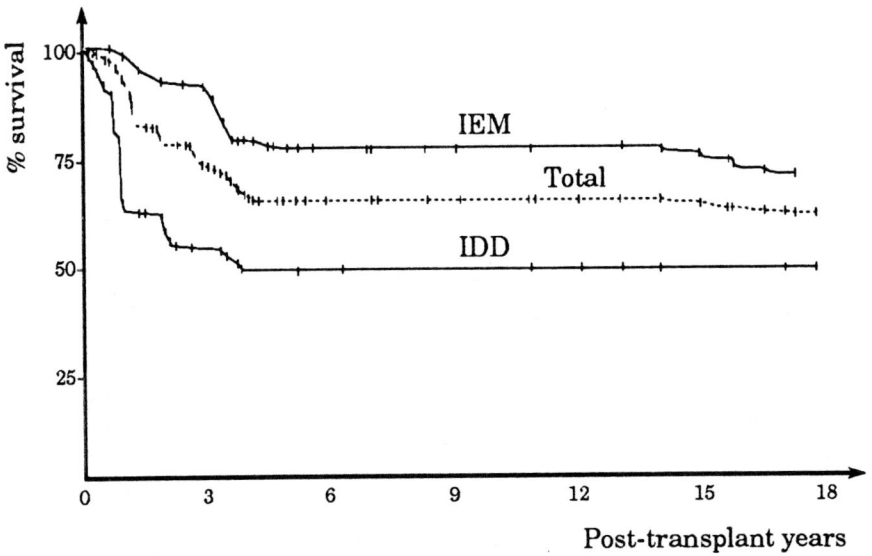

Figure 1. Survival of patients with severe immunodeficiency diseases (IDD) or inborn errors of metabolism (IEM) treated by fetal tissue transplantation. The global survival of all patients from these two groups is shown by the line 'total'.

In utero fetal liver transplantation

Six fetal patients have been treated by *in utero* FLT at 28, 26, 17, 17, 14 and 12 weeks postfertilization. Three patients had immunodeficiencies, two had thalassemia major and the sixth one had Niemann-Pick disease (type A) *(Table I)*. Donor cells were obtained from 7- 13- week-old-fetuses, with conditions approved by the National Committee for Bioethics. Donors and reci-

Table I. Modalities and results of *in utero* transplants in human fetuses.

Patients	Diseases	Age of fetal patients[a]	Age of fetal donors[a]	Date of transplant	Route of cell infusion	Date of birth	Evidence for engraftment	Correction of initial disease	Clinical status
D.T.	BLS[b]	28	7 and 7.5	06.30.1988	I.V.	08.17.1988	HLA markers	Reconstitution of T-cells with normal functions	Alive & well
M.H.	SCID[c]	26	7.5	06.08.1989	I.V.	08.07.1989	HLA markers	Reconstitution of T-cells with subnormal functions	Alive & well
M.R.	TM[d]	12	9.5	10.10.1989	I.P.	03.25.1990	Y chromosome	Presence of HbA coexisting with abnormal Hb	Alive & well
R.M.	TM[d]	17	11.5	04.30.1991	I.V.	------	------	------	Bradycardia & fetal death
A.V.	CGD[e]	17 21	13.5 14	04.22.1992 05.22.1992	I.V. I.V.	------	------	------	Bradycardia & fetal death
C.D.	N-P (A)[f]	14 16	12 13	03.07.1995 03.21.1995	I.P. I.P.	------	N.E.	N.E.	Alive & well

[a] weeks postfertilization
[b] bare lymphocyte syndrome
[c] severe combined immunodeficiency disease
[d] β_0 thalassemia major
[e] chronic granulomatous disease
[f] Niemann-Pick disease (type A)
N.E.: Not Evaluable

pients were not matched. The fetal cells were infused through the umbilical vein of 4 patients and injected intraperitoneally into the 2 other fetuses, under ultrasonic visualization.

The first fetal patient suffered from bare lymphocyte syndrome, a genetically-transmitted form of combined immunodeficiency disease due to lack of expression of HLA antigens [1, 2]. Infections, especially with opportunistic microorganisms, are responsible for the death of these infants, unless they grow up isolated in a fully sterile atmosphere while they are successfully reconstituted with stem cell transplants. When carried out postnatally, however, such a stem cell transplant, in the form of either a bone marrow transplant or a fetal liver transplant, is usually associated with graft failure due to the presence of allogeneic reactions in the host (persisting transplant immunity) and to high susceptibility to infections (defective immunity to infectious antigens). Prenatal diagnosis of bare lymphocyte syndrome could be performed by HLA analysis of lymphocytes in fetal blood [3] and was followed by *in utero* FLT at 28 weeks *(Table 1)*. The transplant was carried out, involving the infusion into the umbilical vein of 7ml of culture medium containing a suspension of 16×10^6 fetal liver and thymic epithelial cells [4-6]. Over the months following the *in utero* transplantation, no adverse effects were observed in the mother or her baby.

The child had evidence of engraftment: initially, 10% of lymphocytes had normal expression of class I HLA antigens and these cells expressed the HLA A9 specificity of donor origin, which made transplanted cells readily detectable in the initial test at birth and in subsequent tests performed. The number of cells deriving from the *in utero* transplant increased up to 26% among peripheral blood lymphocytes at 14 months and stabilized at 17% since the sixth year of age. These results demonstrated the persisting engraftment of the fetal liver cells infused into the sick fetus. In parallel, T cell maturity and immunological reconstitution progressed. T lymphocyte reconstitution is now considered to be virtually complete, and the proliferative responses to antigens (*Candida* antigens, CMV antigens and tetanus toxoid) has occurred and gradually increased to a normal level. Immunoglobulin levels were still relatively low. The child's present condition is excellent. He has not experienced any severe infection and he lives a normal life at home.

After the encouraging results of the first *in utero* fetal liver transplant, a second fetus with a complete form of severe combined deficiency was treated in 1989. Fetal liver transplantation was performed at 26 weeks postfertilization after a prenatal diagnosis of severe immunodeficiency (complete lack of $CD2^+$, $CD3^+$, $CD4^+$, $CD8^+$ lymphocytes but presence of B cells in peripheral blood of this fetus).

The transplant was carried out under the same conditions as the first fetus treated *in utero*. It involved intravenous infusion of 37×10^6 fetal liver cells in the umbilical vein, under ultrasound control *(Table 1)*. There were no side-effects and the child was born normally two months later. Engraftment has therefore been obtained and donor stem cells differentiated into T lymphocytes with adequate immune function *(Table 1)*. Recent analyses confirmed a progressively increasing number of peripheral blood T cells, derived from the cells transplanted *in utero*. Together with the development of a significant population of donor-derived T lymphocytes, satisfactory proliferative responses to various stimuli, including phytomitogens and specific antigens, appeared and grew up to virtually normal levels.

This young girl is now healthy, with a satisfactory immunological reconstitution and lives normally at home, only receiving monthly immunoglobulin infusions.

In 1992, another fetus *(Table 1)* received two fetal liver transplants to treat chronic granulomatous disease. The first transplant was carried out uneventfully by umbilical vein infusion at 17 weeks postfertilization but the number of cells available for infusion was considered insufficient. A second transplant was therefore attempted at 21 weeks but unfortunately resulted in fetal bradycardia (possibly due to relatively rapid infusion of a larger number of cells) and it led to fetal death within one hour.

Due to the results obtained in IDD, we decided to perform *in utero* FLT in fetal patient with severe non-immune hematological disorders. In such conditions, however, graft take may not be facilitated by immune incompetence of the fetal host and we therefore assumed that grafting had to be carried out during the first trimester or the beginning of the second trimester of pregnancy, at a time when normal fetuses have not yet developed cell-mediated immunity [7].

A first young fetus with β^0 thalassemia major was treated in 1989 *(Table I)*. Fetal liver transplantation was carried out at 12 weeks postfertilization. The transplant consisted of intraperitoneal injection of 3×10^8 viable cells under ultrasound control.

Studies performed after birth showed presence of thalassemia. However, there were a few cells of donor origin: PCR gene amplification techniques revealed Y chromosome-specific DNA fragments in peripheral blood lymphocytes of this girl *(Table I)*. In addition, hemoglobin A was found to account for 0.9% of all hemoglobin at six months. No further transplant was needed in this infant who is presently in very good general condition. At one year of age, she had received one blood transfusion, her total hemoglobin level was slightly below normal and the hemoglobin A percentage, 3 months after the blood transfusion, was 30%. These data suggest that the engraftment of a few donor cells has been followed by some cell proliferation, resulting in partial correction of this hematological disorder.

In a further fetal patient in whom a prenatal diagnosis of β^0 thalassemia had also been made, fetal liver cell transplantation was attempted by cord blood infusion at 17 weeks postfertilization. Four ml of blood were drawn, and 10ml of fetal cells containing medium were infused. Unfortunately, fetal bradycardia resulted, possibly related to the relatively rapid infusion, and led to fetal death within one hour.

More recently, 1995, we have performed 2 FLT *in utero* into a fetus with Niemann-Pick disease (type A) *(Table I)*. The mother and her fetus are in excellent condition and we are waiting for birth to perform further investigations.

Tolerance and MHC restriction in human chimeras

Both in patients treated by postnatal FLT and in fetuses receiving FLT *in utero*, the full reconstitution could develop despite a complete mismatch of HLA class I and class II antigens between donor and host. The separation of T and B lymphocyte populations, and the development of cell lines and clones from peripheral blood lymphocytes of these patients, followed by HLA typing, showed that all T lymphocytes were of donor origin, while most B lymphocytes, monocytes and NK cells were shown to be of host type in the reconstituted and now chimeric patients.

Tolerance between donor-derived T cells and host-derived B cells/monocytes was confirmed *in vitro*. Specific unresponsiveness of lymphocytes towards the host cells in a primary mixed leucocyte culture was observed [8]. However, by clonal analysis, $CD4^+$ and $CD8^+$ T cell clones were isolated and shown to be specifically reactive to the HLA class II and class I molecules. The frequency of $CD8^+$ host-reactive T cells was high, in the same range as that found for $CD8^+$ allo-reactive T cells [8]. By contrast, no donor-reactive $CD8^+$ T cells were observed, indicating that in these patients treated with allogeneic FLT, donor-reactive but not host-reactive cells are deleted from the T cell repertoire [8]. Similar findings have been obtained recently in the SCID-hu mouse [9], suggesting tolerance to antigens of the stem cell donor via clonal deletion and tolerance to antigens of the host thymus via clonal anergy.

Tolerance is therefore exerted towards all donor and host antigens, in these patients. In contrast, the HLA restriction of antigen recognition was shown to be imposed upon the patient's T cells by the host determinants only. Antigen-presenting cells of the host could effectively present tetanus toxoid antigens or Epstein-Barr virus antigens to the allogeneic T lymphocytes [10-12]. The antigenic peptide was, as usual, presented in the groove of an HLA molecule but, in this case, it was a different HLA molecule from that of the T lymphocyte itself. The study of numerous clones has demonstrated that T cells from these patients recognize antigen in the context of the allogeneic HLA determinants [10, 12, 13].

Similarly, the *in vivo* defense against virus infections of various kinds has been normal and has not been hindered by the HLA mismatch between infected cells and cytotoxic T lymphocytes able to control the infection. Both *in vivo* and *in vitro* data led us to postulate the "Allo + X" hypothesis, according to which some T lymphocytes can develop a recognition for the X antigen in the context of allogeneic determinants instead of the previously known recognition for "Self + X" [14, 15].

The ontogenetic development of T lymphocytes with such recognition structures takes place primarily in the fetal thymus and might be envisioned schematically to occur as follows. A first degree of diversity develops with a variety of thymocytes which have a primary recognition structure for the histocompatibility antigens (possibly associated with a common peptide). In normal circumstances, only those T cells with recognition for self-histocompatibility antigens are solicited, since the alloantigens are not encountered in the thymus. These cells are induced to proliferate and to develop the full repertoire of antigen recognition in association with self recognition. In chimeric patients, a given set of other histocompatibility antigens is also presented continuously to the differentiating T cells. Those T cells with recognition for the given alloantigens are then solicited, they expand by proliferation and they develop the gene rearrangement leading to the expression of the T cell receptor. In these chimeric patients, T cells that recognize antigen in the context of allo-specificities are positively selected.

A very significant production increase of IL-10 production by cells from these patients has been observed and postulated to play a part in immunological tolerance to alloantigens [16]. Recent measures of the spontaneous production of IL-10 by peripheral blood mononuclear cells from 2 patients treated by FLT *in utero* demonstrated levels significantly higher than in normal controls after 24 hrs of culture: 251pg/ml and 998pg/ml for the 2 patients respectively versus less than 150pg/ml in the controls; and after 48 hrs of culture: 439pg/ml and 1475pg/ml in the patients *versus* less than 150pg/ml in the controls.

Both donor T cells and host accessory cells appeared to contribute to these high IL-10 levels, thus suppressing the activity of host-reactive T cells *in vivo* and participating to clonal anergy of donor-derived T cells to host antigens.

Conclusion

Fetal liver is an efficient source of stem cells for transplantation in children with immunodeficiency diseases or inborn errors of metabolism. Despite HLA mismatch between donor and host, engraftment, chimerism and tolerance are obtained, and immunological reconstitution occurs, with long-term survival in excess of 60%. However, transplantation of stem cells *in utero* should be the optimal therapy for fetuses with a variety of immunological or hematological disorders diagnosed early in gestation. *In utero* fetal liver transplantation has several advantages over postnatal fetal liver transplantation: increased probability of graft take, ideal isolation of the patient (in the uterus), and optimal environment for fetal cell development (in the fetal host). Initial results are promising, and it can now be proposed as a real alternative to therapeutic abortion or to delayed, postnatal transplantation.

Acknowledgments

I am grateful to D Raudrant, A Rebaud, P Cesbron, L Gebuhrer, MG Roncarolo, H Bétuel, C Royo, F Touraine, F Freycon, G Souillet, D Frappaz, N Philippe, F Barbier and MT Zabot for help in these treatments and studies.

References

1. Touraine JL, Bétuel H, Souillet G, Jeune M. Combined immunodeficiency disase associated with absence of cell-surface HLA A and B antigens. *J Pediat* 1978; 93: 47-51.
2. Touraine JL. The bare lymphocyte syndrome. *Lancet* 1981; 1: 319-321.
3. Durandy A, Cerf-Bensussan N, Dumez Y, Griscelli C. Prenatal diagnosis of severe combined immunodeficiency with defective synthesis of HLA molecule. *Prenat Diagn* 1987; 7: 27-31.
4. Berkowitz RL, Chitkara U, Wilkins I, Lynch L, Mehalek K.E. Technical aspects of intravascular intrauterine transfusions: Lessons learned from 33 procedures. *Am J of Obst and Gynecol* 1987; 157, 4-9.
5. Raudrant D, Touraine J-L, Rebaud A. *In utero* transplantation of stem cells in humans: Technical aspects and clinical experience during pregnancy. *Bone Marrow Transplant* 1992; 9 (suppl 1): 98-100
6. Touraine J-L, Raudrant D, Royo C, Rebaud A, Roncarolo M G, Souillet G, Philippe N, Touraine F, Bétuel H. *In utero* transplantation of stem cells in the bare lymphocyte syndrome. *Lancet* 1989; 1: 1382.
7. Royo C, Touraine J-L, de Bouteiller O. Ontogeny of T-lymphocyte differentiation in the human fetus: Acquisition of phenotype and functions. *Thymus* 1987; 10: 57-73.
8. Bacchetta R, Vandekerckhove BAE, Bigler M, Roncarolo M G. Human and mouse SCID models to study tolerance after HLA-mismatched fetal stem cell transplantation. *Exp Hematol* 1992; 20: 722.
9. Vandekerckhove BAE, Namikawa R, Bacchetta R, Roncarolo M G. Human hematopoietic cells and thymic epithelial cells induce tolerance via different mechanisms in the SCID-hu mouse thymus. *J Exp Med* 1992; 175: 1033-1043.
10. Roncarolo M G, Touraine J-L, Bancherau J. Cooperation between major histocompatibility complex mismatched mononuclear cells from a human chimera in the production of antigen-specific antibody. *J Clin Invest* 1986; 77: 673-80.
11. Plotnicky H, Touraine JL. Cytotoxic T cells from a human chimera induce regression of Epstein-Barr virus-infected allogeneic host cells. *Int Immunol* 1993; 5: 1413-1420.
12. Roncarolo M G, Yssel H, Touraine J-L, Bacchetta R, Gebuhrer L, de Vries J.E., Spits H. Antigen recognition by MHC-incompatible cells of a human mismatched chimera. *J Exp Med* 1988; 168: 2139-52.
13. Roncarolo M G, Yssel H, Touraine J-L, Bétuel H, de Vries J, Spits H. Autoreactive T cell clones specific for class I and class II HLA antigens isolated from a human chimera. *J Exp Med* 1988; 167: 1523-1534.
14. Touraine J-L. Bone marrow and fetal liver transplantation in immunodeficiencies and inborn errors of metabolism: Lack of significant restriction of T-cell function in long term chimeras despite HLA-mismatch. *Immunol Rev* 1983; 1: 103-21.
15. Touraine J-L, Bétuel H. Immunodeficiency diseases and expression of HLA antigens. *Human Immunol* 1981; 2: 147-153.
16. Bacchetta R, Bigler M, Touraine J-L, Parkman R, Tovo P A, Abrams J. de Waal Malefyt R, de Vries J E, Roncarolo M G. High levels of interleukin 10 production *in vivo* are associated with tolerance in SCID patients transplanted with HLA mismatched hematopoietic stem cells. *J Exp Med* 1994; 179: 493-502.

Résumé

Après avoir réalisé des greffes de cellules du foie fœtal (GCFF) dans des circonstances post-natales, pendant 19 ans, nous avons développé une nouvelle méthode thérapeutique qui consiste en la greffe *in utero* de cellules souches du foie fœtal humain. Cette greffe très précoce tire bénéfice de la tolérance immunologique qui existe chez le jeune receveur fœtal. Les six fœtus que nous avons traités étaient âgés de 30, 28, 19, 19, 16 et 14 semaines d'aménorrhée. Trois malades avaient des déficits immunitaires, deux autres avaient une thalassémie grave et le dernier avait une maladie de Niemann-Pick de type A. Les cellules greffées provenaient de fœtus donneurs, âgé de 9 à 15 semaines d'aménorrhée, et prélevés dans les conditions définies par le Comité National d'Ethique. Donneurs et receveurs n'étaient pas appariés en terme d'histocompatibilité. Sous contrôle échographique, les cellules fœtales étaient perfusées au niveau de la veine ombilicale, chez 4 fœtus, et injectées par voie intrapéritonéale chez les 2 autres. Chez le premier malade, né en 1988, il existe une prise de greffe prouvée ainsi qu'une reconstitution de l'immunité cellulaire. Cet enfant, qui présentait un syndrome des lymphocytes dénudés, n'a, grâce à cette greffe, pas de manifestation clinique de la maladie et il vit normalement chez lui. Chez le deuxième malade né en 1989, il existe aussi une prise de greffe authentifiée par la présence de cellules ayant un phénotype HLA différent et le déficit immunitaire sévère a pu être en grande partie corrigé. Un fœtus atteint d'une granulomatose chronique est décédé d'une bradychardie après une deuxième greffe *in utero*. Un deuxième fœtus, avec une thalassémie grave, est également décédé d'une bradychardie immédiatement après l'injection intraveineuse. La 5ème malade, greffée à l'âge de 14 semaines par voie intrapéritonéale pour traiter une thalassémie grave, présente des signes de prise de greffe (identification du chromosome Y dans certaines cellules de cette jeune patiente) et la thalassémie a pu être partiellement améliorée avec un taux d'hémoglobine A de 30% à l'âge d'un an. Le dernier patient traité par CGFF *in utero* avait une maladie de Niemann-Pick de type A. Il est actuellement en excellente condition et nous attendons la naissance pour pouvoir évaluer le degré d'efficacité de la greffe dans cette pathologie. Chez les trois enfants nés, aucun effet secondaire ne s'est manifesté chez la mère ou le fœtus. De plus, la greffe *in utero* de cellules souches du foie fœtal présente plusieurs avantages : une meilleure probabilité de prise de la greffe associée au développement d'une tolérance immunologique spécifique ; une isolation parfaite du fœtus dans l'utérus maternel ; enfin, un environnement idéal pour le développement des cellules fœtales (chez le receveur fœtal). Il a été démontré que la tolérance immunologique, dans les lymphocytes T provenant des cellules souches du donneur après « éducation » dans le thymus de l'hôte, s'exerce d'une part *via* une délétion clonale vis-à-vis des antigènes du donneur (délétion induite par les cellules dendritiques et les macrophages du donneur) et d'autre part *via* une anergie clonale vis-à-vis des antigènes du receveur (par l'intermédiaire des cellules épithéliales thymiques de l'hôte). Enfin il a été montré qu'une production importante d'IL-10 persistait de nombreuses années après la greffe et semblait jouer un rôle dans l'établissement d'un chimérisme stable et le maintien de la tolérance.

Allogeneic umbilical cord blood transplantation: report of the international cord blood transplant registry

John E. Wagner

Department of Pediatrics, Division of Bone Marrow Transplantation of the University of Minnesota, School of Medicine, Minneapolis, Minnesota, USA, tel.: (612) 626 2778, fax: (612) 626 2815

Introduction

In an attempt to reduce the morbidity and mortality associated with allogeneic bone marrow transplantation, clinical investigators in Asia, Australia, Europe, North America and South America have evaluated umbilical cord and placental blood as an alternate source of hematopoietic stem and progenitor cells for transplantation. Early successes with the transplantation of umbilical cord blood have prompted considerable investigation in this stem cell source. Numerous laboratory investigators have subsequently confirmed the high frequency of primitive hematopoietic progenitors as well as initiated a description of the functional capacities of the neonatal immune system. As a result of these clinical and laboratory observations, the large scale banking of umbilical cord blood for clinical transplantation has been initiated worldwide. Ontologically, hematopoiesis begins in the primitive yolk sac early after conception, passes through an hepatic phase shortly thereafter and then enters the bone marrow space at the end of the second trimester where it remains almost exclusively throughout adulthood. It has long been known that human umbilical cord and placental blood contain hematopoietic progenitor cells at high frequency. The frequency of granulocyte-macrophage (CFU-GM) progenitor cells equals or exceeds that of adult bone marrow and greatly surpasses that of unmobilized adult peripheral blood. It was for this reason that umbilical cord blood was considered as a potential source of transplantable hematopoietic stem cells in the mid-1980's. While it is has yet to be determined whether a single umbilical cord blood collection contains a sufficient number of hematopoietic stem and progenitor cells to repopulate the bone marrow of an adult-size allogeneic recipient, we now know that 2-4 ounces of umbilical cord blood does contain a sufficient number of primitive hematopoietic progenitors for both early and sustained engraftment in smaller recipients weighing up to 47 kg. In order to minimize the risk of delayed or failed engraftment in all size recipients, investigators are currently exploring techniques for optimizing the collection of umbilical cord blood and expanding the number of primitive and committed hematopoeitic progenitors in the harvested specimen. This article will review what is known about the clinical results with umbilical cord blood transplantation, the characterisitics of hematopoietic progenitor cells in umbilical cord blood, and the functional capacities of the neonatal immune system.

Results

Historical background

The use of human umbilical cord blood as a source of transplantable hematopoietic stem cells was first suggested by EA Boyse in the early 1980's in discussions with HE Broxmeyer and J Bard at the Sloan-Kettering Institute in New York. The initial concept of umbilical cord blood transplantation was supported by the observation that lethally irradiated adult mice could be successfully rescued and completely reconstituted by injections of fetal blood. These results in an animal model in turn led Broxmeyer *et al* to development of a practical umbilical cord blood collection method. Based on results of *in vitro* assays of human umbilical cord blood and the finding that fetal blood from mice could rescue lethally-irradiated adult recipients, Prof E Gluckman (Hôpital St Louis, Paris) performed the first human umbilical cord blood transplant in October 1988 in a patient with Fanconi anemia.

Clinical results

To date, seventy-five patients have been transplanted with umbilical cord blood from sibling or unrelated donors for the treatment of malignant and non-malignant disease. The median age and weight of recipients is 4.1 years and 19.4 kilograms, respectively. Thirty-nine patients received grafts from HLA-identical sibling donors, eleven received grafts from sibling donors disparate at one to three HLA loci and twenty-five received grafts from unrelated donors.

Pretransplant conditioning varied according to disease, disease status and institution; approximately half received irradiation-containing regimens. Prophylaxis for acute GVHD most often consisted of cyclosporine A alone or in combination with methotrexate, methylprednisolone or anti-T cell antibody; prophylaxis was not prescribed for one. Moreover, hematopoietic growth factor was prescribed for approximately half the patients.

Collection and processing of umbilical cord blood. The method of umbilical cord blood collection varied significantly between institutions. In most instances, collections were performed by obstetricians or nurse midwives without prior experience in the large-scale collection of umbilical cord and placental blood. In most cases, the umbilical cord blood graft was cryopreserved without prior red cell depletion. However, red cell depletion of ten grafts was accomplished either by ficollhypaque (n=9) or gelatin-sedimentation (n= 1). The median volume of umbilical cord blood collected was 100 mL (range, 42.1-282 mL) and the median number of nucleated cells and colony forming unitgranulocyte macrophage (CFU-GM) per kilogram recipient weight was 5.2×10^7 (range, 1 to 33) and 2.4×10^4 (range, 0.01 to 100), respectively.

Engraftment. Overall, the probability of hematopoietic recovery was 0.83 ± 0.05. For recipients of HLA-identical or HLA-1 antigen disparate grafts from sibling donors, the probability of hematopoietic recovery was 0.87 ± 0.06 and the median time to neutrophil and platelet recovery was 22.2 days and 51.6 days, respectively. Use of hematopoietic growth factors had no observable effect on time to neutrophil recovery and time to neutrophil recovery did not correlate with the number of nucleated cells or CFU-GM infused, based on recipient body weight.

Notably graft failure occurred almost exclusively in patients with non-malignant disease. All patients with malignant disease and a HLA-identical or HLA- I or 2 antigen disparate donor demonstrated donor derived hematopoietic recovery. In contrast, six patients with non-malignant disease and a HLA-identical or HLA-l antigen disparate donor failed to engraft; three are alive; two with spontaneously autologous hematopoietic recovery and one with hematopoietic recovery after the infusion of cryopreserved autologous marrow. Two patients with leukemia also failed to engraft after the transplantation of HLA-3 antigen disparate sibling donor umbilical cord blood; neither survived.

Graft-versus-host-disease. For patients with HLA-identical or HLA-l antigen disparate sibling donor grafts, the probability of having grade II-IV acute GVHD by 100 days after transplantation was 0.02 ± 0.02 with no patient having grade III-IV acute GVHD. Of patients with HLA-2 or 3 antigen disparate sibling donors or unrelated donors, only one patient with a HLA-3 antigen disparate sibling donor graft developed steroid resistant grade III acute graft-versus-host disease. While grafts were not routinely evaluated for the presence maternal cells, evidence of the non-inherited maternal allele could not be detected in seven of seven grafts evaluated.

For patients with HLA-identical or HLA-l antigen disparate sibling donor grafts, the probability of chronic GVHD at one year after transplantation was 0.06 ± 0.04 with no patient exhibiting extensive disease. Limited chronic GVHD was observed in one patient with a HLAidentical sibling donor and in one patient with a HLA-l antigen disparate sibling donor.

Survival. The probability of survival among the entire group of patients is 0.65 ± 0.08 with a median of 1.5 years follow-up (range, 0.2 to 6.0). For recipients of HLA-identical or HLA-l antigen disparate sibling donor grafts, the probability of survival is 0.73 ± 0.08. Among patients with a HLA-identical or HLA-l antigen disparate sibling donors, the probability of event-free survival for patients with malignant and non-malignant disease was 0.46 ± 0.12 and 0.78 ± 0.10, respectively. Although the rate of engraftment is high and risk of graft-versus-host disease is low, short follow-up for recipients of unrelated umbilical cord blood precludes analysis at this time.

Maternal lymphocyte contamination

While there is evidence indicating that leukocytes, platelets and erythrocytes traverse the placental barrier, the incidence of maternal to fetal transfer of red cells and leukocytes is low (<3%). With the exception of patients with congenital immunodeficiency, maternal lymphocytes have rarely been demonstrated in normal newborns. Nonetheless, maternal T cell contamination of the umbilical cord blood could potentially result in life-threatening graft-versus-host disease. Contact between umbilical cord and placental blood and maternal blood must be strictly avoided. In the cases studied to date, maternal cells have not been detected in the umbilical cord specimens or the patients themselves after transplantation. Kurtzberg *et al* (presented by Broxmeyer *et al*, Wagner *et al* and Vilmer *et al*) have failed to demonstrate maternal T cells in the cord blood grafts by cytogenetic or DNA techniques

Immunological properties of cord blood lymphocytes

It has been hypothesized that umbilical cord blood lymphocytes are "naive" and are "functionally immature". Clinical results thus far would suggest that allorecognition by umbilical cord blood lymphocytes may indeed be decreased. If this is true, then what is the mechanism for this decreased alloreactive response.
Roncarolo *et al* investigated the immunologic properties of umbilical cord blood lymphocytes. In this study, purified umbilical cord blood T cells were found to proliferate vigorously when

activated by allogeneic antigens in primary mixed lymphocyte reactions (MLRs) indicating that umbilical cord blood cells responded normally to activation by alloantigens. In contrast, umbilical cord blood cells had a reduced capacity to stimulate allogeneic cells in primary MLRs. The data suggest that this defect is related to a reduced antigen presenting capacity. The exact mechanism underlying the defect in the antigen presenting capacity of umbilical cord blood, however, remains to be clarified. In addition, umbilical cord blood cells were also impaired in their capacity to generate allogeneic cytotoxic activity in primary MLRs. Whether this defect is intrinsic to the cytotoxic T cells or due to other cells or factors preventing the generation of alloantigen specific cytotoxic T cells is not yet known. Whether these properties account for the reduced capacity of transplanted umbilical cord blood cells tomodulate a graft-versus-host disease remains to be determined.

Umbilical cord blood banking

As a result of the preliminary successes with umbilical cord blood transplantation using sibling donors, pilot programs for the banking of screened, unrelated donor umbilical cord blood have been proposed in many countries worldwide and recently initiated in the United States, France, United Kingdom, Germany and Italy. The first such bank was initiated at the New York Blood Center in February 1993. As of December 1994, more than 4000 umbilical cord blood grafts have been collected, human leukocyte antigen (HLA) typed, tested for transmissible infectious diseases and cryopreserved with an additional fifty umbilical cord blood grafts processed each week. A primary objective of this pilot program is to determine the feasibility of large scale umbilical cord blood collection, testing, and storage. Therefore, it has been necessary to: a) optimize and standardize the umbilical cord blood collection procedure; b) standardize quality assessment procedures (*i.e.,* quantification of hematopoietic progenitors, sterility, detection of genetic and transmissible infectious diseases, c) streamline large scale histocompatibility testing using restricted volumes of the sample from the potential umbilical cord blood graft in mother, d) develop repositories if viable cells, serum and DNA on donor and mother for future testing, e) optimize both the cryopreservation and thawing procedure to reduce cell loss and minimize infusion of DMSO and red cell debrie, and f) establish a computer network for efficient data storage and retrieval. Once completed, the ultimate goal of the New York Blood Center Placental Blood Program as well as the European Cord Blood Banking Project is to provide umbilical cord blood stem cells for transplantation in recipients lacking suitably matched sibling donors.

To date, twenty-five umbilical cord blood grafts from unrelated donors have been used for transplantation. The first unrelated umbilical cord blood transplants were performed in 1993 at the Duke University Medical Center in two children with acute lymphocytic leukemia. In both instances, the patients promptly engrafted and neither had significant acute graft-versus-host disease. With these encouraging results and greater public awareness, the number of search requests facilitated by the New York Blood Center increased significantly. Clinical data are currently being accumulated on the twenty-five patients.

A multi-institutional, international cooperative trial is currently being designed by investigators to determine the safety and efficacy of unrelated umbilical cord blood transplantation in both pediatric and adult recipients. In instances where preliminary search of the unrelated marrow registry identifies a potential unrelated bone marrow donor, the immediate availability of cryopreserved, HLA-compatible umbilical cord blood might justify the use of umbilical cord blood over bone marrow in specific patients, such as those with leukemia, storage diseases, bone marrow failure syndromes or immunodeficiency states at high risk of early death from disease progression or overwhelming infection. While there have been considerable efforts to shorten the time of marrow acquisition from unrelated donors, the median interval from initial search request to bone marrow harvest remains at 4-5 months. Patients with diseases expected to remain stable over a three-six month period of a donor search without relapse or overwhelming infection (*i.e.,* chronic myelogenous leukemia) might be considered ineligible for umbilical cord blood transplantation unless the marrow donor registry fails to identify a suitable donor. As more is learned about the safety of umbilical cord blood transplantation, these restrictive criteria are likely to be modified.

The use of unrelated umbilical cord blood has several known advantages. These include: 1) immediate availability (2 weeks for confirmatory HLA testing), 2) absence of donor risk (collection has no risk; it takes nothing from child or mother), 3) absence of donor attrition (umbilical cord blood units are immediately available whereas 20-30% of marrow donors in registries worldwide are not available for marrow donation at the time of request), 4) a very low risk of transmissible infectious diseases, such as cytomegalovirus (CMV) and Epstein-Barr virus (EBV). Other advantages *potentially* include: 1) lower risk of acute graft-versus-host disease and 2) ability to expand available donor pool in targeted ethnic and racial minorities currently underrepresented in all marrow donor registries.

While the clinical results thus far have been very encouraging, there are potential disadvantages with umbilical cord blood as well: 1) maternal lymphocyte contamination could result in life-threatening graft-versus-host disease, 2) lower risk of graft-versus-host disease might translate into a higher risk of relapse (*i.e.,* absence of graft-versus-leukemia effect), and 3) higher risk of genetic disorder transmission due to inability to observe growth and development of stem cell donor, and 4) an insufficient number of stem and progenitor cells in umbilical cord blood for larger recipients, limiting this stem cell source to pediatric patients.

Conclusion

Several important questions remain to be answered; 1) will the numbers of stem and progenitor cells in umbilical cord blood be sufficient for engraftment and repopulation of the hematopoietic system of larger recipients? 2) will greater HLA disparities between donor and recipient be tolerable? and, 3) will the risk of leukemia relapse be greater after umbilical cord blood transplantation if the risk of GVHD is lower? While the data thus far fail to suggest a higher relapse rate, the limited number of patients, heterogeneity of diseases and disease states and short length of follow-up preclude any definitive statement regarding the "graft-versus-leukemia" effect of umbilical cord blood. In the near future, it is anticipated that answers to these important issues will be satisfactorily resolved and pave the way for defining the broadness of applicability for this newly identified source of transplantable hematopoietic stem cells.

Supported in part by grants from the Childrens Cancer Research Fund, National Institutes of Health Grant No P01-CA21737 and American Cancer Society Career Development Award No 91-56.

Advantages of using foetal and neonatal cells for treatment of hematological diseases in human

E. Gluckman

Service de Greffe de Moelle osseuse, Hôpital Saint-Louis, 1, avenue Claude-Vellefaux, 75475 Paris Cedex 10, France, tel.: (33 1) 42 49 96 44, fax: (33 1) 42 49 96 34

Cord blood hematopoietic stem cells as an alternative source of stem cells

Bone marrow transplantation (BMT) is now recognised as an effective treatment for an increasing number of hematological diseases including malignancies, aplastic anemia and hereditary disorders. Hematopoietic stem cells (HSC) used to reconstitute hematopoiesis after intensive myeloablative therapy are typically obtained from the bone marrow or more recently from peripheral blood after mobilisation by various growth factors [1-3]. Suitable marrow must be provided by an HLA-A, -B and -DR identical related or unrelated donor; unfortunately, such a donor is not always available because of the extreme polymorphism of the HLA system. Even when a donor is available, the inability of current methods of HLA typing techniques to determine all the potential mismatches means that recipients of unrelated bone marrow transplants are at extreme risk for graft versus host disease(GVHD) [4]. Finding new and readily available sources of hematopoietic stem cells will broaden the availibility of this treatment and improve the outcome of the transplant. New sources of HSC currently under investigation are adult cytokine mobilised peripheral blood stem cells and placental blood collected at birth. The first has the advantage of containing a large number of CD34$^+$ progenitor cells and is easily collected, it has the disadvantage of containing a large number of peripheral blood mature lymphocytes which are known to be the effectors of graft versus host disease. Cord blood has the advantage of being easily collected without any risk to the donor, and it contains immature HSC and lymphocytes. These properties should increase the probability of engraftment and diminish the risk of severe graft versus host disease, the disadvantage might be that the number of cells collected in a single cord blood might be insufficient for long term engraftment in the host.

Preliminary analysis of the results of more than 50 cord blood transplants performed throughout the world shows that long-term engraftment has been observed in patients with different diagnoses including both malignant and non malignant disorders [5-9]. The number of cells infused was inferior to the number infused in bone marrow transplants or peripheral blood stem cell transplants (PBSCT), but, despite this small number of cells, the incidence of graft failure was low. Furthermore, there was no correlation between the number of cells and the speed of engraftment, and the addition of *in vivo* growth factors did not modify the speed of engraftment.

This is probably due to the unique properties and growth factor-independence of hematopoietic stem cells from cord blood [10]. It is likely that a limited number of primitive hematopoietic stem cells are sufficient to induce long term engraftment; the present limitation for standardising methods of quantification of HSC, as well as the absence of criteria to identify "stem cells" explain why the minimum number of HSC necessary for engraftment is unknown. It is estimated that long term engraftment can be obtained with 1 5 to 5×10^5 LTC-IC from bone marrow and 2×10^4 LTC-IC from cord blood [11].

Another very important clinical finding is the observation that the incidence of acute and chronic graft versus host disease has been low in family or unrelated matched and mismatched cord blood transplants. To date, the follow-up is not sufficient to know if these cells are able to mount a graft- versus-leukemia (GVL) reactivity.

Cord blood is an abundant source of stem cells that are usually discarded and whose collection is entirely safe to the donor, as the blood is only removed from the placental side of the umbilicus post parturition and clamping. There exists a very large number of potential donors with a possibility of selecting donors according to rare HLA haplotypes. Frozen cells can be tested in advance and can be available at short notice, decreasing the length of the search for donors. Additionally, there is a low prevalence of infectious diseases at birth, particularly cytomegalovirus (CMV), which is a major cause of transplant-related mortality, and thus, cord blood transplants may be associated with lower incidence of post transplant infection.

This has led to an exponential increase in the interest in cord blood transplant and to the development of cord blood banks across the world [12, 13].

Properties of cord blood hematopoietic stem cells

It has been shown that foetal and cord blood hematopoietic stem cells are different from adult blood and marrow hematopoietic stem cells [14]. *In vitro,* clonogenic assays of hematopoietic stem cells from cord blood have demonstrated that colonies are larger and more enriched with immature progenitors than those obtained from adult marrow and peripheral blood [15]. Cord blood stem cells show more potential growth in long-term culture and can be expanded [16, 17]. There are differences in cytokine requirement for growth *in vitro* and for replating capacity, possibly due to autocrine or paracrine production in culture [10]. Stable and long-term engraftment has been observed in SCID mice without the need of additional growth factors [18]. Ontogeny-related changes may be related to the decrease of telomeric length with age [19].

The possible clinical applications of these properties include the use of cord blood hematopoietic stem cells for characterisation of primitive progenitors, selection of cell subsets, *in vivo* expansion and use for gene transfer and gene therapy.

This could be particularly important for the treatment of genetic diseases where the diagnosis can be performed *in utero,* and cord blood can be collected at birth, transfected, and transplanted immediately. On a larger scale, autologous cord blood collection and cryopreservation could be offered in families with an increased risk of cancer, autoimmune disease or infection.

Immunological properties of cord blood cells

Graft-versus-host disease(GVHD) is the major barrier to successful allogeneic bone marrow transplantation. This can be overcome by T-cell depletion, use of immunosuppressive drugs or *in vivo* monoclonal antibodies, but this is often associated with an unacceptable increase of the relapse rate, demonstrating the importance of the graft-versus-leukemia (GVL) activity associated with allogeneic BMT. Early results from unrelated cord blood transplants have provided evidence of lower incidence and severity of acute and chronic GVHD in the recipient than would have been predicted from adult volunteer donor bone marrow transplants. Several hypotheses can explain the decrease of GVHD, some are already known: the incidence of GVHD diminishes with donor and recipient age, with the absence of donor and recipient herpes virus species infections and with a low number of lymphocytes infused. All these requirements are met by cord blood but not necessarily by adult bone marrow or peripheral blood. Other explanations for thedecrease of GVHD can be found in the study of immune function of cord blood cells. It is known that cord blood lymphocytes are enriched in immature progenitors. Lymphoid subsets in cord blood differ from those of adult blood. Immature $CD3^-$ 8^+ or 7^+ cells are present; $CD3^+$ cells have a naive, non activated phenotype ($CD25^-$, DR^-, $CD45RA$ lo); and most $CD3^-$ cells are NK cells ($CD16^+$, $CD56^+$).

Immune deficiency of cord blood lymphocytes might also be explained by the presence of a small number of maternal cells [20]. In a previous study, we used the polymerase chain reaction amplification of 2 minisatellite sequences and found a maternal specific allele in one sample out of 42 cases tested [22]. Using PCR amplification of non-inherited HLA antigens, the New York cord blood bank group has been able to detect maternal cell contamination in 3 cases out of 3000 cord blood samples studied. Using fluorescent in-situ hybridisation, the Seattle group found maternal cells in 6/44 unfractionated cord blood samples at levels ranging from 1/2500 to 1/100. Finally, we used a highly sensitive, allele specific amplification method and have shown that maternal specific alleles were found, in 10 out of 10 samples studied, at a frequency of 10^{-4} to 10^{-5} of cord blood nucleated cells. The presence of maternal cells, at such a low level, in cord blood samples is probably insufficient to induce GVH after transplantation, but it may play a role in the establishment of the foeto-maternal tolerance and in the transmission of infection from the mother to the new-born.

The mechanism of cytotoxicity seems different in cord blood compared to adult peripheral blood. While most of the tests of proliferation and the study of CTL-p and HTL-p seem normal or slightly decreased when compared to adult subpopulations, the study of lymphoid subsets seems to show that there is an increase of $CD 3^-$ subsets mostly, of the NK subset. Cytotoxicity seems mostly dependent on the NK subsets as shown by the study of perforin expression and of the BY55 monoclonal antibody which recognises functional cytotoxic T or NK cells [21, 22].

It remains to be established that the decrease of GVH is an active phenomenon of suppression by these cell subsets [23].

Conclusion

Cord blood banks have been established in several countries for use in family and unrelated transplants. In addition, cord blood cells are widely used for experimental purposes and for the development of cell and gene therapy. For this reason, it is mandatory to organise exchanges between these banks and to develop methods of standardisation of collection, cell separation, purification, quantification of HSC, methods of cryopreservation and thawing. The European Cord Blood Bank (ECBB) group has begun to work on these aspects as well as on the methods of detection of transmissible infectious or genetic diseases. A registry of cord blood transplants has been established within the Immunology working party of the European Blood and Marrow Transplant Group.

References

1. Bensinger WI, Weaver CH, Appelbaum FR, Rowley S, Demirer T, Sanders J, Storb R, Buckner CD. Transplantation of allogeneic peripheral blood stem cells mobilized by recombinant human granulocyte colony stimulating factor. *Blood* 1995; 85: 1655-1658.
2. Korbling M, Przepiorka D, Huh YO, Engel H, Van Biesen K, Giralt S, Andersson AB, Kleine HD, Seong D, Deisseroth AB, Andreeff M, Champlin R. Allogeneic blood stem cell transplantation for refractory leukemia and lymphoma: potential advantage of blood over marrow allografts. *Blood* 1995; 85: 1659-1665.
3. Schmitz N, Dreger P, Suttorp M, Rohwedder EB, Haferlach T, Loffler H, Hunter A, Russell NH. Primary transplantation of allogeneic peripheral blood progenitor cells mobilized by Filgrastim (Granulocyte colony stimulating factor). *Blood* 1995; 85: 1666-1672.
4. Goldman JM for the WMDA executive committee. A special report: bone marrow transplants using volunteer donors-recommendations and requirements for a standardized practice throughout the world-1994 update. *Blood* 1994; 84: 2833-2839.
5. Gluckman E, Broxmeyer HE, Auerbach AD *et al.* Hematopoietic reconstitution in a patient with Fanconi's anemia by means of umbilical cord blood from an HLA identical sibling. *N Engl J Med* 1989; 321: 1174-1178.
6. Vowels MR, Lampotang R, Berdoukas V *et al.* Correction of X linked lymphoproliferative disease by transplantation of cord blood stem cells. *N Engl J Med* 1993; 329: 1623-1625.
7. Issaragrisil S, Visuthisakchai S, Suvatte V, Tanphaichitr VS, Chandanayingyong D, Schreiner T, Kanokpongsakdi S, Siritanaratkul N, Piankijagum A. Brief report: transplantation of cord-blood stem cells into a patient with severe thalassemia. *New Engl J of Med* 1995; 332: 367-369.
8. Wagner JE, Kernan NA, Broxmeyer HE, Gluckman E. Allogeneic umbilical cord blood transplantation: report of the results in 26 patients. *Blood* 1993; 82, Sup 1: 86a. abstract
9. Wagner JE, Broxmeyer HE, Byrd RL *et al.* Transplantation of umbilical cord blood after myeloablative therapy. Analysis of engraftment. *Blood* 1992; 79: 1155-1157.
10. Schibler KR, Li Y, Ohlsrk *et al.* Possible mechanisms accounting for the growth factors independence of hematopoietic progenitors from umbilical cord blood. *Blood* 1994; 84: 3679- 3684.
11. Traycoff C, Kosak ST, Grigsby S, Srour EF. Evaluation of ex-vivo expansion potential of cord blood and bone marrow hematopoietic progenitor cells using cell tracking and limiting dilution analysis. *Blood* 1995; 85: 2059-2068.
12. Rubinstein P, Rosenfeld Re, Adamson Jw, Stevens CE. Stored placental blood for unrelated bone marrow reconstitution. Blood. 1993; 81: 1679-1690.
13. E. Gluckman. European organisation for cord blood banking. Blood Cells.20: 601-608. 1994.
14. Broxmeyer He, Douglas Gw, Hangoc G *et al.* Human umbilical cord blood as a potential source of transplantable stem/progenitor cells. Proc. Natl Acad Sci USA.1989; 86: 3828-3832.
15. Broxmeyer He, Hangoc G, Cooper S *et al.* Growth characteristics and expansion of human umbilical cord blood and estimation of its potential for transplantation in adults. *Proc Natl Acad Sc USA* 1992; 89: 4109-4113.
16. Mayani H, Dragowska W, Lansdorp PM. Cytokine-induced selective expansion and maturation of erythroid versus myeloid progenitors from purified cord blood precursor cells. *Blood* 1992; 79: 2620-2627.
17. Mayani H, Dragowska W, Lansdorp PM. Characterization of functionally distinct subpopulations of CD34+ cord blood cells in serum-free long-term cultures supplemented with hematopoietic cytokines. *Blood* 1993; 82: 2664-2672.
18. Vormoor J, Lapidot T, Pflumio F, Risdon G, Paterson B, Broxmeyer *et al.* Immature human cord blood progenitors engraft and proliferate to high levels in severe combined immunodeficient mice. *Blood* 1994; 83: 2489- 2497.
19. Vaziri H, Dragowska W, Allsopp RC, Thomas TE, Haley CB, Lansdorp PM. Evidence for a mitotic clock in human hematopoietic stem cells: loss of the telomeric DNA with age. *Proc Natl Acad Sci USA* 1994; 91: 9857-9860.
20. Socie G, Gluckman E, Carosella E, Brossard Y, Lafon C, Brison O. Search for maternal cells in human umbilical cord blood by polymerase chain reaction amplification of two minisatellite sequences. *Blood* 1994; 83: 340-344.

21. Bensussan A, Gluckman E, El Marsafy S *et al.* By55mAb delineates within human cord blood and bone marrow lymphocytes distinct cell subsets mediating cytotoxic activity. *Proc Natl Acad Sci USA* 1994; 91: 9136-9140.
22. Berthou C, Legrosmaida S, Soulier A, Wargnier A, Guillet J, Rabian C, Gluckman E, Sasportes M. Cord blood lymphocytes lack constitutive perforin expression in contrast to adult peripheral blood T lymphocytes. *Blood* 1995; 85: 1540-1546.
23. Risdon G, Gaddy J, Horie M, Broxmeyer HE. Alloantigen priming induces a state of unresponsiveness in human umbilical cord blood T cells. *Proc Natl Acad Sci USA* 1995; 92: 2413-2417.

Résumé

La greffe de moelle osseuse allogénique est un traitement efficace d'un grand nombre de maladies hématologiques malignes ou non. De nouvelles sources de cellules souches hématopoïétiques sont actuellement à l'étude. Elles sont isolées, soit du sang après mobilisation par des cytokines chez l'adulte, soit du sang placentaire prélevé à la naissance. L'analyse des résultats de plus d'une cinquantaine de greffes de cellules souches hématopoïétiques du sang placentaire a montré une prise à long terme dans la majorité des cas, malgré le faible nombre de cellules injectées. Par ailleurs, l'incidence et la gravité de la réaction du greffon contre l'hôte a été faible même lorsque le donneur n'était pas totalement HLA compatible. Le recul est insuffisant pour savoir si la fonction *graft versus leukemia* est maintenue. La facilité d'obtention de ces cellules explique le développement de banques de sang placentaire.

Les propriétés des cellules souches hématopoïétiques du sang placentaire sont originales avec un enrichissement en cellules immatures et une plus grande capacité d'expansion *in vivo* et *in vitro*. Cela est particulièrement important pour la thérapie cellulaire et la thérapie génique.

Le déficit immunitaire du nouveau-né est caractérisé par un accroissement de populations T immatures, un enrichissement en cellules NK et la présence de cellules naïves non activées suppressives. L'ensemble de ces caractéristiques peut expliquer la diminution de la GVH et la possibilité de faire des greffes non strictement HLA identiques. Cela devrait aboutir à la diminution du pool de donneurs nécessaires pour traiter un plus grand nombre de patients.

II. APLASTIC ANEMIA

II. APLASIES MÉDULLAIRES

1) Mechanisms of aplastic anemia

1) *Mécanismes des aplasies médullaires*

The pathophysiology of acquired aplastic anemia

Neal S. Young, Jaroslaw P. Maciejewski, Carmine Selleri, Tadatsugu Sato, Antonia Nisticò, Kevin E. Brown, Spencer W. Green, Susan Wong, and Stacie Anderson

Hematology Branch, National Heart, Lung, and Blood Institute, Bethesda, MD 20892-1652, USA, tel.: (301) 496 5093, fax: (301) 496 8396

Summary

Aplastic anemia probably has two major etiologies: type I, direct toxicity as observed with high doses of irradiation, myelotoxic drugs, and perhaps chemicals like benzene and some insecticides; and type II, immune-mediated community-acquired disease. We focus here on type II aplastic anemia. This disease may be considered in three phases: 1. incitement by the presentation of drug metabolites or viral antigens to the immune system; 2. immune pathophysiology, mediated predominantly by activated cytotoxic lymphocytes and soluble lymphokines; and 3. evolution to clonal hematologic diseases like paroxysmal nocturnal hemoglobinuria after effective immunosuppressive therapy. Most is known about the second phase of the disease, to which treatment is directed. γ-interferon is an important mediator of hematopoietic suppression in aplastic anemia. Expression of the γ-interferon gene can be detected in most aplastic anemia patients' marrow and not in controls. This cytokine and also tumor necrosis factor inhibit a spectrum of hematopoietic cells from stem cells to late progenitors. γ-interferon and tumor necrosis factor-α induce Fas receptor expression on $CD34^+$ cells, which allows for triggering of apoptosis by monoclonal antibodies in vitro *and presumably Fas ligand* in vivo. *Fas antigen expression is increased on $CD34^+$ cells from aplastic anemia patients. Local production of γ-interferon is more inhibitory than the addition of interferon to progenitor and stem cell generation in long-term marrow cultures. Endogenous production by stromal cells engineered by gene transduction to secrete 20 u/ml of γ-interferon was as inhibitory as 500 U/ml of exogenous interferon added weekly. Type II aplastic anemia appears to be related to other human T cell mediated diseases-type I diabetes mellitus and multiple sclerosis- in which cytotoxic lymphocytes that secrete γ-interferon effect organ specific destruction, and all of which respond to immunosuppressive therapies.*

The etiology of aplastic anemia is confusing (for reviews, see [1, 2]). Aplastic anemia, defined as pancytopenia with a predominantly fatty marrow, may be difficult to distinguish diagnostically from other diseases, especially hypocellular myelodysplasia and sometimes also acute leukemia in children or the elderly. The marrow morphology is identical in constitutional aplastic anemia, in which multiple severe physical anomalies accompany the blood disease as in acquired aplasia, a purely hematologic process. Acquired aplastic anemia has many clinical associations, including histories of exposure to benzene or pesticides; medicinal drug use; and preceding viral illnesses like hepatitis and infectious mononucleosis. Aplasia can accompany pregnancy and may resolve with its termination. The acquired genetic disease paroxysmal nocturnal hemoglobinuria, now defined as resulting from alterations in a specific gene in the hematopoietic stem cell, is closely related to aplastic anemia. Aplastic marrow failure is the cause of death in the fatal syndrome of transfusion-associated graft-versus-host disease. Unsurprisingly, aplastic anemia has been regarded as a highly heterogenous syndrome, in which multiple different pathways lead to a common final marrow pathology.

Despite such diverse associations, in other respects acquired aplastic anemia appears a simple process. The pathologic picture is fairly consistent. Fatty replacement of hematopoiesis dominates, although the estimated total cellularity and proportion of residual lymphocytes may vary. Dysplastic features are usually minimal: megaloblastoid erythroid differentiation is common. Some hemophagocytosis may be observed. Cytogenetic analysis of marrow chromosomes is normal. Clinically, "classical" cases are stereotypical: previously well children, adolescent, or young adults with the onset over several days to weeks of thrombocytopenic bleeding symptoms with fatigue and lassitude due to anemia. Demographically, men and women are about equally affected, but in referrals to tertiary hospital centers there is a prominent peak in the rate at age 20-25 years, a paucity of middle-aged patients, and a second peak among the elderly. Most striking is the response of patients with aplastic anemia to therapies (for review, see [3] and Bacigalupo, Deeg, this volume). Bone marrow transplantation is successful in a large majority of patients with suitable matched sibling donors. Although the rate of graft rejection or failure may be higher than for other transplantable conditions, aggressive conditioning regimens increase the probability of engraftment. In contrast to the leukemias, death after transplant for aplastic anemia is usually due to complications of the procedure rather than return of the primary disease. Success with marrow transplantation has been interpreted to imply that patients suffer a deficit of stem cells and not a lesion of the hematopoietic microenvironment, stroma, or growth factor production. Patients who are not candidates for transplant also show a very high response rate to nonreplacement therapy with antilymphocyte globulins and cyclosporine. Recent intensive immunosuppressive regimens have produced hematologic response rates of 70-80% and good long-term survival. These observations suggest the unity of aplastic anemia as a disease entity.

The hematopoietic cell compartment in marrow failure

The CD34$^+$ cell compartment, which contains progenitor and stem cells, is severely reduced in blood and marrow [4]. Functional assays of hematopoietic colony forming cells, applied early to aplastic anemia, always show a marked decrease in blood and marrow progenitor cell numbers, of all lineages and stages of differentiation—CFU-GM, BFU-E, CFU-E, CFU-Meg, and CFU-GEMM. Human stem cells resisted direct measurement until the recent development of the long-term culture initiating cell (LTCIC) test as a surrogate assay; LTCIC also are greatly reduced in aplastic anemia [5] (and our unpublished data). On recovery, CD34$^+$ cells and colon-forming cell numbers increase, but not to normal levels; remarkably, LTCIC remain severely reduced even with restoration of near normal hematopoiesis (our unpublished data). These phenotypic and functional measurements support the inference from morphology that aplastic anemia results from a deficit in stem and progenitor cells. They further suggest that stem cell loss may be permanent but compensated by increased production in the later progenitor compartment.

In contrast, studies of support functions have been largely normal. In long-term bone marrow culture (LTBMC), aplastic adherent cells show normal stroma formation and support nonadherent cells from normal donors (whereas nonadherent cells from patients fail to grow on normal stroma) [6]. In general, circulating levels of hematopoietic growth factors and the production of hematopoietins are normal or high in patients' serum samples or tissue culture of patient cells. Two exceptions are production of interleukin-1 by monocytes, which is low in severe aplastic anemia [7, 8], and stem cell factor levels in blood, which are depressed in many patients [9, 10]. The pathophysiologic significance of these findings is uncertain, especially as patients do not appear to respond hematologically to therapeutic attempts to replace these factors. Fibroblast-colony formation is low in some patients [11], but this assay has not been shown to correlate with stromal cell function.

Clues from epidemiology

A remarkable feature of aplastic anemia is its geographic distribution. The impression that the disease was more common in the Far East was confirmed in a formal epidemiologic study in Bangkok, where the annual incidence was 4/million [12] compared to 2/million in Europe [13]; the rate may be even higher, about 6 in rural northeast Thailand and in Ho Chi Minh City, Vietnam. Even within restricted geographic areas, aplastic anemia may vary considerably from city to city (as in Europe and Israel) and among suburban areas of Bangkok (see Issaragrisil, this volume).

Case control studies have been performed in both Europe and Thailand. In Europe, about one third of cases can be attributed to drug exposure (mainly nonsteroidal anti-inflammatory agents, sulfonamides, thyrostatics, psychotropic drugs, penicillamine, allopurinol, and gold). In Thailand, only 15% of cases have suspect medication histories. Significant risk factors in Thailand are low socioeconomic status, exposure to industrial solvents and agricultural pesticides, and, independently, grain farming, essentially rice farming (Issaragrisil and colleagues, unpublished data).

Toxicity from radiation and chemicals

Irradiation, γ-rays externally, α-particles internally, and radiomimetic drugs, all of which effect dose-dependent damage to marrow are the most frequent causes of aplastic anemia, usually in the setting of medical therapy for cancer and occasionally accidentally. The busulfan-treated mouse is an animal model of this type of aplastic anemia, and long-term bone marrow culture can reproduce some drug and radiation effects [14]. Remarkably, the true LD50 of radiation in humans remains uncertain. Occasional patients have recovered autologous marrow function after presumed myeloablative treatment and graft failure, evidence of the influence of supportive care on survival as well as the recuperative capacity of the stem cell compartment.

Direct toxicity to the marrow, through DNA damage and the subsequent induction of the apoptotic program, is the mechanism for radiation effects. Direct toxicity may partly underlie aplastic anemia due to organic chemicals like benzene and pesticides and perhaps also some drug effects, in which genotoxic drug intermediates may be generated by a patient's unique metabolic machinery. Chloramphenicol, because of its structural similarity to amidopyrine, also was thought to act directly on marrow, but decades of study have not established a logical mechanism for the generation of a cytotoxic compound from this drug in selected patients [15]. For most drugs marrow toxicity effects would need to be more potent than those obtained with high doses of chemotherapeutic drugs specifically designed for their ability to kill proliferating cells.

Viruses and drugs as antigens

In community acquired aplastic anemia, drug exposure is usually to only modest quantities of medication, not to extreme doses or long duration. Inciting viral infections may be uncomplicated hepatitis or infectious mononucleosis. How can these ordinarily innocuous stimuli cause extensive marrow destruction? The response of aplastic anemia patients with suspicious drug and viral exposure histories has suggested that the immune system might be activated by exposure to antigens presented as part of a chemical or viral structure (see below). However, remarkably little is known of the nature of such antigens.

For drugs, reactive intermediates of metabolism might conjugate to host proteins and then serve as haptens. Studies of antibodies in agranulocytosis support this mechanism for some drugs. Cell-mediated immune responses are practically much more difficult to investigate in the laboratory, For viruses, pathophysiologic cell-mediated immune responses underlie several animal models of disease, such as lymphocytic choriomeningitis virus neurotoxicity and coxsackie virus myocarditis. For human disease, Epstein-Barr virus can be found in the marrow of a few patients with aplastic anemia [16], and infection generally is associated with lymphocyte activation. Other members of the herpesvirus family, cytomegalovirus and human herpes virus 6, have suppressive effects on hematopoiesis *in vitro* and *in vivo* [17-20]. The hepatitis/aplasia syndrome is a clear example of an apparent viral illness in which marrow failure is a delayed effect. However, the virus that causes the non A non B non C hepatitis that precedes aplastic anemia (and causes also the fulminant hepatitis associated with aplastic anemia after liver transplantation) has yet to be identified [21, 22].

Immune pathophysiology

Mathé and others observed autologous reconstitution of hematopoiesis in some patients who failed to engraft donor marrow, suggesting effective treatment of an autoimmune process by anti-lymphocyte globulin or cyclophosphamide used in the conditioning regimens [23]. In coculture experiments, lymphocytes from the blood or marrow of patients suppressed normal hematopoietic colony formation, and lymphocyte depletion could improve progenitor growth [24]. Separation and quantitation of these observations was confounded by possible allosensitization influences in heavily transfused patients. Inhibition was also produced by supernatants of aplastic marrow or blood cell tissue cultures, generated in the absence of foreign antigens [25]. These suppressor molecules were identified as γ-interferon and lymphotoxin (tumor necrosis factor-β), produced by activated cytotoxic lymphocytes in mass culture or after cell cloning [26-29].

The mechanism of cytokine effects on hematopoietic cells has been elucidated by *in vitro* studies with normal cells. Both γ-interferon and tumor necrosis factor inhibit in a dose-dependent fashion hematopoietic colony formation across a wide spectrum of progenitor cells, including

CD34$^+$CD38$^+$ late progenitors, more immature CD34$^+$CD38$^-$ cells, and LTCIC [30]. In highly purified CD34$^+$ cells exposed to these cytokines, target cells undergo programmed cell death, as detected by agarose gel electrophoresis and enzymatic assay for DNA degradation. γ-Interferon and tumor necrosis factor induce expression of Fas antigen on CD34$^+$ cells [31]. Fas is a member of the tumor necrosis factor receptor family, and its triggering by binding of Fas ligand or some monoclonal antibodies signals the cell to undergo apoptosis. Fas antigen expression is ordinarily low on normal marrow CD34$^+$ cells but is elevated on fresh samples from aplastic marrow, consistent with continuing immune-mediated apoptosis in the hematopoietic cell compartment. Studies with transgenic animals have suggested that immune-mediated damage occurs either by activation of the Fas receptor or the perforin\granzyme pathways; the role of granzymes in aplastic anemia has not yet been investigated.

Recent data from our laboratory has suggested that the important immune events in aplastic anemia occur locally, in the marrow. Here, activated T cells may be localized even when they are not detected in blood; natural killer cells and $\gamma\delta$-T cells may also be abnormally high in marrow [32]. Expression of the gene for γ-interferon can be measured by modifications of the polymerase chain reaction for gene amplification: gene activity was not detected in normal marrow or among hematologic controls but in a high proportion of aplastic anemia patients, especially among patients who would later respond to cyclosporine [33, 34]. Macrophage inflammatory protein-1α and tumor necrosis factor-β gene expression have also been reported as increased compared to their levels in normal marrow [8, 35, 36].

The concentrations of interferon needed to affect colony formation *in vitro* are substantial, in our hands, approximately 500 U/ml for 50% inhibition. Patients and animals can also tolerate high doses of interferon *in vivo* without marked marrow suppression. To test the effect of local production, we engineered human stromal cells to constitutively synthesize γ-interferon by retrovirus-mediated gene transfer [37]. These cells formed a normal cobble-stone adherent cell layer and grossly produced several hematopoietic growth factors. However, generation of both progenitor cells, CFU-GM and BFU-E, and stem cells, LTCIC, was markedly inhibited, despite the low levels of γ-interferon in the culture supernatants, about 20 U/ml. CD34$^+$ cells in the nonadherent cell layer undergo both apoptosis and retardation of mitotic cycle. These results suggest that local production of interferon alone is sufficient to inhibit hematopoiesis *in vitro* and probably also *in vivo*.

Identification of specific cytokines and their receptors has implications for intracellular events in target cells. Interferon regulatory factor-1 (IRF-1), an important transcriptional regulator for a wide variety of genes, is induced in CD34$^+$ cells on exposure to γ-interferon, and antisense experiments suggest that the importance of IRF-1 in the process of hematopoietic colony suppression by this cytokine [38]. Nitric oxide synthase is also inducible by interferon, and this enzyme too is present in CD34$^+$ cells; NO is a potent inhibitor of hematopoiesis *in vitro* [39]. Downstream effects of γ-interferon might contribute to certain aspects of bone marrow failure, including not only cell death but retardation of mitosis, dysplasia, and mutagenesis.

Why do so few individuals develop aplastic anemia in response to drug or viral antigens? The host factors responsible for an appropriate immune response to a foreign antigen as well as for maintenance of self tolerance are poorly understood. However, susceptibility to aplastic anemia, as with other autoimmune diseases, has been linked to certain histocompatability types, especially HLA-DR2 [40, 41], and responsiveness to cyclosporine therapy among Japanese and German patients has been associated with a specific haplotype [42].

Clonal evolution

Although bone marrow failure can be successfully treated with immunosuppression, some patients develop late clonal hematologic diseases years after antilymphocyte globulin administration ([43] and reviewed in [44]; see also Socié, this volume). Most commonly laboratory evidence of paroxysmal nocturnal hemoglobinuria (PNH) is detected on routine screening, either by complement-mediated hemolysis in the Ham test or the more sensitive assay of cell surface expression of glycosylphosphoinositol-linked proteins by flow cytometry [45]. Myelodysplasia and acute myelogenous leukemia also occur [46]. Analysis of granulocyte and monocyte surface proteins have also shown that a very high proportion of aplastic patients have subtle evidence of the specific PNH defect on presentation with marrow failure [47,48]. In both pure paroxysmal nocturnal hemoglobinuria and PNH that arises out of aplastic anemia, mutations in a single gene called PIG-A have been detected by molecular analysis.

How the PIG-A gene relates to hematopoiesis is uncertain. In knock-out mice, PIG-A- stem cells do not have a proliferative advantage and their progeny represent a minor proportion of blood cells. From total human blood and marrow cells also PNH cells grow poorly in tissue culture. The selective advantage conferred by a nonfunctioning PIG-A gene may intrinsically enhance hematopoiesis only in patients, as for example by affecting cell-cell adhesion or matrix interactions; the absence of proteins that mediate immune system interactions, for example binding of a target cell to a lymphoycte, might also benefit these defective cells in an autoimmune host.

Leukemia or myelodysplasia might develop in aplastic anemia because the disease is primarily malignant; for example, the immune response might be an attempt to contain proliferation of a transformed cell population and directed against an aberrant protein expressed by a genetically altered gene. Although mutations in ras and other oncogenes have been detected after clinical transformation for some cases, they have not been found in samples obtained on presentation with aplasia. Immunosuppression itself might contribute to failed immune surveillance. Finally, the contracted, oligoclonal stem cell compartment itself may predispose to secondary malignant events or favor proliferation of leukemic cells.

Conclusions

Aplastic anemia may develop from direct damage to marrow cells by physical and chemical agents (Type I) or mediated through the immune system as a response to drug metabolites, viruses, or self antigens (Type II). In both types of disease, the full spectrum of hematopoietic cells from stem cells to late progenitors is targeted. A second common feature is apoptotic cell death, leading to loss of stem cells which is reflected in both the functional failure to produce blood cells and the morphology of the marrow, showing loss of cells in the absence of inflammation . Most community-acquired aplastic anemia is probably type II. Immune aplastic anemia resembles other human diseases like type I diabetes mellitus and multiple sclerosis in which tissue specific organ damage is mediated by cytotoxic T cells that secrete γ-interferon and other cytokines, resulting in apoptotic cell destruction. Viruses have been implicated in the pathogenesis of these diseases, which occur predominantly in children and young adults, and cyclosporine and other immunosuppressive regimens are often effective. Identification of new hepatitis viruses and clarification of the function of the PIG-A gene will help in understanding the ultimate pathogenesis of aplastic anemia.

References

1. Aplastic Anaemia. London: Baillière Tindall, 1989.
2. Young NS, Alter BP. Aplastic Anemia, Acquired and Inherited. Philadelphia: Saunders, 1994.
3. Young NS, Barrett AJ. The treatment of severe acquired aplastic anemia. *Blood* 1995; in press.
4. Maciejewski JP, Anderson S, Katevas P, Young NS. Phenotypic and functional analysis of the bone marrow progenitor cell compartment in aplastic anemia. *Br J Haematol* 1994; 87: 227-234.
5. Schrezenmeier H, Gerok M, Heimpel H, Raghavachar A. Assessment of frequency of hematopoietic stem cells in aplastic anemia by limiting dilution type long term marrow culture [abstract]. *Exp Hematol* 1992; 20: 806.
6. Marsh JCW, Chang J, Testa NG, Hows JM, Dexter TM. In vitro assesssment of marrow 'stem cell' and stromal cell function in aplastic anaemia. *Br J Haematol* 1991; 78: 258-267.
7. Nakao S, Matsushima K, Young N. Deficient interleukin 1 production by aplastic anemia monocytes. *Br J Haematol* 1989; 71: 431-436.
8. Holmberg LA, Seidel K, Leisenring W, Torok-Storb B. Aplastic anemia: analysis of stromal cell function in long-term marrow cultures. *Blood* 1994; 84: 3685-3690.
9. Wodnar-Filipowicz A, Yancik S, Moser Y, dalle Carbonare V, Gratwohl A, Tichelli A, Speck B, Nissen C. Levels of soluble stem cell factor in serum of patients with aplastic anemia. *Blood* 1993; 81: 3259-3264.
10. Nimer SD, Leung DHY, Wolin MJ, Golde DW. Serum stem cell factor levels in patients with aplastic anemia. *Int J Hematol* 1994; 60: 185-189.
11. Juneja HS, Gardner FH, Minguell JJ, Helmer RE,III. Abnormal marrow fibroblasts in aplastic anemia. *Exp Hematol* 1984; 12: 221-230.
12. Issaragrisil S, Sriratanasatavorn C, Piankijagum A, Vannasaeng S, Porapakkham Y, Leaverton PE, Kaufman DW, Anderson TE, Shapiro S, Young NS. The incidence of aplastic anemia in Bangkok. *Blood* 1991; 77: 2166-2168.
13. Kaufman DW, Kelly JP, Levy M, Shapiro S. The Drug Etiology of Agranulocytosis and Aplastic Anemia. New York: Oxford, 1991.
14. Hellman S, Botnick LE, Hannon EC, Vigneulle RM. Proliferative capacity of murine hematopoietic stem cells. *Proc Natl Acad Sci USA* 1978; 75: 490-494.
15. Yunis AA. Chloramphenicol toxicity: 25 years of research. *Am J Med* 1989; 87: 3-44N-3-48N.
16. Baranski B, Armstrong G, Truman JT, Quinnan GV, Straus SE, Young NS. Epstein-Barr virus in the bone marrow of patients with aplastic anemia. *Ann Intern Med* 1988; 109: 695-704.
17. Apperley JF, Dowding C, Hibbin J, Buiter J, Matutes E, Sissons PJ, Gordon M, Goldman JM. The effect of cytomegalovirus on hemopoiesis: *in vitro* evidence for selective infection of marrow stromal cells. *Exp Hematol* 1989; 17: 38-45.
18. Simmons P, Kaushansky K, Torok-Storb B. Mechanisms of cytomegalovirus-mediated myelosuppression: Perturbation of stromal cell function versus direct infection of myeloid cells. *Proc Natl Acad Sci USA* 1990; 87: 1386-1390.
19. Yoshikawa T, Suga S, Asano Y, Nakashima T, Yazaki T, Sobue R, Hirano M, Fukuda M, Kojima S, Matsuyama.T. . Human herpesvirus-6 infection in bone marrow transplantation. *Blood* 1991; 78: 1381-1384.
20. Carrigan DR, Knox KK. Human herpesvirus 6 (HHV-6) isolation from bone marrow: HHV-6-associated bone marrow suppression in bone marrow transplant patients. *Blood* 1994; 84: 3307-3310.
21. Pol S, Driss F, Devergie A, Brechot C, Gluckman E. Is hepatitis C virus involved in hepatitis-associated aplastic anemia? *Ann Intern Med* 1990; 113: 435-437.
22. Hibbs J, Rosenfeld S, Feinstone SM, Kojima S, Bacigalupo A, Locasciulli A, Tzakis AG, Alter HJ, Young NS. Hepatitis/aplasia syndrome: non A, non B, non C? *JAMA* 1992; 267: 2051-2054.
23. Mathé G, Amiel JL, Schwarzenberg L, Choay J, Trolard P, Schneider M, Hayat M, Schlumberger JR, Jasmin Cl. Bone marrow graft in man after conditioning by antilymphocytic serum. *Br Med J* 1970; 2: 131-136.
24. Kagan WA, Ascensao JA, Pahwa RN, Hansen JA, Goldstein G, Valera EB, Incefy GS, Moore MAS, Good RA. Aplastic anemia: presence in human bone marrow of cells that suppress myelopoiesis. *Proc Natl Acad Sci USA* 1976; 73: 2890-2894.

25. Bacigalupo A, 'Podesta M, Frassoni F, Piaggio G, van Lint MT, Raffo MR, Repetto M, Marmont A. Generation of CFU-C suppressor T cells *in vitro* V. A multistep process. *Br J Haematol* 1982; 52: 421-427.
26. Zoumbos N, Gascon P, Trost S, Djeu J, Young N. Circulating activated suppressor T lymphocytes in aplastic anemia. *N Engl J Med* 1985; 312: 257-265.
27. Zoumbos N, Gascon P, Djeu J, Young NS. Interferon is a mediator of hematopoietic suppression in aplastic anemia *in vitro* and possibly *in vivo*. *Proc Natl Acad Sci USA* 1985; 82: 188-192.
28. Laver J, Castro-Malaspina H, Kernan NA, Levick J, Evans RL, , Moore MAS. *In vitro* interferon-gamma production by cultured T-cells in severe aplastic anaemia: Correlation with granulomonopoietic inhibition in patients who respond to anti-thymocyte globulin. *Br J Haematol* 1988; 69: 545-550.
29. Tong J, Bacigalupo A, Piaggio G, Figari O, Sogno G, Marmont A. *In vitro* response of T cells from aplastic anemia patients to antilymphocyte globulin and phytohemagglutinin: Colony-stimulating activity and lymphokine production. *Exp Hematol* 1991; 19: 312-316.
30. Selleri C, Anderson S, Young N, Maciejewski J. Interferon-gamma and tumor necrosis factor-alpha suppress both early and late stages of hematopoiesis and induce programmed cell death [abstract]. *Blood* 1994; 84: 215a.
31. Maciejewski J, Selleri C, Young NS. Fas antigen expression on CD34$^+$ human marrow cells is induced by interferon-gamma and tumor necrosis factor-alpha and potentiates hematopoietic suppression *in vitro*. *Blood* 1995; in press.
32. Maciejewski JP, Hibbs JR, Anderson S, Katevas P, Young NS. Bone marrow and peripheral blood lymphocyte phenotype in patients with bone marrow failure. *Exp Hematol* 1994; 22: 1102-1110.
33. Nakao S, Yamaguchi M, Shiobara S. Interferon gamma gene expression in unstimulated bone marrow mononuclear cells predicts a response to cyclosporine therapy in aplastic anemia. *Blood* 1992; 79: 2532-2535.
34. Nisticò A, Young NS. Gamma-interferon gene expression in the bone marrow of patients with aplastic anemia. *Ann Intern Med* 1994; 120: 463-469.
35. Maciejewski J, Liu J, Green S, Walsh C, Plumb M, Young NS. Expression of a stem cell inhibitor (SCI/LD78) gene in patients with bone marrow failure. *Exp Hematol* 1992; 20: 1112-1117.
36. Katevas P, Maciejewski J, Sorrentino B, Young NS. Increased expression of TNF-beta in patients with aplastic anemia. *Blood* 1993; 82 (Suppl. 7): 345a.
37. Selleri C, Young NS, Maciejewski J. Interferon-gamma and tumor necrosis factor-alpha broadly suppress human hematopoiesis and induce apoptosis in purified hematopoietic cells. *Exp Hematol* 1995; Submitted:
38. Sato T, Selleri C, Young NS, Maciejewski J, Jaroslaw P. Hematopoietic inhibition by interferon-_ is partially mediated through interferon regulatory factor-1. *Blood* 1995; Submitted:
39. Maciejewski JP, Selleri C, Sato T, Cho HJ, Keefer LK, Nathan CF, Young NS. Nitric oxide suppression of human hematopoiesis *in vitro*: contribution to inhibitory action of interferon-_ and tumor necrosis factor-α. *J Clin Invest* 1995; in press.
40. Nimer SD, Ireland P, Meshkinpour A, Frane M. An increased HLA DR2 frequency is seen in aplastic anemia patients. *Blood* 1994; 84: 923-927.
41. Nakao S, Yamaguchi M, Saito M, Yasue S, Shiobara S, Matsuda T, Nitta M, Sasaki M. HLA-DR2 predicts a favorable response to cyclosporine therapy in patients with bone marrow failure [letter]. *Am J Hematol* 1992; 40: 239-240.
42. Nakao S, Takamatsu H, Chuhjo T, Ueda M, Shiobara S, Matsuda T, Kaneshige T, Mizoguchi H. Identification of a specific HLA class II haplotype strongly associated with susceptibility to cyclosporine-dependent aplastic anemia. *Blood* 1994; 84: 4257-4261.
43. Tichelli A, Gratwohl A, Wursch A, Nissen C, Speck B. Late haematological complications in severe aplastic anaemia. *Br J Haematol* 1988; 69: 413-418.
44. Young NS. The problem of clonality in aplastic anemia. Dr. Dameshek's riddle, restated. *Blood* 1992; 79: 1385-1392.
45. Schubert J, Alvarado M, Uciechowski P, Zielinska-Skowronek M, Freund M, Vogt H, Schmidt RE. Diagnosis of paroxysmal nocturnal haemoglobinuria using immunophenotyping of peripheral blood cells. *Br J Haematol* 1991; 79: 487-492.

46. Socié G, Henry-Amar M, Bacigalupo A, Hows J, Tichelli A, Ljungman P, McCann SR, Frickhofen N, Van't Veer-Korthof EV, Gluckman E. Malignant tumors occurring after treatment of aplastic anemia. *N Engl J Med* 1993; 329: 1152-1157.
47. Schrenzenmeier H, Hertenstein B, Wagner B, Raghavachar A, Heimpel H. A pathogenetic link between aplastic anemia and paroxysmal nocturnal hemoglobinuria is suggested by a high frequency of aplastic anemia with a deficiency of phosphatidylinositol glycan proteins. *Exp Hematol* 1995; 23: 81-87.
48. Bennaceur-Griscelli A, Gluckman ML, Scrobohaci P, Jonveaux T, Bazarbachi A, Carosella ED, Sigaux F, Socié G. Aplastic anemia and paroxysmal nocturnal hemoglobinuria: search for a pathogentic link. *Blood* 1995; 85: 1354-1363.

Résumé

L'aplasie médullaire a probablement deux causes majeures : type 1, toxicité directe liée à une exposition à une irradiation à forte dose, des drogues myélotoxiques ou des agents chimiques comme le benzène ou certains insecticides ; et type 2, d'origine autoimmune. Dans le type 2, la maladie peut évoluer en 3 phases : 1) déclenchement par la présentation au système immunitaire d'un métabolite chimique ou d'un antigène viral, 2) pathologie immune liée à l'activation des cellules T et des lymphokines et, 3) évolution vers une maladie clonale comme l'hémoglobinurie paroxystique nocturne. La seconde phase est la plus connue. L'interféron (INF) gamma est un important médiateur de la suppression de l'hématopoïèse, il est détecté chez les aplasiques et pas chez les normaux. Cette cytokine ainsi que le *tumor necrosis factor* (TNF) inhibe les progéniteurs hématopoïétiques à tous les stades de leur différenciation. Tous deux induisent l'expression du récepteur de Fas sur les cellules $CD34^+$, ce qui entraîne l'apoptose par l'anticorps monoclonal *in vitro* et probablement par le ligand de Fas *in vivo*. L'expression de l'antigène Fas est augmentée sur les cellules $CD34^+$ des malades aplasiques. La production locale d'INF gamma est plus inhibitrice que l'addition d'INF dans les cultures à long terme. La production endogène par les cellules stromales après transduction pour produire 20u/ml d'INF gamma est aussi inhibitrice que 500 U/ml d'INF exogène rajouté chaque semaine aux cultures. L'aplasie médullaire de type auto-immun semble donc apparentée à d'autres maladies liées à la cytotoxicité des cellules T comme le diabète de type 1 ou la sclérose en plaques où les cellules cytotoxiques T sécrètent de l'INF responsable de la destruction spécifique de l'organe cible ; toutes ces maladies répondent aux traitements immunosuppresseurs.

Mobilization of peripheral blood hemopoietic progenitors (PBHP) from patients with severe aplastic anemia (SAA) after prolonged administration of G-CSF

A. Bacigalupo[1], G. Piaggio[1], M. Podesta[1], M. Valbonesi[2], G. Lercari[2], O. Figari[1], G. Sogno[1], E. Tedone[1], M.R. Raffo[1], L. Grassia[1], M.T. Van Lint[1] and A.M. Marmont[1]

[1] *Divisione di Ematologia;* [2] *Centro Trasfusionale, Ospedale San Martino, 16132 Genova, Italy, tel.: (39 10) 35 54 69, fax: (39 10) 35 55 83.*

Summary

Seven patients with severe aplastic anemia (SAA), 11-46 years old, 4 at diagnosis of their disease and 3 patients failing previous immunesuppression were treated with antilymphocyte globulin (ALG) (day 1-5), cyclosporin A (CyA) (5 mg/kg/day p.o) (day 6-90) and G-CSF 5 ug/kg/day (day 6-90). A total of 26 leukapheresis were performed, (range 2-6/patient), between day +10 and +168 of G-CSF treatment. WBC count at the time of harvest ranged from 1.2 t 18.1 x10^9/l. The results can be summarized as follows: the median number of cells collected/patient was 2.9x10^8/kg (range 2.6-10.4), the median number of CD34+cells was 1.8x10^6/kg (range 0.27-3.8) and the median number of CFU-GM was 2.6x10^4/kg (range 0-39). Ten leukapheresis performed between day +33 and +59 of G-CSF treatment, grew granulocyte macrophage (GM) and erythroid colonies in vitro. *No colony growth was obtained from 16 leukapheresis performed before day+33 or after day+60.*

In four patients the total number of CFU-GM recovered were in the range described for autologous PB stem cell grafts (2.6-39x10^4/kg).

In conclusion this study suggests that circulating hemopoietic progenitors can be recovered after ALG priming and after at least one month of G-CSF treatment in a proportion of patients with SAA. Whether these cells will be suitable for autologous transplantation remains to be determined.

It is now recognized that large numbers of PBHP can be recovered after high dose chemotherapy [1, 2] and more so with the use of growth factors [3-5]. This work was prompted by a study of Haas and coworkers [6], showing that GM-CSF priming could mobilize peripheral blood hemopoietic progenitors (PBHP) also in lymphomas with chemo-radiotherapy induced hypo/aplasia.

Similarly to the latter, the majority of patients with acquired aplastic anemia (SAA) have residual hemopoietic progenitors, and their number is usually understimated by current in vitro culture techniques [7-9]. This assumption seems to e supported by hematologic reconstitution following antilymphocyte globulin treatment in the majority of SAA patients [10-13], and by enhanced growth in the presence of stem cell factor (SCF) [14].

If SAA patients have residual stem cells, it may be possible to mobilize hemopoietic progenitors with the use of in vivo growth factors and then collect them by leukapheresis for cryopreservation.

We are now reporting 7 SAA patients who were treated with ALG for 5 days, followed by cyclosporin and G-CSF for 3 months.

Materials and methods

Patients. Seven patients were admitted to our Department with the diagnosis of aplastic anemia: main clinical data are outlined in *Table I*.
All seven were transfusion dependent at the time of G-CSF treatment, according to an ongoing EBMT (European Group for Bone Marrow Transplantation) trial designed for patient presenting with less than 0.5×10^9 PMN/l. This protocol includes horse antilymphocyte globulin (HALG) (Merieux, Lyon France), 15 mg/kg/day on days 1,2,3,4,5; 6-methylprednisolone 5 mg/kg/day i.v. on days 1-5, then 2.5 mg/kg/day/i.v. on days 6-10 then tapering the dose untill discontinuation on day +30,; cyclosporin A 5 mg/kg/day/p.o. from day +6 to day +90 and G-CSF 5 ug/kg/day (i.v for 15 days then subcutaneous) from day +6 to day +90 One patient (N.2) was not eligible for this study (PMN 0.9×10^9/l), so he received the same regimen without G-CSF. He underwent a leukapheresis immediately after ALG , and then , because of deteriorating PB counts he was started on G-CSF on day +51.

Leukapheresis. Each patient underwent 2 to 6 leukapheresis using a continous flow cell separator Fenwal CS 3000.

Cell surface markers. PB cells recovered from leukapheresis were processed with a workstation Coulter Q-Prep, without further separation. Cell surface antigens were detected by a direct immunoluorescence (IFA), using a panel of conjugated FITC/PE monoclonal antibodies (MoAbs): Cyto-stat Coulter Clone CD3, CD4, CD8, for T-lymphocytes, CD19, HLA-DR, for B lymphocytes, CD13, CD14, CD33, for myelo-monocytic cells (Coulter, Hieleah, FL USA) and CD34 HPCA-2, for progenitor cells (Becton Dickinson, Mountain View, CAL USA). Fluorescence was analyzed with a Coulter EPICS Profile II. Isotypically matched mouse immunoglobulins, directly conjugated to FITC or PE, were used as negative controls in all experiments.

In vitro colony growth. Peripheral blood cells recovered from leukapheresis (10^5) were plated unfractionated in 1 ml of IMDM containing 30% FCS, in 0.9% methylcellulose, for CFU-GM growth with 100 ng/ml of rhGM-CSF (Sandoz). In the attempt of improving colony formation, peripheral blood cells from 3 leukapheresis were kept in liquid culture (10^6 cells /ml) for 5 days in the presence of Stem Cell Factor (SCF) (Genzyme, USA) 100 ng/ml.

Cells from the first 18 leukapheresis were further separated as follows: after a Ficoll Hypaque gradient (1077 gm/cm^2) and plastic adherence (2 hours at 37oC) cells were T depleted (with CAMPATH1M 1 ug/10^6 cells+ autologous complement 20%, or E-rosetting with neuraminidase treated sheep red blood cells) and plated for CFU-GM growth as described above.

CD34+ cells were positively selected by incubating 10×10^6 T cell depleted cells with CD34 Mab (HPCA-2, Bekton-Dickinson) for 30' at 4oC and then for 30' at 4oC with anti-mouse Ig coated Dynabeads (DYNAL, Oslo, Norway): thereafter the CD34-negative and CD34-positive fractions were plated in 0.9% methylcellulose for CFU-GEMM growth with IMDM containing 30% FCS, $2/10^{-4}$ M Hemin, $5\backslash10^{-5}$ beta mercaptoethanol, 1% BSA (Fraction V, SIGMA), in the presence of 2U/ml recombinant human erythropoietin (rhEpo Cilag,Milan,Italy) 100 ng of

rhGM-CSF (Sandoz Basle), 100 ng/ml rhIl3 (kindly provided by Sandoz,Basel) with or without SCF (20 ng/ml) (Genzyme, USA).
The cultures were incubated for 14 days in a 37^C, 5% CO2 humidified incubator. Colonies were counted with an Olympus IM inverted microscope. Cryopreservation. PB cells were cryopreserved in culture medium (TC 199) containing 10% DMSO and 5% autologous heparinized plasma, by means of a freezing flow rate unit (Planer 203). Cryopreserved samples were stored in gas phase of liquid nitrogen

Results

Patients. All patients completed the designed course of treatment. Two patients (N2,N3) died on day +150 and +200 of infection: we were unable to collect from these patients peripheral blood cells capable of colony formation *in vitro*. The other 5 patients are surviving between day 100 and day 365 from G-CSF treatment: 3 are transfusion dependent, and 2 are transfusion independent. The number of patients is too small to draw any conclusions on the efficacy of G-CSF administration on hematologic response.
Leukapheresis. A total of 26 leukapheresis were performed. There were no major problems in carrying out the procedures, also with low leukocyte counts.
Leukapheresis were performed when possible, at intervals of 7-15 days.
The median number of cells collected/procedure was 2.9 x10^8/kg (range 2.6-10.4).
Cell phenotype. The surface phenotype of recovered cells was as follows: CD3: 47+18, CD4:32+3, CD8:26+4, CD19:20+6, CD13:5+6, CD14:15+14, DR:16+9, CD33+:34-: 7+2, CD33-34+: 0.24+0.15, CD33+34+: 0.52+0.35.
We saw no major increment of circulating CD34+ cells during treatment with G-CSF. The median number of CD34+ cells collected /leukapheresis was 1.8 (range 0.27-3.8)
Colony formation *in vitro*. 16/26 leukaheresis performed before day+30 or after day+60, grew no colonies. Ten leukapheresis performed between day +30 and day +60 yielded a large number of GM and erythroid colonies. PB cells from two apheresis (patient N.1) also grew large numbers of BFU-E : 17 and 37x10^4/kg Patients N1 and N4 underwent two additional leukapheresis on days +74 and +90 respectively, but there was no colony formation at this time.
T cell depletion and colony formation. T cell depletion did not seem to enrich for hemopoietic progenitors, and indeed had a detrimental effect on 3 leukapheresis from which large number of colonies had been grown from unseparated cells. Two of these cell populations had been treated with CAMPATH-1M and one with E-rosetting. There was one exception: the last leukapheresis from patient N1, which grew no colonies before or after TCD, but did grow 35 mixed colonies (CFU-GEMM) from 10^5 CD34+ positively selected cells.

Discussion

These results suggest that prolonged administration of G-CSF and cyclosporin A to patients with aplastic anemia, following treatment with ALG, can result in mobilization of large numbers of hemopoietic progenitors. It confirms that some patients with SAA still have a stem cell reservoir, in spite of pancytopenia [14]. It is further supported by previous work showing an increased number of BFU-E in the peripheral blood after ALG therapy [8]. Our finding is also in keeping with data obtained in animals showing that treatment with G-CSF alone mobilized pluripotent stem cells in the peripheral blood, which could be successfully used for autografts [15].

This may also suggest that "response" of SAA patients to ALG with o without G-CSF may be dependent on circulation in the peripheral blood and re-seeding of hemopoietic progenitors.

Many questions remain to be answered :the timing of PB cell collection, the quality of cells collected,their ability to allow sustained hematologic recovery if used for autologous transplantation. As to the first question, our data would indicate that circulation of hemopoietic progenitors in the peripheral blood occurs in the first and second month of G-CSF treatment. Because T cells have been implicated in the pathogenesis of aplastic anemia [16], because a large proportion of PB cells are T cells (mean 47%), and because "treatment" implies the use of high dose cyclophosphamide as a potent lymphotoxic agent, we thought that it would be perhaps undesirable to "re-infuse" a large number of autologous T cells. We have been confronted with the detrimental effect of T cell depletion on PB hemopoietic progenitors. This is somehow similar to cord blood, where cell separation leeds to significant loss of colony formation capacity [17]. Untill this problem is sorted out we will cryopreserve unseparated cells. Finally, we do not know at present whether these cells will be capable of sustained hematologic recovery if infused after high dose cyclophopshamide. There are several in vitro studies suggesting that hemopoietic progenitors from SAA patients are abnormal: in particular J Marsh recently showed with elegant long term cultures that they have a reduced capacity of proliferation and survival also when grown on normal stromal layers [18]. The finding of a high proportion of female patients with "clonal" hemopoiesis [19, 20] would also leed to the same conclusion. However, a recent review has pointed out that abnormalities of hemopoietic progenitors from SAA patients, and particularly clonality, may not necessarily indicate an intrinsic defect, or a pre-leukemic disorder [21]. In keeping with this view is a recent contribution showing the lack of point mutation of N-ras oncogene in marrow cells from SAA patients [22]. We would like to favour this view, and interpret the high incidence of leukemia and myelodysplasia seen in long term survivors after ALG [23], as the expression of long lasting stressed hemopoiesis. If we were capable of modifying the accessory cell circuits, as known to occurr after high dose cyclophosphamide, and if we then reinfused autologous hemopoietic progenitors, this may allow better hematologic recovery than seen with ALG alone, and thus reduce the risk of late clonal disease.

Acknowledgements

This work was supported by the Associazione Ricerca Trapianto Midollo Osseo (**ARITMO**), and Associazione Italiana Ricerca contro il Cancro (**AIRC**).

References

1. Bell AJ, Jamblin TJ, Oscier DG. Peripheral blood stem cell autografting. Hematol Oncol 5:45,1987
2. Juttner CA, To LB, Haylock Dn, Dyson PG, Thorp D, Dasrt GW, Ho JQK, Horvath N, Bardy P. Autologous stem cell transplantation. *Transpl Proc* 21: 2929, 1989.
3. Siena S, Bregni M, Brando B, Ravagnani F, Bonadonna G, Gianni AM. Circulationof CD34+ Hematopoietic Stem Cells in the Peripheral Blood of High-Dose Cyclophosphamide-Treated Patients: Enhancement by Intravenous Recombinant Human Granulocyte-Macrophage Colony-Stimulating Factor. *Blood,* (Vol 74, No 6) 1905: 1914, 1989.
4. Siena S, Bregni M, Brando B, Belli N, Ravagnani F, Gandola L, Stern AK, Lansdorp M, Bonadonna G, Gianni AM. Flow cytometry for clinical estimation of circulating hemopoietic progenitors for autologous transplantation in cancer patients. *Blood,* 77: 400, 1991.

5. Tarella C, Ferrero D, Bregni M, Siena S, Gallo E, Pileri A, Gianni M. Peripheral blood expansion of early progenitor cells after high dose cyclophosphamide and rhGM-CSF. *Eur J Cancer* 27: 22, 1991.
6. Haas R, Ho AD, Bredthauer U, Cayeux S, Egerer G, Knauf W, Hunstein W. Sucessful autologous transplantation of blood stem cells mobilized with recombinant human granulocyte-macrophage colony-stimulating factor. *Exp Hematology,* (Vol 18 No 2) 94: 98, 1990.
7. Nissen C (1989) Pathophysiology of aplastic anaemia. *Bailliere's Clinical Haematology* 2: 37.
8. Torok Storb BJ. T cell effects on in vitro erythropoiesis: immune regulation and immune reactivity In: Young NS, Levine A, Humphries RK, eds. Aplastic Anemia:stem cell biology and advances in treatment. New York: Alan R Liss. 1984:163-172.
9. Bacigalupo A, G Piaggio, O Figari, J Tong, G Sogno, E Tedone, A Sette*, P Caciagli*, S Badolati*, Marmont AM. Response of CFU-GM to increasing doses of rhGM-CSF in patients with Aplasti Anemia. *Exp Hematol* 19: 829-832, 1991.
10. Speck B, Gluckman E, Haak, HL, Van Rood JJ. Treatment of aplastic anemia by antithymocyte globulin with and without allogeneic bone marrow infusions. *Lancet* 1977; ii: 1145-47.
11. Camitta B, O'Reilly RJ, Sensenbrenner L, Rappeport J, Champlin R, Doney K, August C, Hoffman RG, Kirkpatrick D, Stuart R, Santos G, Parkman R., Gale RP, Storb R, Nathan D. Antithoracic duct lymphocyte globulin therapy of severe aplastic anemia. *Blood* 1983; 62: 883-887.
12. Doney KC, Weiden PL, Buckner CD, Storb R, Thomas ED. Treatment of severe aplastic anemia using antithymocyte globulin with or without an infusion of HLA haploidentical marrow. *Exp Hematol* 1981; 9: 829-33.
13. Frickhofen N et al. Treatment of aplastic anemia with antilymphocyte globulin and methylprednisolone with or without cyclosporine. *New England Journal of Medicine* 1991, 324 (19): 1297.
14. Bagnara GP, Strippoli P, Bonsi L, Brizzi MF, Avanzi GC, Timeus F, Ramenghi U, Piaggio G, Tong J, Podesta' M, Paolucci G, Pegoraro L, Gabutti V, Bacigalupo A. Effect of stem cell factor on colony growth from acquired and constitutional (Fanconi) aplastic anemia. *Blood* 1992 (in press).
15. Molineux G, Pojda Z, Hampson IN, Lord BI, Dexter TM. Transplantation Potential of Peripheral Blood Stem Cells Induced by Granulocyte Colony-Stimulating Factor. *Blood,* (Vol 76) 2153: 2158, 1990.
16. Young NS. The pathogenesis and pathophysiology of aplastic anemia, in Hoffman R, Benz EJ, Shattil SJ, Furie B, Cohen HJ (eds): Hematology. Basic principles and practice. New York, NY, Churchill Livingstone 1991, p122.
17. Thiery D, Hervatin F, Treiman R, Brossard Y, Stock R, Benbunan M, Gluckman E. Hemopoietic progenitor cells in cord blood. *Bone Marrow Transp* 1992 9: (suppl 1); 101-104.
18. Marsh JCW, Chang J, Testa N, Hows JM, Dexter TM. The hemopoietic defect in aplastic anemia. *Blood* 76: 1748, 1990.
19. Van Kamp H, Landegent JE, Jansen RPM, Willemze R, Fibbe WE. Clonal hemopoiesis in patients with acquired. *Blood* 78: 3209-3214, 1991.
20. Josten KM, Tooze JA, Borthwick Clarke C, Gordon Smith EC, Rutheford TR. Acquired aplastic anemia and paroxysmal nocturnal hemoglobinuria: studies on clonality. *Blood* 78: 3162-3167, 1991.
21. Young N. The problem of clonality in aplastic anemia. Dr Dameshek's riddle, restated. *Blood* 79; 1385, 1992.
22. Shinoara K, Yuiri T, Kamel S, Ayame H, Tanaka M, Ando S, Tairi M. Absence of point mutation of N-ras oncogene in bone marrow cells from patients with aplastic anemia. *Int J Cell Cloning* 10: 94-98, 1992.
23. De Planque M, Bacigalupo A, Wursch A, Hows J, Devergie A, Frickhofen N, Brand A, Nissen C. Long-term follow-up of severe aplastic anaemia patients treated with antithymocyte globulin. *British Journal of Haematology* 73: 121, 1989.

Résumé

Sept malades atteints d'aplasie médullaire ont été étudiés ; l'âge était de 11 à 46 ans ; 4 ont été étudiés au diagnostic et 3 après échec d'une immunosuppression ; ils ont été traités par sérum anti-lymphocytaire (ALG) (jours 1 à 5), ciclosporine A (CyA) (5 mg/kg/j po) (jours 6-90) et G-CSF 5ug/kg/j (j 6-90). Un total de 26 leucophérèses a été fait, soit 2-6 par patients, entre le jour 10 et le jour 168 du traitement par G-CSF. Le taux de globules blancs au moment du prélèvement était de 1,2 à $18,1 \times 10^9$/l. Le nombre médian de cellules recueillies par malade a été de $2,9 \times 10^8$/kg, (2,6-10,4) ; de $CD34^+$ $1,8 \times 10^6$/kg, (0,27-3,8) et de CFU-GM $2,6 \times 10^4$ /kg (0-39). Dix leucophérèses effectuées entre le jour 33 et 59 de G-CSF ont permis d'obtenir des colonies de GM et d'érythroblastes *in vitro*. Aucune colonie n'a été obtenue de 16 leucophérèses faites avant le jour 33 ou après le jour 60. Chez 4 malades, le nombre total de CFU-GM obtenu était au voisinage de celui utilisé pour une greffe de cellules souches périphériques autologues (2,6- 39×10^4/kg). En conclusion, cette étude semble démontrer que des cellules souches circulantes peuvent être recueillies après traitement par ALG et au moins 1 mois de G-CSF chez certains malades atteints d'aplasie médullaire. Il reste à démontrer que ces cellules peuvent être utilisées pour une greffe autologue.

Stroma derived hemopoietic progenitors: cell cycle dependent proliferation and differentiation

Ralf Huss[1], Cynthia A. Hoy[2], H. Joachim Deeg[2]

[1] Institute of Immunology, University Hospital, Virchowstr. 171, D-45122 Essen, Germany, tel.: (49 201) 723 4200, fax: (49 201) 723 5936; [2] Fred Hutchinson Cancer Research Center, 1124 Columbia St, M318, Seattle, WA 98104, USA

Summary

The canine marrow derived CD34⁻, DR⁻ stromal cell line D064 is able to differentiate into cells with characteristics of hemopoietic progenitors. While differentiating, these cells start to express CD34 and DR. Differentiation can be induced by the addition of exogenous canine recombinant stem cell factor (SCF). Addition of Interleukin-6 (IL-6) on the other hand, is able to inhibit differentiation of D064 cells, but rather promotes adherent growth and proliferation. Both factors, SCF and IL-6 are produced by the D064 cells themselves, suggesting an autocrine regulatory function. The influence of SCF or IL-6 on differentiation or proliferation, respectively, is also reflected in the DNA content of D064 cells during the cell cycle. SCF increases the number of D064 cells in G_1/G-phase during differentiation, while IL-6 induces cell mitosis (increased $S/G_2/M$-phase). The analysis of the cyclin dependent kinase (cdk) inhibitor p27 reveals that SCF induces the expression of p27 over time, while no p27 is detectable in the presence of IL-6 or an anti-SCF monoclonal antibody. The accumulation of intracellular p27 preceeds the detachment of D064 cells and their differentiation. But, as the cells differentiate and more commited progenitors emerge (clonal expansion), p27 is no longer expressed. These data suggest that SCF and IL-6 are two essential factors in the marrow microenvironment in regards to cell cycle progression and the differentiation and proliferation of early hematopoietic stem cells. Although, they have opposing funtions, they are both essential for the survival / proliferation and differentiation of stromal cells and hemopoietic progenitors.

Stroma-derived fibroblasts

We have recently described a fibroblast-like cell derived from canine bone marrow which is able to differentiate into cells with hematopoietic characteristics [1]. The cell line D064 was established according to standard procedures [2], cloned and grown in culture as adherent fibroblast-like cells. D064 cells maintained their function as marrow stromal cells and were able to support hematopoietic growth in standard Dexter cultures [1]. These cells are CD34⁻, DR⁻ and transcribe a variety of hematopoietic growth factors while still adherent [3]. With time in culture, some D064 cells detach, but remain in culture as viable, small lymphocyte-like cells. This differentiation appears to be due to the accumulation of endogenous autocrine factor, *eg* stem cell factor (SCF). The spontaneously differentiating cells start to express CD34, DR and c-kit on the surface [1].

Differentiation and proliferation

D064 cells differentiate not only spontaneously in culture. Differentiation into cells with hemopoietic characteristics also occurs when recombinant canine stem cell factor (SCF, c-kit ligand) is added at concentrations of 100 ng/ml [1]. The emerging cells change their morphology and the surface expression of surface markers (CD34$^+$, DR$^+$). When the non-adherent D064 cells are plated in a colony-forming-unit (CFU) assay, they produce a variety of CFUs, mainly CFU-GM (granulocyte-monocyte), but also CFU-F (fibroblast) and CFU-mix. The clonal growth of differentiated D064 cells can also be maintained in long-term cultures over several weeks. The presence of an anti-MHC class II monoclonal antibody in this assay, reduces the yield of CFUs by 50% or more, which is in agreement with previous observations [4], suggesting that the expression of MHC class II (DR) is a differentiation marker. Differentiation is reversible, either when non-adherent cells are taken out of the D064 cell culture and placed into fresh culture medium or when interleukin-6 (IL-6) is added to the culture. IL-6 does not only inhibit the differentiation of D064 cells in culture, but induces the proliferation of D064 cells, while still adherent [1].

Cell cycle

The induction of differentiation by SCF (non-adherence) and the promotion of proliferation by IL-6 (adherence) is also reflected in the cell cycle as measured by DNA content of D064 cells. In the presence of SCF, the number of D064 cells in S-phase decreased by approx. 10-30%, as compared to D064 cells growing in tissue culture without the addition of growth factors, and the number of D064 cells in G_1-phase increased, respectively [5]. The DNA content was measured by the analysis of DNA in propidium iodide stained cell nuclei and flow cytometry (FACscan, Becton-Dickinson). The adherent growing D064 cells showed no alteration in the cell cycle when IL-6 was added at any concentration, suggesting that proliferation occurs predominantely in adherent growing cells, while differentiating cells are arrested in G_1.

p27^{kip1} analysis

A link between cell cycle progression and adherent growth has been shown in other models [6]. In our model, hemopoietic differentiation can be induced by SCF and occurs when the D064 cells are arrested in G_1-phase. IL-6, on the contrary, induces progression of the cell cycle into S-phase, while D064 cells are still adherent. We tried to correlate these findings with the intracellular expression of the cyclin dependent kinase (cdk) inhibitor $p27^{kip1}$. When p27 is expressed, the cell is arrested in G_1-phase and can not progress into S-phase and cell division [7]. We incubated D064 cells with SCF (100 ng/ml) from 0 (zero) to 48 hours, and harvested the adherent as well as the non-adherent cells. Cell lysates were separated by a SDS-polyacrylamide gel electrophoresis and transfered for Western blot analysis. After blotting, the membrane bound proteins were visualized with a polyclonal antibody, directed against human p27. As shown in *Figure 1*, the expression of p27 in D064 cells increased over time in the presence of SCF, while the non-adherent differentiating cells expressed hardly any p27. This suggests, that hemopoietic differentiation is initiated in progenitor cells in the presence of p27 during G_1-phase arrest. When D064 cells lose their ability to adhere and are committed to hemopoietic differentiation, then p27 is no longer present and clonal expansion can occur. The initiation of hemopoietic differentiation and expression of p27 is under the control of SCF as shown in *Figure 2*. Neutralization of SCF [8] or the addition of IL-6 completely inhibits the intracellular expression of p27. In summary, the expression of p27 in D064 cells correlates with differentiation and proliferation. The initiation of hemopoietic differentiation is induced by SCF and occurs in the pre-

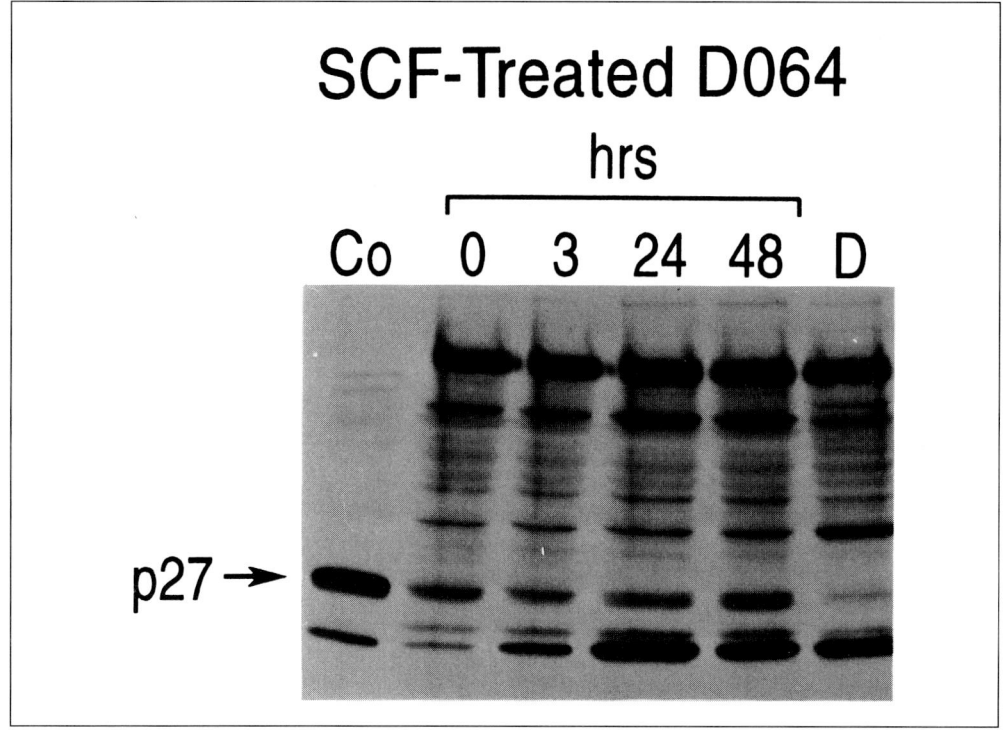

Figure 1. Western blot analysis of SCF-treated D064 cells. D064 cells were incubated with SCF (c-kit ligand) for 0, 3, 24 and 48 hours. The adherent cells were harvested at these time points and the cellular proteins were run in a SDS-plyacrylamide gel electrophoresis. After blotting, the membrane was incubate with a polyclonal anti-p27 antibody (generously provided by J.M. Roberts). Non-adherent differentiating cells (D) were also used as well as human peripheral blood lymphocytes (Co).
The presence of SCF in culture induced the expression of p27 over time (0-48 hours); differentiating cells no longer show p27. ("Co" served as a control for p27.)

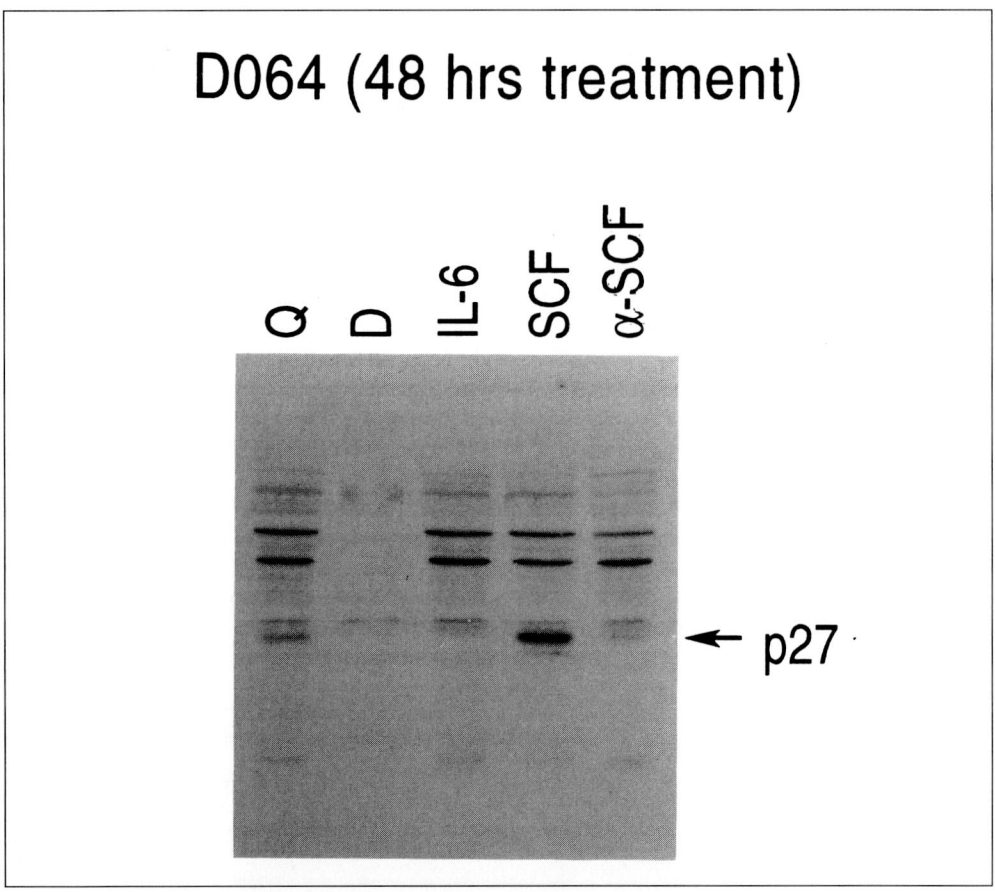

Figure 2. Western blot analysis of D064 cells with an anti-p27 polyclonal antibody. The level of p27 in D064 cells is increased by SCF and inhibited by Interleukin-6 and anti-SCF monoclonal antibody. Differentiating D064 cells (D) have no p27 expression, while untreated, adherent D064 cells (Q) show some p27 expression.

sence of p27 expression. Proliferation and clonal expansion, on the contrary, occurs under the control of IL-6 and in the absence of p27. This model of early hemopoietic differentiation shows an absolute correlation between growth factors and cell cycle progression in differentiation and proliferation.

Acknowledgement

We thank Eduardo Firpo and James M Roberts for their advice and the p27 analysis. This work was supported by PHS grants CA 18029, HL-36444, CA 31787 and CA 18222. RH was also supported by a grant from the Deutsche Forschungsgemeinschaft, Bad Godesberg, Germany.

References

1. Huss R, Hong DS, McSweeney PA, Hoy CA, Deeg HJ. Differentiation of canine marrow cells with hemopoietic characteristics from an adherent stromal cell precursor. *Proc Natl Acad Sci USA* 1995; 92: 748-752.
2. Singer JW, Charbord P, Keating A, Nemunaitis J, Raugi G, Wight TN, Lopez JA, Roth GJ, Dow LW, Fialkow PJ. Simian virus 40-transformed adherent cells from human long-term marrow cultures: Cloned cell lines produce cells with stromal and hematopoeitiec characteristics. *Blood* 1987, 70: 464-474.
3. Huss R, Hong DS, Storb R, Deeg HJ. Alteration of growth factor expression in marrow stromal cells by MHC class II corsslinking. In: Abraham N, Shadduck RK, Levine AS, Takaku T, eds. *Molecular Biology of Hematopoiesis*, Vol. 3. Andover, UK: Intercept Ltd, 1994: 719-25.
4. Huss R, Deeg HJ. MHC antigens and hemopoiesis. *Transplant Immunol* 1994, 2: 257-261.
5. Huss R, Hoy CA, Deeg HJ. Contact and growth factors involved in proliferation and differentiation in a canine marrow stromal cell line. *Blood* 1995 (in press)
6. Guadagno TM, Ohtsubo M, Roberts JM, Assoian RK. A link between cyclin A expression and adhesion-dependent cell cycle progression. *Science* 1993, 262: 1572-75.
7. Polyak K, Kato JY, Solomon MJ, Sherr CJ, Massagne J, Roberts JM, Koff A. $p27^{kip1}$, a cyclin-cdk inhibitor links transforming growth factor-beta and contact inhibition to cell cycle arrest. *Genes Develop* 1994, 8(1): 9-22.
8. Huss R, Hong DS, Beckham C, Kimball L, Myerson D, Storb R, Deeg HJ. Ultrastructural localization of stem cell factor in canine marrow-derived stromal cells. *Exp Hematol* 1995, 23: 33-40.

Résumé

La lignée stromale canine DO64 CD34⁻, DR⁻ peut se différencier en cellules ayant les caractéristiques des cellules souches hématopoïétiques. Au cours de la différenciation, ces cellules commencent à exprimer CD34 et DR. La différenciation peut être induite par l'addition de *stem cell factor* (SCF) canin exogène. Par ailleurs, l'addition d'IL-6 peut inhiber la différenciation des cellules DO64 et faciliter la croissance et la prolifération. Les deux facteurs sont produits par les cellules de la lignée elles-mêmes faisant penser à une fonction régularisatrice autocrine. L' influence du SCF et de l'IL-6 sur la différenciation ou la prolifération se retrouve par l'étude du contenu en DNA des cellules pendant le cycle cellulaire. SCF augmente le nombre de cellules en G1/G pendant la différenciation alors que l'IL-6 induit la mitose (augmentation de la phase S/G2/M). L'analyse de l'inhibiteur p 27 kinase cycline-dépendant montre que SCF induit l'expression de p27 alors que p27 n'est pas détectable en présence d'IL-6 ou d'un anticorps monoclonal anti-SCF. L'accumulation intracellulaire de p27 précède le détachement des cellules DO64 et leur différenciation. Mais, alors que ces cellules se différencient et que des précurseurs plus différenciés apparaissent (expansion clonale), la p27 n'est plus exprimée. Ces résultats signifient que SCF et IL-6 sont 2 facteurs essentiels du microenvironnement impliqués dans la progression du cycle cellulaire, la différenciation et la prolifération des précurseurs précoces de l'hématopoïèse. Bien qu'ayant des fonctions opposées, ils sont tous les deux essentiels pour la survie, la prolifération et la différenciation des cellules stromales et des cellules souches hématopoïétiques.

2) Clonality

2) *Clonalité*

Is aplastic anemia a preleukemic disorder? Facts and hypotheses

G. Socié

Service de Greffe de Moëlle et Unité de Recherche sur la Biologie des Cellules Souches, LIRB-CEA, DSV Hôpital Saint-Louis, avenue Claude-Vellefaux, Paris Cedex 10, France, tel.: (33 1) 42 49 98 24, fax: (33 1) 48 03 19 60

Abstract

"AA, PNH and hypoplastic leukemia might have a common denominator in the form of an insult to the marrow" (Dameshek, 1967).

Evidences for a link between these 3 diseases are reviewed.

*1) **Clinical clues:** Clonal disorders may complicate congenital or acquired AA. The commonest congenital disorder is Fanconi's anemia, in which leukemia occurs in at least 10% of cases. In acquired AA, the Basel group first drew attention to a high incidence of myelodysplastic syndrome (MDS) in patients with AA seemingly cured of their aplasia by ALG. In a recent survey of the EBMT the 10-year cumulative incidence rates were 9.6% for MDS, 6.6% for AL (a 115 fold increased incidence as expected from the general population). In multivariate analysis, 5 factors affected the risk of MDS/AL: addition of androgens to ALG (RR=0.28), older age (RR=1.03), treatment in 1982 or later (RR=3.01), splenectomy (RR=3.65) and 2 or more ALG courses (RR=2.26).*

*2) **Biological clues:** The borderland between MDS and AA is also found at the marrow morphology level since some degree of dysmyelopoiesis is not unusual in AA. Cytogenetic analyses in AA are scarce but data from the Seattle group and from the EBMT showed that some patients with otherwise typical AA have clonal cytogenetic abnormalities at diagnosis. Recently, flow cytometry has been used to assess the GPI molecule defect in PNH. Our group, as others, have now clearly shown that a significant proportion of patients with otherwise typical AA have in fact a GPI defect due to alterations within the PIG-A gene. Finally, in the recent years, AA patients were reported to have molecular evidences of clonal hematopoiesis. This latter aspect must now be discuss in the light of recent clonality studies in normal individuals.*

These clinical and biological clues lead to the description of models of AA as a preleukemic disorder. A Model that tentatively includes all these clinical and biological aspects is described.

As early as 1967 Dr Dameshek stated in an editorial that *"Aplastic Anemia [AA], Paroxysmal Nocturnal Hemoglobinuria [PNH] and hypoplastic leukemia might have a common denominator in the form of an insult to the marrow"* [1]. In the past few years the inter-relationship between AA, PNH, and the myelodysplastic syndrome [MDS] have been restated in two editorials by Marsh and Geary, in 1991 [2] and by N.S.Young in 1992 [3]. The later editorial specifically discussed the recent problem of clonality studies using X-chromosome polymorphism markers [3]. In this review we will thus focus on most recent aspects of this problem. We will first review main clinical studies, and summarize a recent analysis on risk factors for developing MDS and acute leukemia [AL] after treatment for AA. In the second part we will review biological evidences showing that, in at least some cases, AA might represent a pre-malignant states.

Clinical clues

Clonal disorders may complicate congenital or acquired AA [4]. In acquired AA, the Basel group first drew attention, in 1986, to a high incidence of MDS in patients with AA seemingly cured of their aplasia by Antilymphocyte Globulins [ALG] [5]. This group then published two follow-up studies showing that following ALG the projected incidence of clonal diseases (MDS and/or PNH) might be as high as 42% at fifteen years post treatment with ALG (26%+/– 8 for MDS alone) [6, 7]. This incidence seems high when compared to that described in older series of patients treated with androgens (5.3% crude incidence) [8, 9]. However, since the median onset of MDS after ALG is 5 years, and since long term survivor series after androgen therapy include patients with less disease, any real comparison with these older series are difficult to draw. More recently other single centers studies have been published on MDS/AL after ALG treatment of AA [10, 11]. The reported projected incidences lies in the 10% range at ten years. Thus, the true incidence of MDS/AL following immunosuppressive therapy was thought to lie between 10 and 42%, and the reason for such wide differences in the reported incidence was not clear (low numbers of patients at risk and/or few malignant events). Two consecutive multicenter studies of the Severe Aplastic Anemia Working Party of the European Group for Blood and Bone Marrow Transplantation [EBMT] shed some light on this issue [12, 13]. The first one, published in 1989, included 468 patients. Eleven MDS cases and 1 case of AL were reported, leading to a 7-year projected MDS/AL incidence of 15% [12]. The second one included 860 patients who were treated with immunosuppressive therapy (and 748 patients who underwent bone marrow transplantation) [13]. On April 1992, the mean follow up of the immunosuppressive therapy group was 39 months (range 1 month to 14 years). All myelodysplastic syndromes and 15/17 cases of acute leukemia occurred within the immunosuppressive therapy group. Fifteen patients developed an acute leukemia (9 with pre-existing myelodysplastic syndrome). Overall, the 10-year cumulative incidence rate was 18.8% (95% confidence limits (CL): 12.6-27.4) after immunosuppressive therapy. According to the type of malignancy, the 10-year cumulative incidence rates were 9.6% (95%CL: 5.5-16.5) for myelodysplastic syndrome not followed by an acute leukemia and 6.6% (95% CL: 3.6-11.8) for acute leukemia after immunosuppressive therapy. Relative to general population, the observed to expected ratio for acute leukemia after immunosuppressive therapy was 115 ($P < 0.001$), 4 times higher than that after bone marrow transplantation (observed to expected = 28.6, $P < 0.001$). In multivariate analysis, 5 factors significantly affected the risk for developing myelodysplastic syndrome or acute leukemia after immunosuppressive therapy: the addition of androgens to antithymocyte globulin plus methylprednisolone (relative risk = 0.28, $P = 0.016$), older age at diagnosis (relative risk = 1.03,

P = 0.023) with age considered as a continuous variable and risk increasing with age, calendar time (relative risk = 3.01, P = 0.024), splenectomy (relative risk = 3.65, P = 0.026), and 2 or more immunosuppressive therapy courses (relative risk = 2.26, P = 0.030). When myelodysplastic syndrome was taken as the end-point, the same factors remained significant. However, in this analysis splenectomy emerged as the most prognostic factor (relative risk = 5.56, P = 0.005), followed by calendar period (relative risk = 4.11, P = 0.013), 2 or more immunosuppressive therapy courses (relative risk = 2.77, P = 0.015), the addition of androgens to antithymocyte globulin plus methylprednisolone (relative risk = 0.25, P = 0.020), and older age at diagnosis (relative risk = 1.03, P = 0.020). More recently cyclosporine A has been used in patients with AA [see N Frickhofen chapter in this issue]. To date there is no quatification of MDS/AL risk in patients who were treated with cyclosporine A alone. Hematopoietic growth factors have also been used either alone or in combination with immunosuppressive therapy, mostly in patients who relapsed from their disease. Reported MDS/AL incidence in patients surviving more than 2 years after the use of growth factor is 14.3% [14, 15].

The incidence of acute myeloblastic leukemia in patients with Fanconi's anemia is more than 15000 times that expected in the general population [16]. A recent analysis on 388 patients of the International Fanconi Anemia Registry stated that the actuarial risk of clonal cytogenetic abnormalities was 67% and that the actuarial risk of MDS/AML was 52% [17]. However, the real significance of such cytogenetic abnormalities have recently been the subject of some debate [18, 19].

Biological clues

The borderland between MDS and AA is also found at the marrow morphology level since some degree of dysmyelopoiesis is not unusual in AA [20]. In a recent study A Tichelli *et al* showed that ALG treated patients retain a reduced number of megakaryocytes and the persistence of atypical monocytes. Patients who later develop MDS are not different from the total population on the marrow morphological basis but show an increased number of ring sideroblasts and atypical monocytes during regeneration [21].

Cytogenetic analyses in AA are scarce but data from the Seattle group showed that 7/176 patients with otherwise typical, bone marrow biopsy confirmed, AA have clonal cytogenetic abnormalities at diagnosis [22]. Monosomy 7, the most frequent abnormality in chemo-radiotherapy-induced MDS, was found in 3 out of the 7 patients with clonal cytogenetic abnormalities in this study. Monosomy 7 is also the most frequent clonal cytogenetic abnormalities in patients developing MDS after ALG [7, 10, 11]. A preliminary analysis of a still ongoing survey of the EBMT on cytogenetic data, at diagnosis, in patients with AA show that 6% (11/179) of the patients with otherwise typical AA have clonal cytogenetic abnormalities [A. Tichelli, personal communication].

Recently, flow cytometry has been used to assess the GPI molecule defect in PNH. Our group [23], as others [24, 25], has now clearly shown that a significant proportion of patients with otherwise typical AA have in fact a GPI defect due to alterations within the *PIG*-A gene. In these series, the proportion of aplastic patients with a GPI-defect syndrome represent 30 to 50% of the cases and included untreated as well newly diagnosed patients. A recent suvey of the EBMT-SAA working party showed that 35/101 newly diagnosed patients with AA have a GPI-linked molecule defect in at least one lineage. Finally, recent advances in the biology of PNH [see L Luzzatto, chapter in this issue] allowed to prove, that in most cases, MDS/AL develop in the PNH clone in patients with PNH [26-29].

Finally, in the recent years, AA patients were reported to have molecular evidence of clonal hematopoiesis. This latter aspect must now be discuss in the light of recent clonality studies in normal individuals. First clonality series using X-chromosome inactivation studies were published in 1991. In the Leiden group study 13/18 patients with aplastic anemia were shown to have an unilateral X-inactivation pattern compatible with monoclonality [30]. By contrast only one out of the 6 patients with AA had such a profile in the St. Georges Hospital study [31], a proportion similar to that found recently in a pediatric population (2 out of 18 patients with monoclonal pattern) [32]. It should be noted that in the two early studies no somatic DNA controls were included to rule out constitutional skewed methylation pattern [30, 31]. More recent studies from the Ulm group [see A Ragavashar chapter this issue] and from a joint Basel/Cardiff study [33] raised however some problems about the interpretation of such clonality analyses. In the first one no correlation was found between clonality results and those of flow cytometry in patients with a GPI- molecule defect. In the second one of two patients with molecularly sequenced *N-ras* point mutations one exhitbits a monoclonal pattern but the other one a polyclonal pattern using the X-chromosome inactivation analysis techniques. Furthermore recent RE Gales and coworkers' clonality studies in normal individuals raised important questions with respect to the clonality of normal hematopoiesis since these authors demonstrated: 1) that nearly 20% of normal women exhibit an X-chromosome inactivation pattern compatible with monoclonality, 2) that there is a tissue specificity of X-chromosome inactivation pattern and 3) that the proportion of normal women with a monoclonal pattern increase with age (33% of the females over the age 75 as compared to 6% between 20-58 years of age). [34-36].

In Fanconi's anaemia a study by the International Fanconi Anemia Registry showed that one out of 7 female patients in the AA stage of the disease had an X-chromosome inactivation pattern compatible with monoclonality and that none of 18 patients studied had *N-ras* or *p53* gene mutation [37].

Hypothesis

Current hypotheses on the physiopathogeny of MDS have been recently reviewed by List and Jacobs and lead to a model where MDS follow the more general process of multistep carcinogenesis [38]. These authors stated that toxic insult, aging or other non-identified factors lead to clonal expansion of a clone bearing *N-ras, fms, p53* or other non-identified gene, mutations. Abnormal clonal cytogenetic abnormalities, such as monosomy 7 then lead to the progression of the mutated clone and clinical emergence of MDS. A Model stating that AA may be a pre-pre-leukemic disorder, tentatively including all the clinical and biological aspects reviewed previously, may thus be draw within the more general multisep carcinogenesis hypothesis. First there is growing evidences that hematopoiesis is not only quantitatively, but also qualitatively abnormal in AA. This abnormal hematopoiesis seems to be clonal in some cases (through *PIG-A* gene alteration, for example). This clone has a growth advantage over the aplastic marrow (*"clonality as escape"* as stated by NS Young [3]). Then accumulation of mutational events through *N-ras, fms, p53* or other non-identified gene, mutations, and abnormal clonal cytogenetic abnormalities, such as monosomy 7, may lead to the progression of the mutated clone and clinical emergence of a MDS and then AL, following the more general process described above. In this model AA could be compared to polyposis, the first step of colo-rectal carcinogenesis.

References

1. Dameshek W. What do aplastic anemia, paroxysmal nocturnal hemoglobinuria and "hypoplastic" leukemia have in common? *Blood* 1967; 30: 251-4.
2. Marsh JCW, Geary CG. Is aplastic anaemia a pre-leukaemic disorder? *Br J Haematol* 1991; 77: 447-52.
3. Young NS. The problem of clonality in aplastic anemia: Dr Damesheh's riddle, restated. *Blood* 1992; 79: 1385-92.
4. Deiss A. Non-neoplastic diseases, chemical agents, and hematological disodres that may precede hematological neoplasms in Lee GR, Bithell TC, Foerster J, Athens JW and Lukens JN (eds): *Wintrobe's Clinical Hematology, 9th Edition*. Philadelphia: Lea and Febiger, 1993: 1946-68.
5. Speck B, Gratwohl A, Nissen C, Osterwalder B, Würsch A, Tichelli A, Lori A, Reusser P, Jeannet M, Signer E. Treatment of severe aplastic anemia. *Exp Hematol* 1986; 14: 126-32.
6. Tichelli A, Gratwohl A, Würsch A, Nissen C, Speck B. Late haematological complications in severe aplastic anaemia. *Br J Haematol* 1988; 69: 413-8.
7. Tichelli A, Gratwohl A, Nissen C, Speck B. Late clonal complications in severe aplastic anaemia. *Leuk Lym* 1994; 12: 167-75.
8. Najean Y. L'anémie aplastique est elle un état préleucémique? *Nouv Presse Med* 1981; 10: 3775-8.
9. Najean Y, Haguenauer O. Long term (5 to 20 years) evolution of nongrafted aplastic anemias. *Blood* 1990; 76: 2222-8.
10. De Planque MM, Kluin-Nelemans HC, Van Krieken HJM, Kluin PM, Brand A, Beverstock GC, Willemze R, Van Rood JJ. Evolution of acquired severe aplastic anaemia to myelodysplasia and subsequent leukaemia in adults. *Br J Haematol* 1988; 70:55-62.
11. Paquette RL, Tebyani N, Frane M, Ireland P, Ho WG, Champlin RE, Nimer SD. Long-term outcome of aplastic anemia in adults treated with antithymocyte globulin: comparison with bone marrow transplantation. *Blood* 1995; 85: 283-90.
12. De Planque MM, Bacigalupo A, Würsch A, Hows JM, Devergie A, Frickhofen N, Brand A, Nissen C. Long-term follow-up of severe aplastic anemia patients treated with antithymocyte globulin. *Br J Haematol* 1989; 73: 121-6.
13. Socié G, Henry-Amar M, Bacigalupo A, Hows J, Tichelli A, Ljungman P, Mc Cann SR, Frickhofen N, Van't Veer-Korthof E, Gluckman E. Malignant tumors occurrring after treatment of aplastic anemia. *N Engl J Med* 1993; 329: 1152-7.
14. Imashuku S, Hibi S, Morimoto Y, Yoshihara T, Ikushima S, Morioka Y, Todo S. Myelodysplasia and acute myeloid leukaemia in cases of aplastic anaemia and congenital neutropenia following G-CSF administration. *Br J Haematol* 1995; 89: 188-90.
15. Imashuku S, Hibi S, Nakajima F, Mitsui T, Yokoyama S, Kojima S, Matsuyama T, Nakahata T, Ueda K, Tsukimoto I, Hanawa Y, Takaku F. A review of 125 cases to determine the risk of myelodysplasia and leukemia in pediatric neutropenic patients after recombinant G-CSF. *Blood* 1994; 84: 2380-1.
16. Auerbach AD, Allen RG. Leukemia and preleukemia in Fanconi anemia patients.*Cancer Genet Cytogenet* 1991; 51: 1-12.
17. Butturini A, Gale RP, Verlander PC, Alder-Brecher B, Gillio A, Auerbach AD. Hematologic abnormalities in Fanconi anemia: An International Fanconi Anemia Registry study. *Blood* 1994; 84: 1650-5.
18. Alter BP, Scalise A, Mc Combs J, Najfeld V. Clonal chromosomal abnormalities in Fanconi's anaemia: what do they really mean? *Br J Haematol* 1993; 85: 627-30.
19. Alter BP. Hematologic abnormalities in Fanconi anemia. *Blood* 1995; 85: 1148-9.
20. Young NS and Alter BP (eds). Aplastic anemia acquired and inherited. Philadelphia: WBS Saunders, 1994.
21. Tichelli A, Gratwohl A, Nissen C, Signer E, Stebler-Gysi C, Speck B. Morpology in patients with severe aplastic anemia treated with antilymphocyte globulin. *Blood* 1992; 80: 337-45.
22. Appelbaum FR, Barrall J, Storb R, Ramberg R, Doney K, Sale GE, Thomas ED. Clonal cytogenetic abnormalities in patients with otherwise typical aplastic anemia. *Exp Hematol* 1987; 15: 1134-9.
23. Griscelli-Bennaceur A, Gluckman E, Scrobohaci ML, Jonveaux P, Vu T, Bazarbachi A, Carosella ED, Sigaux F, Socié G. Aplastic anemia and paroxysmal nocturnal hemoglobinuria: search for a pathogenetic link. *Blood* 1995; 85: 1354-63.

24. Schreznmeier H, Hertenstein B, Wagenr B, Ragavashar A, Heimpel H. A pathogenetic link between aplastic anemia and paroxysmal nocturnal hemoglobinuria is suggested by a high frequency of aplastic anemia patients with a deficiency of phosphatidylinositol glycan anchored proteins. *Exp Hematol* 1995; 23: 81-7.
25. Scubert J, Vogt HG, Skowronek M, Freund M, Kaltwasser JP, Hoelzer D, Schmidt RE. Development of the glycosylphosphatidylinositol-anchoring defect characteristic for paroxysmal nocturnal hemoglobinuria in patients with aplastic anemia. *Blood* 1994; 83: 2323-28.
26. Van Kamp H, Smit JW, Van der Berg E, Halie MR, Vellenga E. Myelodysplasia following paroxysmal nocturnal hemoglobinuria: evidence for the emergence of a separate clone. *Br J Haematol* 1994; 87: 399-400.
27. Stafford HA, Nagarajan S, Weinberg J, Medof ME. PIG-A, DAF and proto-oncogene expression in paroxysmal nocturnal hemoglobinuria-associated acute myelogenous leukaemia blasts. *Br J Haematol* 1995; 89: 72-8.
28. Longo L, Bessler M, Beris P, Swirsky D, Luzzatto L. Myelodysplasia in a patient with pre-existing paroxysmal nocturnal hemoglobinuria: a clonal disorder originating from within a clonal disease. *Br J Haematol* 1994; 87: 401-3.
29. Shichima T, Terasawa T, Hashimoto C, Ohto H, Takahashi M, Shibata A, Maruyama Y. Discordant and heterogeneous expression of GPI-anchored membrane proteins on leukemic cells in a patient with paroxysmal nocturnal hemoglobinuria. *Blood* 1993; 81: 1855-62.
30. Van Kamp H, Landegent JE, Jansen RPM, Willemze R, Fibbe WE. Clonal hematopoiesis in patients with acquired aplastic anemia. *Blood* 1991; 78: 3209-14.
31. Josten KM, Tooze JA, Borthwick-Clarke C, Gordon-smith EC, Rutherford TR. Acquired aplastic anemia and paroxysmal nocturnal hemoglobinuria: studies on clonality. *Blood* 1991; 78: 3162-7.
32. Tsuge I, Matsuoka H, Abe T, Kamachi Y, Torii S, Matsuyama T. Clonal haematopoiesis in children with acquired aplastic anaemia. *Br J Haematol* 1993; 84: 137-43.
33. Padua RA, Petterson T, Taylor C, Culligan D, Warren N, Wagstaff M, Pollard P, Kapelko K, Tichelli A, Jacobs A. Ras mutations in patients with aplastic anemia. *Blood* 1992; 80 (suppl 1): 657a
34. Gale RE, Wheadon H, Goldstone AH, Burnett AK, Linch DC. Frequency of clonal remission in acute myeloid leukaemia. *Lancet* 1993; 341: 138-42.
35. Gale RE, Linch DC. Interpretation of X-chromosome inactivation patterns. *Blood* 1994; 84: 2376-7.
36. Gale RE, Wheadon H, Boulos P, Linch DC. Tissue specificity of X-chromosome inactivation patterns. *Blood* 1994; 83: 2899-905.
37. Venkatraj VS, Gaidano G, Auerbac AD. Clonality studies and N-ras and p-53 mutation analysis of hematopoietic cells in fanconi anemia. *Leukemia* 1994; 8: 1354-8.
38. List AF, Jacobs A. Biology and pathogenesis of the myelodysplastic syndromes. *Seminars Oncol* 1992; 19: 14-24.

Résumé

Un lien entre la physiopathogénie de l'aplasie médullaire, de l'hémoglobinurie paroxystique nocturne et des sydromes pré-leucémiques a été suggéré par le Dr Dameshek dès 1967. Ce(s) lien(s) sont revus à la lumière de données récentes, cliniques et biologiques. Tenant compte de ces éléments récents, un modèle est proposé, qui suggère que certaines aplasies médullaires pourraient être des syndromes pré-leucémiques.

Tyrosine kinase receptors and their ligands in aplastic anemia

A. Wodnar-Filipowicz, C.Y. Manz, E. Schklovskaya, M. Slanicka Krieger, A. Gratwohl, A. Tichelli, B. Speck and C. Nissen

Research Department and Hematology Clinic, Kantonsspital Basel, Hebel Street 20, 4031 Basel, Switzerland, tel.: (41 61) 265 42 54, fax: (41 61) 265 44 50

Abstract

The tyrosine kinase receptors play a role in regulating growth, survival and differentiation of a number of cell types. Within the hematopoietic system, two closely related transmembrane receptors c-kit and flk-2/flt-3 are primarily expressed on stem and progenitor cells. Their respective ligands: stem cell factor (SCF) and the recently identified flt3 ligand are involved in regulation of the early stages of hematopoiesis. Our work focuses on the role of these receptor/ligand systems in the pathophysiology of aplastic anemia (AA), a disease characterized by multilineage failure of the bone marrow. We have: (i) characterized the progenitor cell compartment in AA by immunophenotypic analysis of cell surface early antigens CD34 and c-kit (analysed additionally at the mRNA level); (ii) determined the hematopoietic effects of SCF and flt3 ligand on AA bone marrow progenitors in vitro in clonogenic and long-term proliferation assays; and (iii) characterized the expression of SCF by bone marrow microenvironmental cells. We have found a deficiency of hematopoietic progenitor cells in AA, which was frequently associated with depressed growth of bone marrow stroma and decreased production of SCF by stroma cells. SCF and flt3 ligand had distinct stimulatory effects on AA marrow progenitors, SCF enhancing growth and flt3 ligand prolonging survival of colony-forming cells. Our results indicate a role of the two tyrosine kinase receptor ligands for in vitro or in vivo expansion of the reduced progenitor cell pool in aplastic anemia and, therefore, suggest a potential of these cytokines in treatment of the disease.

Aplastic anemia (AA) is characterized by multilineage bone marrow failure resulting in pancytopeniA Although certain viruses, drugs and chemicals have been implicated in the etiology of the disorder, its actual cause remains poorly understood. An intrinsic defect or immune-mediated injury to early hematopoietic progenitors have been proposed as major pathogenic mechanisms of the disease. A defective stromal microenvironment in the bone marrow may contribute to the hematopoietic lesion in some AA cases [1, 2]. Bone marrow transplantation offers virtually the only chance of cure. Immunosuppressive therapy with antilymphocyte globulin (ALG) and cyclosporin A has substantially improved prognosis [3, 4] but leaves the patient with residual disease activity prone for relapse and development of late clonal disorders of hematopoiesis [5, 6]. Hematopoietic growth factors like erythropoietin (Epo), granulocyte-macrophage colony-stimulating factor (GM-CSF), granulocyte colony-stimulating factor (G-CSF) and interleukin-3 (IL-3) are now in clinical use for the treatment of AA. They improve survival of severely neutropenic patients but their effects have been transient, and there is no evidence that growth factors can correct the underlying stem cell defect in AA [7].

The cytokines currently in clinical use act at a relatively late stage of hematopoiesis. However, improvement of bone marrow function in AA would rather be expected from growth factors influencing more primitive stages of hematopoietic development. Recent studies have identified a novel group of hematopoietic growth factors which act at a very immature level of hematopoiesis: stem cell factor (SCF) and flt3 ligand which bind and activate cells via tyrosine kinase receptors.

SCF is produced by bone marrow stromal cells and has been implicated in the maintenance of an optimum hematopoietic microenvironment [8, 9]. The factor interacts with *c-kit* receptors expressed at high levels on primitive and commited progenitors [10]. SCF exists in two biologically active forms: soluble and membrane-bound, the latter playing an important role in cell-cell interaction between stroma and hematopoietic stem cells [11]. Naturally occuring murine mutations of both SCF and *c-kit* are associated with lethal hematopoietic and developmental phenotypes, called *steel (Sl)* and *white spotting (W)*, respectively [12, 13]. *Sl* mutations result in abnormal expression of SCF gene locus, while *W* mutations severely impair the tyrosine kinase activity of *c-kit* receptors. In human blood diseases, abnormal expression of *c-kit* protein has been found in acute myeloblastic leukemia [14].

flt3 ligand is a recently cloned hematopoietic cytokine [15, 16], which interacts with transmembrane tyrosine kinase receptors designated *flk-2* in the mouse and *flt-3* in humans [17, 18]. flt-3 receptors are structurally related to *c-kit* receptors and, together with *c-fms* receptors for macrophage colony-stimulating factor, belong to the subclass of tyrosine kinase receptors with five immunoglobulin-like repeats in the extracellular receptor domain [19]. Although flt3 ligand is ubiquotously expressed, a highly restricted expression of its receptors narrows the population of target cells to early hematopoietic progenitors in human bone marrow [20].

Identification of early-acting hematopoietic growth factors has greatly contributed to the recently achieved progress in characterisation, isolation and functional analysis of cells at early developmental stages. Analysis of hematopoietic progenitors in aplastic anemia is hampered by hypocellularity of the bone marrow limiting the amount of cells available for experimental use. We have recently reported results on the proliferative efficacy of SCF in AA *in vitro* and of studies on SCF expression in this disease [21-23]. Effects of flt3 ligand on AA bone marrow cells have not yet been described. Here, we summarize our recent data on quantitative and qualitative analysis of hematopoietic progenitors and the biological effects of SCF and flt3 ligand in short- and long-term cultures of AA bone marrow cells. The aim of this work is to establish the role of early-acting cytokines in pathophysiology of AA and to investigate their hematopoietic potential for treatment of hypoproliferative marrow disorders.

Hematopoietic effect of SCF in AA *in vitro*

Formation of hematopoietic colonies by AA bone marrow cells is grossly reduced. The proliferative defect persists long after immunosuppressive therapy and, to a lesser degree, also after bone marrow transplantation. Poor colony growth *in vitro* cannot be overcome by high doses of Epo, IL-3, GM-CSF and G-CSF. We have demonstrated that SCF is the most efficient among

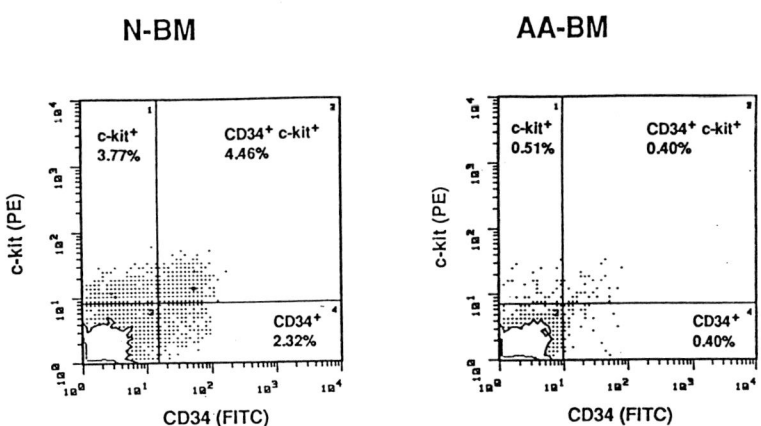

Figure 1. Flow cytometric analysis of bone marrow progenitor cells stained with antibodies against CD34 and *c-kit* surface antigens.

known hematopoietic cytokines in stimulating proliferation of colony-forming cells from AA bone marrows [21]. The highest number of colonies formed in methylcellulose corresponded to 30% of the level observed with normal marrows and proliferation of cells in liquid cultures approached 70% of control values. The most marked effect of SCF was on generation of erythroid colonies.

Response to SCF varies widely among individual patients and several bone marrows virtually do not respond to stimulation. In order to find out whether differences in growth response are due to differences in the content of colony-forming cells, we have quantitated hematopoietic progenitors in patients marrows by flow cytometric cell analysis. Multipotent progenitors can be identified by the surface expression of CD34 antigen [24]. CD34$^+$ cells represent a heterogenous population of cells that includes primitive, uncommitted stem cells as well as more mature subsets committed to myeloid, lymphoid or erythroid progeny [25]. A primitive subset of CD34$^+$ cells, negative for lineage specific markers expresses *c-kit* receptors on its surface [26]. We found that AA bone marrow cells are deficient in CD34$^+$ and CD34$^+$*c-kit*$^+$ cell subpopulations. Their frequency was 2-30 fold below normal levels. An example of FACScan analysis of normal and AA cells immunostained with monoclonal antibody against CD34 and *c-kit* surface antigens is given in *Figure 1*. Using bone marrow cells from a group of AA patients, we have purified CD34$^+$ cells by FACSort and compared their proliferative response to SCF before and after fractionation. Before sorting, formation of hematopoietic colonies was significantly below normal levels (67±24 versus 420±39 colonies/10^5 mononuclear cells). When purified CD34$^+$ cells were plated into methycellulose, the mean difference between AA normal colony numbers was less apparent (61±18 *versus* 153±23 colonies/10^3 cells). However, large differences were observed between individual bone marrow samples. Responsiveness to SCF correlated with disease severity: growth impairment was more pronounced in patients with prolonged severe pancytopenia.

Expression of SCF in AA

To evaluate the role of the hematopoietic microenvironment and stroma-derived cytokines in the etiology and clinical manifestation of AA, we have characterized stroma function in AA in terms of expression of SCF. The serum concentration of soluble SCF was determined assuming that it reflects factor production *in vivo* [22]. In comparison with normal sera which contained SCF at 3.3±1.0 ng/ml, factor levels in AA were moderately reduced to an average of 2.5±0.2 ng/ml *(Table I)*. The difference was statistically highly significant (p=0.0001). Abnormally low SCF serum levels in the severe phase of the disease at diagnosis appeared to normalize years after immunosuppressive therapy. It should be emphasized that high SCF levels were associated with a favourable clinical outcome, while SCF serum levels in patients who died in the course of treatment were considerably below normal. Deficiency of SCF in AA is not associated with abnormalities at the gene expression level, since we found normal levels of expression of SCF mRNA and a normal proportion between mRNA species encoding the soluble and the membrane-bound isoforms of SCF [23]. Rather, SCF protein production in low due to suboptimal proliferation of SCF-producing cells. We have observed poor growth of bone marrow microenvironmental cells in cultures of heterogenous adherent stroma cells and have confirmed growth defects in homogenous cultures of stromal fibroblasts. Proliferative abnormalities of stroma *in vitro* persist for years after immunuppressive therapy and are associated with relapse of AA *(Table II)*. Stroma growth *in vitro* could be enhanced by addition of SCF in combination with other stroma-derived cytokines: IL-11, leukemia inhibitory factor and basic fibroblast growth factor *(Figure 2)*. We conclude that AA may be associated with inadequate proliferation of marrow microenvironmental cells leading to SCF deficiency, but stromal defects in AA do not resemble defects in *Sl* mice having alterations at the SCF gene locus.

Table I. SCF serum levels in AA (ng/ml).

N	mean value	(n = 267)	3.3 ± 1.0
AA {p = .0001}	mean value	(n = 128)	2.5 ± 0.2
AA	at presentation	(n = 32)	2.5 ± 0.2
	1m - 1y post ALG	(n = 63)	2.3 ± 0.2
	1m - 1y post BMT	(n = 9)	2.2 ± 0.4
	> 1y post ALG	(n = 22)	3.2 ± 0.5
AA	alive	(n = 87)	2.8 ± 0.2
	died	(n = 41)	1.9 ± 0.1

Table II. Stroma growth and incidence of late complications after ALG treatment.

	Stroma confluence	
	≤ 30%	> 30%
Total AA patients	29	25
PNH/MDS	4	7
Relapse {p=0.028}	8	1

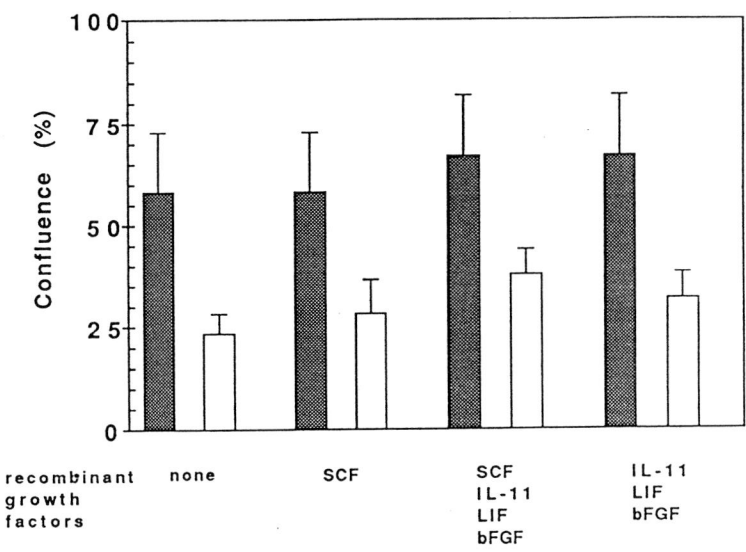

Figure 2. Effect of SCF and other stroma-derived cytokines on proliferation of adherent cells in stroma cultures. Growth of normal (n=4; dark columns) and aplastic (n=14; open columns) bone marrow is presented as a mean cell confluence ± SEM.

c-kit receptors in AA

To investigate the possibility that, in analogy to *W* mutants, abnormalities of *c-kit* gene are responsible for hematopoietic failure in AA we have analysed *c-kit* locus and its expression at the mRNA and protein levels. PCR analysis gave no evidence for the presence of deletions or rearrangements within the extracellular, transmembrane and kinase portions of *c-kit* coding region [27]. In search for point mutations which could alter the signalling activity of the receptor, we have performed the SSCP analysis of DNA isolated from bone marrow cells of 4 patients who showed no *in vitro* response to SCF and were, therefore, considered as candidates for the presence of abnormalities within the SCF *c-kit* receptors. In one of the analysed bone marrows, we found two point mutations: G → C in position 2607 (exon 18) and A - C in position 1642 (exon 10), the latter resulting in a met → leu substitution in the transmembrane domain (unpublished results; in collaboration with CM. deCastro, R.E Kaufman). Similar polymorphic mutations have been, however, observed in control bone marrow cells and are probably of little or no functional consequence to receptor activity. Normal expression of *c-kit* receptors has also been found by FACS analysis of purified progenitor CD34$^+$ cells *(Table III)*. The mean proportion of

Table III. CD34$^+$c-kit$^+$ bone marrow progenitor cells (in % of CD34$^+$ cells).

N (n = 5)	51.6 ± 8.9%	(range 28.7-76.9%)
AA (n = 10)	45.7 ± 7.7%	(range 1.4-78.9%)

CD34+c-kit+ progenitors in AA was about 50% and did not differ from normal. We conclude that hematopoietic abnormalities in AA and lower than normal proliferative responsiveness of cells to SCF is not associated with abnormalities in *c-kit* in marrow progenitors.

Hematopoietic effect of flt3 ligand in AA *in vitro*

flt3 ligand had a week mitogenic effect on normal and AA bone marrow cells analysed in suspension cultures when used alone, and had a synergistic effect when used together with other hematopoietic growth factors. For example, the proliferative cell response to SCF was enhanced by the ligand by 2-5 fold. Cell clonogenicity assayed in liquid cultures at weekly intervals, has revealed that flt3 plays a role in the maintenance of colony-forming cells *in vitro*. While in the presence of SCF an increase of colony formation during the first week in culture was followed by rapid exhaustion of colony-forming cells, flt3 prolonged survival of hematopoietic progenitors which reached their maximum level at week 3. The effect of flt3 in AA cultures resembled the pattern observed with normal cells, except that numbers and survival time of colony-forming cells were lower in AA *(Table IV)*. FACS analysis of CD34+ cell content showed an approximately 3 fold increase of progenitors during the first week in suspension cultures containing the flt3 ligand; thereafter CD34+ cells declined in AA, but were maintained for up to 4 weeks in cultures of normal bone marrows (not shown). flt3 ligand stimulated the granulocyte/macrophage, rather than the erythroid lineage.

Table IV. Effect of flt3 ligand on survival of colony-forming cells in suspension cultures (colonies/1 ml culture).

	N 1*	N 2*	AA 1**	AA 2**
week 0	86 ± 7	81 ± 9	39 ± 8	20 ± 5
week 1	413 ± 130	255 ± 8	48 ± 4	80 ± 9
week 2	455 ± 25	309 ± 40	42 ± 15	15 ± 4
week 3	301 ± 10	349 ± 32	27 ± 10	0
week 4	523 ± 52	285 ± 63	11 ± 10	0

* Cultures initiated with 5×10^4 cells/ml
** Cultures initiated with 1×10^5 cells/ml

Clinical prospects of SCF and flt3 ligand in AA

The discovery of the tyrosine kinase receptors *c-kit* and *flt-3* and their ligands, SCF and flt3 ligand, has been of great importance for studies on AA Identification of these molecules has provided tools to characterize early hematopoietic precursor cells, analyse their frequency, growth requirements and potential defects. A number of *in vitro* hematopoietic assays have shown that SCF and flt3 ligand are able to stimulate proliferation and clonogenic differentiation of AA bone marrow cells. While both cytokines appear to act on primitive hematopoietic cells, their biological activities differ in many aspects. SCF is a potent inducer of cell growth and colony formation by hematopoietic precursors. Its strongest stimulatory effect is on the erythroid progenitor cells. In contrary, flt3 ligand only modestly influences proliferation of cells, but has an ability to expand and prolong the survival of hematopoietic colony-forming cells. The ligand stimulates cells of the myeloid lineages and has little or no effect on the erythroid pathway. It appears, that despite structural similarities between SCF and flt3 ligand and between c-kit and flt-3 receptors, the two cytokines play distinct roles in the hematopoietic system. Differences in the biological activities of the ligands are likely to have their basis in the differences in the signalling pathways from the two tyrosine kinase receptors.

Although early-acting growth factors are not expected to correct the stem cell deficiency in AA, the behaviour of cells in culture provides several arguments for the potential therapeutic benefit of SCF and flt3 ligand. Efficacy of cytokines *in vitro* depends largely on the severity of the disease. Cells from patients with very severe AA have virtually not responded to SCF and flt3 ligand, predicting that the use of these factors will be disappointing in patients with no residual bone marrow function, as described previously for GM-CSF [28]. Most of our *in vitro* studies have been performed with bone marrow cells from patients who recovered some bone marrow function after therapy with ALG. Despite hematological remission and clinical improvement, cells of patients after immunosuppression retain a profound proliferative defect as a sign of residual disease. The factors may, therefore, have a place as a supportive measure in the context of ALG therapy. Such an adjuvant effect is known for G-CSF [29]. It is conceivable that SCF could be used as its erythropoietic analogue. Since SCF and flt3 ligand act synergistically with each other and with a variety of other hematopoietic cytokines, one may envisage their role in a growth factor combination therapy. An advantage of flt3 ligand, compared to SCF, is its apparent lack of an effect on mast cells thus avoidance of inflammatory allergic reactions which are a hazard of large therapeutic doses of SCF. Currently, the most promising clinical application of SCF [30] and of flt3 ligand is their use in *ex vivo* expansion of hematopoietic progenitors from bone marrow or peripheral blood for autologous or allogeneic transplantation.

References

1. Young NS. The pathogenesis and pathophysiology of aplastic anemia, in Hematology. Basic principles and practice, Hoffman K (ed) Churchill-Livingstone, New York-Tokyo, 1991, p122.
2. Nissen-Druey C. Pathophysiology of aplastic anema. *Seminars in Hematology* 28: 313, 1991.
3. Speck B, Gratwohl A, Nissen C, Leibundgut V, Ruggero D, Osterwalder B, Burrie HP, Corru P, Jeannet M. Treatment of severe aplastic anemia with antilymphocyte globulin or bone marrow transplantation. *Br Med J* 282: 860, 1981.
4. Frickhofen N, Kaltwasser JP, Schrezenmeier, Raghavachar A, Vogt HG, Herrmann F, Freund M, Meusers P, Salama A, Heimpel H. Treatment of aplastic anemia with antilymphocyte globulin and methylprednisolone with or without cyclosporin. *N Engl J Med* 19: 1297, 1991.
5. Tichelli A, Gratwohl A, Wursch A, Nissen C, Speck B. Late hematological complications in severe aplastic anemia. *Br J Hematol* 69: 413, 1988.
6. Moore MAS, Castro-Malaspina H. Immunosuppression in aplastic anemia – postponing the inevitable? *N Engl J Med* 324: 1358, 1991.
7. Marsh J, Socie G, Schrezenmeier H, Tochelli A, Gluckman E, Ljungman P, McCann SR, Raghavachar A, Marin P, Hows JM, Bacigalupo A. Haemopoietic growth factors in aplastic anaemia: a cautionary note. *The Lancet* 344: 172, 1994.
8. Martin FH, Suggs SV, Langley KE, Lu HS, Ting J, Okino KH, Morris CF, McNiece IK, Jakobsen FW, Mendiaz EA, Birkett NC, Smith KA, Johnson MJ, Parker VP, Flores JC, Patel AC, Fisher EF, Erjavec HO, Herrera CJ, Wypych J, Sachdev RK, Pope JA, Leshe I, Wen D, Lin CH, Cupples RL, Zsebo KM. Primary structure and functional expression of rat and human stem cell factor DNAs. *Cell* 63: 203, 1990.

9. Williams DE, Eisenman J, Baird A, Rauch C, Van Ness K, March CJ, Park LS, Martin U, Mochizuki DY, Boswell HS, Burgess GS, Cosman D, Lyman SD. Identification of a ligand for the *c-kit* proto-oncogene. *Cell* 63: 167, 1990.
10. Huang E, Nocka K, Beier DR, Chu TY, Buck J, Lahm HW, Wellner D, Leder P, Besmer P. The hematopoietic growth factor KL is encoded by the Sl locus and is the ligand of the *c-kit* receptor, the gene product of the W locus. *Cell* 63: 225, 1990.
11. Toksoz D, Zsebo KM, Smith KA, Hu S, Brankow D, Suggs SV, Martin FH, Williams DA. Support of human hematopoiesis in long-term bone marrow cultures by murine stromal cells selectively expressing the membrane-bound and secreted forms of the human homolog of the steel gene product, stem cell factor. *Proc Natl Acad Sci USA* 89: 7350, 1992.
12. Geissler EN, Ryan MA, Housman DE. The dominant white-spotting (W) locus of the mouse encodes the c-kit proto-oncogene. *Cell* 55: 185, 1988.
13. Flanagan JG, Leder P. The *kit* ligand: a cell surface molecule altered in Steel mutant fibroblasts. *Cell* 63: 185, 1990.
14. Ikeda H, Kanakura Y, Tamaki T, Kuriu A, Kitayama H, Ishikawa J, Kanayama Y, Younezawa T, Tarui S, Griffin JD. Expression and functional role of the protooncogene c-kit in acute myeloblastic leukemia cells. *Blood* 78: 2962, 1991.
15. Lyman SD, James L, Vanden Bos T, de Vries P, Brasel K, Gliniak B, Hollingsworth LT, Picha KS, McKenna HJ, Splett RR, Fletcher FA, Maraskovsky E, Farah T, Foxworthe E, Williams DE, Beckmann MP. Molecular cloning of a ligand for the flt3/flk-2 tyrosine kinase receptor: a proliferative factor for primitive hematopoietic cells. *Cell* 75: 1157, 1993.
16. Hannum C, Culpepper J, Campbell D, McClanahan T, Zurawski S, Bazan JF, Kastelein R, Hudak S, Wagner J, Mattson J, Luh J, Duda G, Martina N, Peterson D, Menon S, Shanafelt A, Muench M, Kelner G, Namikawa R, Rennick D, Roncarolo MG, Zlotnik A, Rosnet O, Dubreuil P, Birnbaum D, Lee F. Ligand for flt3/flk2 receptor tyrosine kinase regulates growth of haematopoietic stem cells and is encoded by variant RNAs. *Nature* 368: 643, 1994.
17. Matthews W, Jordan CT, Wiegand GW, Pardoll D, Lemischka IR. A receptor tyrosine kinase specific to hematopoietic stem and progenitor cell-enriched populations. *Cell* 65: 1143, 1991.
18. Rosnet O, Schiff C, Pebusque MJ, Marchetto S, Tonnelle C, Toiron Y, Birg F, Birnbaum D. Human flt3/flk2 Gene: cDNA cloning and expression in hematopoietic cells. *Blood* 82: 1110, 1993.
19. Ulrich A, Schlessinger J. Signal transduction by receptors with tyrosine kinase activity. *Cell* 61: 203, 1990.
20. Small D, Levenstein M, Kim E, Carow C, Amin S, Rockwell P, Witte L, Burrow C, Ratajczak M, Gewirtz AM, Civin CI. Stk-1, the human homolog of flk-2/flt3, is selectively expressed in CD34$^+$ human bone marrow cells and is involved in the proliferation of early progenitor/stem cells. *Proc Natl Acad Sci USA* 91: 459, 1994.
21. Wodnar-Filipowicz A, Tichelli A, Zsebo KM, Speck B, Nissen C. Stem cell factor stimulates the in vitro growth of bone marrow cells from aplastic anemia patients. *Blood* 79: 3196, 1992.
22. Wodnar-Filipowicz A, Yancik S, Moser Y, dalle Carbonare V, Gratwohl A, Tichelli A, Speck B, Nissen C. Levels of soluble stem cell factor in serum of patients with aplastic anemia. *Blood* 81: 3259, 1993
23. Slanicka Krieger M, Nissen C, Wodnar-Filipowicz A. Stem cell factor in aplastic anemia: in vitro expression in bone marrow stroma and fibroblast cultures. *Eur J Haematol* in press, 1995.
24. Civin CI, Strauss LC, Brovall C, Fackler MJ, Schwartz JF, Shaper JH. A hematopoieitc progenitor cell surface antigen defined by a monoclonal antibody raised against KG-1 cells. *J Immunol* 133: 157, 1984.
25. Huang S, Terstappen LW. Lymphoid and myeloid differentiation of single human CD34$^+$, HLA$^-$DR$^+$, CD38$^-$ hematopoietic stem cells. *Blood* 83: 1515, 1994.
26. Bernstein ID, Andrews RG, Zsebo KM. Recombinant Human stem cell factor enhances the formation of colonies by CD34$^+$ and CD34$^+$lin$^-$ cells, and the generation of colony-forming cell progeny from CD34$^+$lin$^-$ cells cultured with interleukin-3, granulocyte colony-stimulating factor, or granulocyte-macrophage colony-stimulating factor. *Blood* 77: 2316, 1991.
27. Wodnar-Filipowicz A, Speck B, Nissen C. Effect of sctem cell factor (c-kit ligand) on in vitro proliferation of bone marrow cells from aplastic anemia patients in Aplastic anemia: Currecnt perspectives on the pathogenesis and treatment. (Raghavachar A, Schrezenmeier H, Frickhofen N, eds) Blackwell-MZV, Vienna, pg.77, 1993.

28. Nissen C, Tichelli A, Gratwohl A, Speck B, Milne A, Gordon-Smith EC, Schaedelin J. Failure of recombinant human granulocyte/macrophage colony-stimulating factor therapy in aplastic anemia patients with severe neutropenia. *Blood* 72: 2045, 1988.
29. Kojima S, Fukuda M, Matsuyama T, Horibe K. Treatment of aplastic anemia in children with recombinant human granulocyte colony-stimulating factor. *Blood* 77: 937, 1991.
30. Sheridan WP, Foote MA, Morstyn G. Stem-cell factor. *Focus on Growth Factors* 5: 5, 1994.

Résumé

Les récepteurs de type tyrosine kinase (TK) sont présents sur un grand nombre de cellules de différents tissus. Ils règlent leur croissance, leur survie et leur différenciation. Dans la moelle osseuse, on sait que les cellules souches expriment deux récepteurs du type TK : c-kit et flk-2/flt-3. Ces deux récepteurs transmembranaires apparentés et leurs ligands, *stem cell factor* (SCF) et flt-3 ligand, jouent un rôle important dans la régulation de l'hémopoïèse primitive. Notre travail se concentre sur le rôle de ces récepteurs et leurs ligands dans la physiopathologie de l'anémie aplastique (AA), maladie caractérisée par une insuffisance médullaire touchant toutes les lignées hématopoïétiques. Nous avons (*i*) caractérisé le compartiment des progéniteurs des AA par analyse immunophénotypique des antigènes CD34 et *c-kit* (supplémentée par l'analyse de *c-kit* au niveau ARNm), (*ii*) analysé les effets hématopoïétiques de SCF et flt3 ligand sur les progéniteurs de patients aplastiques en cultures à court et à long terme, et (*iii*) recherché l'expression de *c-kit* par les cellules du stroma de la moelle osseuse. Nous avons trouvé une forte réduction des cellules souches dans le AA, souvent accompagnée d'une croissance faible du stroma, et une production abaissée de SCF par le stroma. SCF et flt3 ligand ont des effets stimulateurs différents sur les progéniteurs : tandis que SCF plutôt augmente leur croissance, flt3 ligand prolonge surtout leur survie. Nos résultats montrent que les deux ligands pour les récepteurs type TK sont importants comme stimulateurs de l'hémopoïèse primitive. Nous suggérons qu'ils pourraient être utiles en stimulant l'expansion du réseau de progéniteurs fortement diminué dans les AA, donc être intéressants pour l'usage clinique.

The aplastic anemia-paroxysmal nocturnal hemoglobinuria syndrome

Aruna Raghavachar and Hubert Schrezenmeier

Department of Medicine III, University of Ulm, Robert-Koch Street 8, D-89081, Ulm, Germany, tel.: (49 73) 15 02 44 02, fax: (49 73) 15 02 43 93

Summary

There is a close association between aplastic anemia (AA) and clonal disorders of hematopoiesis, in particular paroxysmal nocturnal hemoglobinuria (PNH), suggesting a pathogenetic link between these disorders. Clonality of blood cells in AA was analysed on the basis of polymorphic X-linked loci inactivation. In addition, the failure to express phosphatidylinositol glycan-anchored proteins (PIG-AP) on blood cells of AA patients was used as an indirect marker for the molecular PNH defect. Clonal hemopoiesis was observed in 13% of AA patients. On the contrary, a PIG-AP deficient population was identified in > 50% of AA patients. Patients with a PIG-AP deficiency had poor response to immunosuppressive therapy and thus constitute a distinct subtype of AA-patients. This will be discussed in the context of our observation of the transient emergence of PIG-AP deficient T-cells being observed after in vivo *application of Campath-1H antibody for treatment of refractory B-cell lymphomas. We hypothesize that clonal hemopoiesis or PIG-AP deficient hemopoiesis are indicative for severe bone marrow failure and ongoing hemopoietic stress rather than for a molecular event in terms of hemopoietic neoplasia. Clonal hemopoiesis may be selected by an immune attack.*

Aplastic anemia is a disease characterized by pancytopenia and marrow aplasia. There is a close clinical association between AA and PNH: Patients with AA might evolve to PNH and vice versa [1]. The pathophysiological basis of AA is heterogeneous, resembling a T-cell mediated disease in some patients [2]. For PNH it has been shown that an acquired deficiency of the phosphatidylinositol-glycan PIG anchor (PIG-AP) on hemopoietic cells is the cause of the disease. The PIG-AP deficiency in PNH arises through somatic mutations in the X-linked gene PIG A, which encodes for a protein required for an early step in the biosynthesis of the PIG-anchor [3]. The AA-PNH syndrome encompasses patients with AA and a PIG-AP deficiency as well as patients with PNH and bone marrow failure. The pathogenetic relationship between AA and PNH has been evaluated by different experimental approaches: [1]. Using X-inactivation analysis at the DNA level as a means for clonal analysis in females with AA [2] looking for PIG-AP deficient blood cells in patients with AA [3] describing mechanisms which result in the selection of PIG-AP deficient cells in other experimental systems *in vivo* [4] following normal versus PIG-AP deficient hemopoiesis during the course of the disease and with different therapeutic interventions.

Clonal hemopoiesis in AA

We have conducted a large study on X-inactivation analysis in 30 female patients with AA, using a PCR-based analysis of phosphoglycerate kinase (PGK_1)-restriction fragment length polymorphisms (RFLPs) [4]. Granulocytes and mononuclear cells (MNC) were studied in parallel, and a population with an imbalanced X-inactivation pattern was defined as clonal if the hybridisation pattern was different for both cell populations, or if there was a changing X-inactivation pattern over time. This strict definition of clonality takes into account the known limitations of the methodology i.e. skewed Lyonization and tissue specific X-inactivation patterns. Consequently, only 4 (13%) of our patients demonstrated a true clonal pattern of hemopoiesis. The presence of clonal hemopoiesis detected by X-inactivation analysis was not predictive for later clonal evolution to myelodysplasia, acute myeloid leukemia or PNH in our patients with AA. On the other hand, the demonstration of polyclonal hemopoiesis in 6 patients who later developed clonal disorders may indicate either the lack of prognostic value of clonality analysis or the failure of the technique to detect small clonal populations of cells. In PNH it has been clearly shown by X-inactivation studies that PIG-AP deficient cells are clonal [5]. We therefore re-analysed cell fractions in 2 patients with AA and PIG-AP deficient granulocytes with a polyclonal X-inactivation pattern. After sorting for PIG-AP deficient cells we found that the PIG-AP deficient cells were clonal and that they were being obscured by normal cells, producing the polyclonal pattern on analysis of unsorted cells. We found no correlation between the size of the PIG-AP deficient cell population in AA and the observed X-inactivation patterns in unseparated granulocytes and MNC populations.

PIG-AP deficient hemopoiesis in AA

We used immunophenotyping for PIG-AP on peripheral blood cells of AA patients to analyse whether PIG-AP deficient peripheral blood cells can be detected in patients with AA at diagnosis and during follow-up [6]. The quantification of the expression of PIG-AP was performed by flow cytometry using the monoclonal antibodies CD16 and CD66b for granulocytes, CD14 and CD48 for monocytes, CD48 and CD52 for lymphocytes, and CD55 and CD59 for erythrocytes. We analysed cells from 63 patients with acquired AA. A PIG-AP deficient population was identified in 33 of 63 patients (52 %) in at least one cell lineage, whereby granulocytes were the mostly affected cell population as compared to lymphocytes and red cells. Thus, the proportion of AA patients who show features of typical acquired AA along with a PNH phenotype (i.e., the AA/PNH syndrome) is substantially higher than previously recognized. PIG-AP deficiency in AA was not related to age, gender of the patient or severity of bone marrow failure *(Table I)*. However, the analysis of bone marrow recovery in response to immunosuppressive treatment showed a significantly higher response rate in the group of patients without a PIG-AP-deficient population than in patients with a PIG-AP-deficient population in at least one cell lineage (76 *vs* 28.8%) *(Table I)*. This strong association between good response to immunosuppressive treatment and absence of a PIG-AP-deficient population has to be validated by prospective studies.

Table I. Clinical characteristics of the AA patients stratified for the presence or absence of a PIG-AP deficient population.

	Expression of PIG-AP		p
	normal (n = 30)	PIG-AP deficient population in ≥ 1 lineage- (n = 33)	
Age (years) (median, range)	32.5 (15 – 74)	32 (18 – 80)	0.34*
Gender: male / female	14 / 16	15 / 18	0.92**
Severity: vSAA	9	6	
SAA	11	16	
nSAA	10	11	0.49**
Response to IS (3 months): (n = 53)			
NR	6	20	
PR or CR	19	8	< 0.001***

* Mann-Whitney-Test
** k^2-Test
*** Fisher's exact test

However, the pattern of PIG-AP expression in AA might identify a subgroup with a AA/PNH syndrome with different course of the disease due to a different pathogenetic mechanism.

Emergence of PIG-AP deficient lymphocytes in lymphoma patients treated with a monoclonal antibody *in vivo*

CD52 (the Campath-1 antigen) is a PIG-AP expressed on normal T and B-Lymphocytes, monocytes and the majority of B-cell Non Hodgkin Lymphomas. We observed the emergence of CD52 negative CD3 positive lymphocytes in three patients receiving the humanized monoclonal antibody Campath-1H for treatment of refractory chronic lymphocytic leukemia [7]. The results of immunophenotypic analysis are summarized in *Table II*. In addition to the absence of CD52, the PIG-AP CD48 and CD59 were not detectable on the CD52-negative T cells in two patients. PIG-AP deficient cells were not observed in granulocytes and erythrocytes. This discordant results in different hemopoietic lineages can be explained by the expression of the CD52 antigen and as a result of a different selection pressure. PIG-AP deficient T-cell clones, established from patient 1 and patient 3 were analysed for PIG-A mRNA by RT-PCR. In all T-cell clones without PIG-AP deficiency we obtained a normal amplification product (3), while in all PIG-AP deficient clones from patient 1 the full length transcript was missing, suggesting that a

Table II. Emergence of CD52-negative, PIG-AP deficient T-lymphocytes after Campath-1H treatment of refractory B-NHL.

	Proportion of lymphocytes (%) staining for			
	CD3	CD8	CD52	CD3$^+$CD52$^-$
NHL01				
before Campath	38	13	99	nd
4 months*	98	77	0	97
6 months	84	63	63	32
9 months	64	43	78	19
NHL02				
before Campath	24	11	99	nd
4 months	87	48	27	69
5 months	70	30	82	11
7 months	34	17	97	2
NHL03				
before Campath	71	10	98	nd
2 months	58	40	35	24
4 months	90	69	3	90
10 months	39	14	72	15

* months from starting Campath-1H. Patients received Campath-1H three times weekly for a total treatment period of 12 weeks.

mutation of the PIG-A gene was the cause of the expression defect of PIG-AP. These demonstrates (a) that a selection of PIG-AP deficient cells is possible and (b) that a survival advantage for PIG-AP deficient cells was caused by the selection pressure of the antibody therapy. This survival advantage disappeared after end of treatment *(Table II)*.

Differential expansion of PIG-AP deficient cells *in vivo* in patients with the AA/PNH syndrome

The follow-up study in one female with acquired AA who developed a positive Ham's test 53 mo. later (AA/PNH syndrome), exemplifies one possibility *(Table III)*: the patient was treated with cyclosporine and the pancytopenia gradually improved. In parallel there was a close monitoring of the expression of PIG-AP on her blood cells. The expression of PIG-AP remained essentially absent indicating that the marrow repopulating cells were derived from a PNH clone. One might speculate that in this case an immune attack sparing the PNH clone may have existed which allowed for the outgrowth of PNH-type cells. The role of cyclosporine in this selection process remains unclear. At the moment we are collecting prospectively samples from our patients to identify typical patterns of reconstitution in responding patients and compare them to non-responders in terms of the proportion of PIG-AP deficient versus normal hemopoiesis. So far, two out of 12 patients with AA and normal PIG-AP expression at diagnosis developed a PIG-AP-deficient population, whereas in 8 out of 20 patients with a PIG-AP deficiency at diagnosis this defect disappeared over time.

Table III. *In vivo* expansion of PG-AP deficient hemopoiesis in patient he developing PNH after aplastic anemia.

Days from diagnosis	PMN (G/l) CD16⁻	CD66b⁻	Monocytes (G/l) CD48⁻	Erythrocytes (T/l) CD55⁻
2969	0.65	nd	0.09	0.72
3189	1.01	0.88	0.27	0.89
3258	1.41	1.34	0.29	1.77
3427	1.92	1.80	0.40	1.86

References

1. Marsh J, Geary CG. Is aplastic anemia a pre-leukemic disorder? *Br J Haematol* 1991; 77: 447-452.
2. Young NS. The problem of clonality in aplastic anemia: Dr Dameshek's riddle, restated. *Blood* 1992; 79: 1385-1392.
3. Miyata T, Yamada N, Iida Y, Nishimura J, Takeda J, Kitani T, Kinoshita T. Abnormalities of PIG-A transcripts in granulocytes from patients with paroxysmal nocturnal hemoglobinuria. *New Engl J Med* 1994; 330: 249 - 255.
4. Raghavachar A, Janssen JWG, Schrezenmeier H, Wagner B, Bartram CR, Schulz AS, Hein C, Cowling G, Mubarik A, Testa NG, Dexter TM, Hows JM, Marsh JCW. Clonal hematopoiesis as defined by polymorphic X-linked loci occurs infrequently in aplastic anemia. *Blood*, in press.
5. Ohashi H, Hotta T, Ichikawa A, Kinoshita T, Taguchi R, Kiguchi T, Ikezawa H, Saito H. Peripheral blood cells are predominantly chimeric of affected an normal cells in patients with paroxysmal nocturnal hemoglobinuria: Simultaneous investigation on clonality and expression of glycophosphatidylinositol-anchored proteins. *Blood* 1994; 83: 853-859
6. Schrezenmeier H, Hertenstein B, Wagner B, Raghavachar A, Heimpel H. A pathogenetic link between aplastic anemia and paroxysmal nocturnal hemoglobinuria is suggested by a high frequency of aplastic anemia patients with a deficiency of phosphatidylinositol glycan anchored proteins. *Exp Hematol* 1995; 23: 81-87.
7. Hertenstein B, Wagner B, Bunjes D, Duncker C, Raghavachar A, Arnold R, Heimpel H, Schrezenmeier H. Emergence of CD52 negative, phosphatidylinositolglycan (PIG)-anchor deficient T-lymphocytes after *in vivo* application of Campath-1H for refractory B-cell Non Hodgkin Lymphoma. *Blood*, in press.

Résumé

L'association étroite entre l'aplasie médullaire et des désordres clonaux de l'hématopoïèse, comme l'hémoglobinurie paroxystique nocturne (HPN), établit un lien entre ces maladies. La clonalité des cellules de l'aplasie a été analysée par l'inactivation du locus polymorphe lié à l'X . Par ailleurs, le défaut d'expression des protéines d'ancrages phosphatidylinositol glycan (PIG-AP) présent sur les cellules des patients atteints d'aplasie est utilisé comme un marqueur du défaut moléculaire de l'HPN. Une hématopoïèse clonale a été observée dans 13% des cas d'aplasie médullaire. Une population déficiente en PIG-AP a été identifiée dans plus de 50% des cas d'aplasie médullaire. Les malades déficients en PIG-AP ont une mauvaise réponse au traitement par immunosuppresseurs et constituent une catégorie distincte. Cela est discuté dans le contexte de l'émergence transitoire de cellules T déficientes en PIG-AP après administration de l'anticorps monoclonal Campah-1H pour le traitement de lymphomes B réfractaires. Nous formulons l'hypothèse que l'hématopoïèse clonale ou le défaut de PIG-AP témoignent d'une insuffisance médullaire et d'un stress hématopoïétique persistant plus qu'un événement moléculaire précurseur d'une néoplasie. Une hématopoïèse clonale pourrait être sélectionnée par une attaque immune.

3) Fanconi anemia

3) Anémie de Fanconi

Fanconi's anemia: clinical aspects and diagnosis

Blanche P. Alter

Division of Pediatric Hematology/Oncology, Children's Hospital C3.270, University of Texas Medical Branch, 301 University Boulevard, Galveston, Texas 77555-0361, USA, tel.: (409) 772 2341, fax: (409) 772 4599

Summary

Fanconi's anemia (FA) is the most frequent inherited bone marrow failure syndrome, with ~1000 cases reported in the literature. The diagnosis is made by analysis of chromosome breakage or cell cycle arrest; <20% of patients are in complementation group C. In vitro hematopoietic culture growth correlates with clinical classification according to hematologic severity. Hematopoietic growth factors such as stem cell factor may be stimulatory in vitro. In vivo GM-CSF, IL-3 or G-CSF increase myelopoiesis, while G-CSF also increases platelets and hemoglobin in a few patients. Patients with FA are at risk of leukemia (~10% frequency), myelodysplastic syndrome (MDS) and/or clonal hematopoiesis (~3%), solid tumors (~5%), or liver disease (~4%). The leukemia is primarily myeloid. Cytogenetic abnormalities in leukemics most frequently involve chromosomes 7 or 5. In patients without leukemia we found ~30% to have clonal cytogenetic markers, which vary over time, and do not involve any specific chromosome. Squamous carcinomas occur most often in the oropharyngeal, gastrointestinal, or gynecologic areas, with an excess of females in all categories. In particular, the risk of tongue cancer may be increased following bone marrow transplantation. Liver tumors are more frequently hepatomas than adenomas, but are not themselves usually fatal. In ~10% of those patients with malignancies more than one primary was present. The mean age for development of complications was in the teens for leukemia, liver disease, and clonal hematopoiesis or MDS, and in the mid-20's for solid tumors. The median survival for all patients is 19 years of age, although it is 30 for those reported in the last 5 years.

Fanconi's anemia (FA) is the most frequent of a group of inherited disorders associated with bone marrow failure; there are approximately a thousand cases reported in the literature. The other inherited marrow failure syndromes, in order of the numbers of cases reported, include Diamond-Blackfan anemia or congenital pure red cell aplasia (~500 cases); dyskeratosis congenita, ie ectodermal dysplasia, reticulated hyperpigmentation, and leukoplakia, with ~ 50% developing aplastic anemia (~200 cases); Shwachman-Diamond syndrome, which is neutropenia and exocrine pancreatic insufficiency, in which ~25% develop aplastic anemia (~200 reported cases); thrombocytopenia with absent radii, who have only the single cytopenia (<200 cases); Kostmann's syndrome, severe congenital neutropenia, who do not develop aplastic anemia (<200 cases); and amegakaryocytic thrombocytopenia without overt birth defects, half of whom may develop aplastic anemia (<100 cases). Because most countries do not have mandatory reporting of these diagnoses and disease-based registries are voluntary, these numbers must be construed as rough estimates only, and not true measures of prevalence. Details regarding these disorders can be obtained from 2 recent reviews [1, 2].

Among the close to 1000 cases of FA that have been reported, the ratio of males to females was 1.3:1. The inheritance of FA is clearly autosomal recessive, despite the slight excess of males [3, 4]. The mean age at diagnosis (usually associated with aplastic anemia) was approximately 8 years in males and 9 in females. While less than 5% were under one year, 10% were 16 or older, and thus FA must be considered in patients with aplastic anemia at almost any age. Approximately 20% had no birth defects, and thus were only diagnosed because they were members of an affected family, or because of a high index of suspicion. The physical anomalies which may be present, in descending order of frequency, include café au lait spots and/or hyperpigmentation (~60%), short stature (~60%), upper limb deformities involving thumbs alone or also radii (~50%), hypogonadism (~40%), microcephaly (~25%), microphthalmia or strabismus (~25%), and structural renal anomalies (~25%). Less frequent (~10-15%) are low birth weight, developmental retardation, deformities of the lower limbs, and abnormal hearing. Other neurologic, skeletal, cardiopulmonary, and gastrointestinal anomalies have also been reported in 5-10% of the cases.

The diagnosis of FA depends on suspicion in patients with characteristic anomalies, or young patients (although not just children) with aplastic anemia, refractory anemia or myelodysplasia, myeloid leukemia, or gastrointestinal or gynecologic malignancy at an unusually early age. The traditional diagnostic test involves detection of increased chromosome breakage in peripheral blood lymphocytes, initially noted spontaneously [5], and more recently following clastogenic stress with mitomycin C [6] or diepoxybutane [7]. There is also a cell cycle delay with arrest at G2/M following culture with nitrogen mustard [8, 9]. Both of these tests presumably relate to an as yet unidentified defect in DNA repair. Molecular approaches are now becoming available, beginning with the cloning of the gene mutated in FA patients of complementation group C [10]; less than 20% of the cases are in this group, however [11-13].

In an effort to correlate *in vitro* hematopoietic culture data with clinical information, we classified the patients into groups related to their hematologic status [14]. Group 1 have severe aplastic anemia, failed all therapy, and are on transfusions only. Group 2 are similar but still on androgens. Group 3 are responding to treatment with androgens or growth factors. Group 4 are severe enough to be ready for treatment. Group 5 are stable without treatment but have one or more sign of marrow malfunction, such as anemia, leukopenia, thrombocytopenia, macrocytosis, and/or elevated fetal hemoglobin. The best group, group 6, have no evidence of hematologic disease, or perhaps only subtle changes in MCV or Hb F.

We examined *in vitro* erythropoiesis from marrow progenitors in the presence of various cytokines [15]. The most effective additive was stem cell factor (SCF, kit-ligand), which increased the numbers of CFU-E-derived and BFU-E-derived colonies (colony forming units-erythroid and burst forming units-erythroid) in cultures from 21 of 28 patients studied to date, although only 5 reached normal levels. SCF was more effective than interleukin-3 (IL-3), which enhanced BFU-E growth in only 4 cultures, and resulted in normal levels in only 2. There was some relationship between the clinical group number and the *in vitro* results, in that the BFU-E growth from both marrow and blood was higher from group 6 and some group 5 patients than from the other groups. In addition, we have seen the colony-forming efficiency decline as a patient moved from group 6 to group 5.

Cytokine treatment has been employed in a limited number of patients with a small number of growth factors. Guinan et al treated 7 with GM-CSF; 6 had an increase in neutrophils, but there were no red cell or platelet responses [16]. A similar number of patients were treated with IL-3 by Gillio, with a similar neutrophil-only effect (data unpublished). We are participating in a G-CSF trial organized by Rackoff and sponsored by Amgen [17], in which all of 10 patients had a neutrophil response, 3 had a platelet response, and 4 showed a red cell effect. The "standard of care" remains the use of androgens combined with steroids, which has a more than 50% short term response rate. Bone marrow transplant is recommended for those who have a matched related donor, although the use of unrelated donors remains complex; this will be discussed by others.

I would like to turn now to the problem of malignant complications in FA *(Table I)*. If we assume a denominator of approximately 1000 cases, the literature contains reports of ~150 patients with one or more malignancy (~15%), and ~160 types of malignancies. These figures are probably minimal and certainly rough estimates, since there are clearly many unreported cases of malignancies. There are 83 leukemias, 31 patients with myelodysplastic syndromes (MDS, not yet a malignancy) and/or preleukemia, 44 with other cancers, and 28 with liver tumors. The ages at diagnosis of FA are slightly higher in those with MDS and other cancers than for the entire group. The mean age at diagnosis of the complication is 14 years for leukemia, 16 for liver disease, 17 for MDS, and 23 for other cancers. In particular, the other cancers seem to be occur-

Table I. Complications in Fanconi's anemia.

	Leukemia	MDS	Other Cancer	Liver Disease
Number of cases	83	31	44	37
Male:female ratio	1.31	1.07	0.33	1.64
Age at diagnosis of FA (yrs)				
Mean	10	13	13	9
Median	9	12	10	6
Range	0.13-28	1-31	0.1-32	1-48
Percentage ≥ 16	20	32	31	11
Age at complication (yrs)				
Mean	14	17	24	16
Median	14	17	26	13
Range	0.13-29	4.5-31	0.3-38	2.5-48
Interval from diagnosis to complication (yrs)				
Mean	4	7	11	7
Median	3	2	11	5
Range	0-19	0-31	0-29	0-24
Number without pancytopenia	20 (24%)	13 (42%)	7 (16%)	1 (3%)
Number without androgens	39 (47%)	19 (61%)	16 (36%)	1 (3%)
Number reported deceased	65 (78%)	23 (74%)	26 (59%)	32 (86%)

147 patients had one or more malignancy; the number of malignancies was 155. MDS cases include 6 who developed leukemia; the others are not included in the total. 4 patients with tumors after BMT are not included.

ring in an older subset of FA patients. Furthermore, the interval from diagnosis of FA to the complication is longer in that group (11 years). Androgens probably do not have a role in the process in those with leukemia, MDS, or other cancers, since more than 40% of the patients never received that treatment. Among those with liver tumors, only one patient did not have androgen therapy, and thus the combination of androgens plus FA may exacerbate a malignant predisposition. Mortality is high in all categories, reflecting the problems of chemotherapy and/or radiation therapy in patients with an underlying defect in DNA repair.

Among the 83 cases of leukemia more than half were either acute myeloblastic or myelomonocytic, followed by monocytic or erythroleukemia. The more rare leukemias include 3 with acute lymphoblastic, 2 chronic myelomonocytic, and 1 acute megakaryoblastic. Five of those with leukemia also had liver tumors, and 1 had an astrocytoma. Approximately 80% were reported to have died, and in fact I am aware of only 1 long time survivor (>5 years). The majority of the leukemias thus involve the myeloid lineage, a type of cancer which has only a 20% survival rate even in children without FA.

We are attempting to understand the relation, if any, between detection of a clonal cytogenetic marker in the marrow of an FA patient who does not have leukemia, and the potential for leukemic transformation [18]. Literature reports include 30 such patients, as well as one with MDS. Six of these (20%) went on to develop leukemia at 0.3 to 1.3 tears, while 15 died without development of leukemia at up to 12 years, and 10 were alive without leukemia at up to 3 years. The chromosomes reported to be involved in clonality in FA patients with leukemia are primarily 7 (50%) and 1 (25%) [19], while in MDS there is no overwhelming propensity for any single chromosome, and cases have been reported with 1, 2, 3, 5, 6, 7, 8, 9, 12, 13, 16, 17, 18, 21, and markers.

Three FA patients without leukemia were reported to have had transient clonal abnormalities (see [18] for details). One patient had trisomy 21 initially, which was replaced by del(3), del(12), + markers at 1.5 years, and evolved into leukemia after another year. A second patient had normal chromosomes, developed i(7q) at 3 months, had a normal study at 6 months, and i(7q) again at 14 months. The third began with trisomy 8, developed a derivative Y at 1.5 years, and 4 months later had only trisomy 8. Neither of the latter 2 had developed leukemia when reported.

To further explore the significance of clonal anomalies, particularly in light of the possibility of fluctuation, we initiated a prospective study of FA bone marrows. The first 17 patients are reported elsewhere [18]. We recommend a bone marrow at diagnosis, one annually, and one at the time of any substantial hematologic change. We have studied 22 patients so far, with samples adequate for cytogenetic analysis in 15 cases. Six patients had clonal findings: 1 of 7 with aplastic marrows, 2 of 2 who were initially aplastic but then developed MDS, 1 of 6 with MDS from the onset, 1 of 4 with a normal marrow, and 1 of 2 whose marrows were normal and then became myelodysplastic. There was no apparent association between marrow morphology and clonality. Three of the 6 had transient clones. The first initially had der dup(1) in half the cells, and der(18) in 10%; at 1 year neither of those were seen, and almost all cells were der(4). The next year only a del(1) was found. Six months later, however, the der(18) which was a minor clone in the first study now predominated; the marrow had evolved from a normal morphology to myelodysplasia, and within 6 months leukemia (AML) developed. This was the only leukemia in our patients. The second case began with del(3), which was absent 3 months later, but returned by 8 months. The third had der(2) at first, to which was added a second clone with der(1) 1.5 year later. The remaining 3 patients had der(X), +X+8+21, and dup(1) respectively. Only one has had follow-up studies with no fluctuations.

Thus we have confirmed the observations of clonal transience in FA, the fact that monosomy 7 is not the most frequent finding (there were none of our 6, and 4 of 25 in the literature without leukemia), and that approximately one-third of FA patients have clonal anomalies when marrow chromosomes are examined. One of the 3 literature cases was normal when first studied, while none of our 6 were, giving a frequency of 1 in 9 in which a normal marrow was documented to evolve into one with a clonal abnormality (and none of these involved chromosome 7). A major problem with any of these analyses is the statistical problem with an assay in which anywhere from 12 to 100 cells are examined. Since a "clone" requires only the minimum of 2 cells, it might be easy to miss a minor clone. Additional prospective monitoring is needed to determine the significance of clones, clonal transience, and their relevance for leukemia if any. Since so many patients do have clones, and do not have or apparently develop leukemia, if seems premature to advocate unrelated donor bone marrow transplants for patients in whom clones are detected.

A possible explanation for clonality and for clonal fluctuation is derived from the clonal model for hematopoiesis. If at any given time the marrow is constituted from the progeny of a very small number of stem cells, then any uncorrected errors which are manifest as overt chromosomal aberrations will lead to a "clone". The relative proportion of the clone will reflect the relative number of progeny from the stem cell in which the event occurred. At a later time, the phenomenon of "clonal evolution" may have occurred, and the stem cells which are driving the marrow at that time are different, with either no or different chromosomal anomalies. Since FA is due to a defect in DNA repair, there may be more stem cells with chromosomal errors such as deletion, duplication, or rearrangement in FA than in non-FA marrows.

In addition to leukemia (whether related to myelodysplasia or not), FA patients have a high rate of development of other malignancies. Forty-four patients in the literature had a total of 54 tumors. Eleven had 2 or more primaries, including 2 with liver cancer and 1 with leukemia. Forty-three of the 54 tumors were in females; 33 females had cancer compared to only 11 males. When the 11 gynecologic cancers (vulva, breast, and cervical) are excluded, there is still an unexplained two-fold excess of females in this group. Oropharyngeal (primarily tongue and gingiva) and gastrointestinal (mainly esophageal and anal) cancers are the most common, with 15 and 16 of each respectively. Four brain tumors were reported, 3 astrocytomas and 1 probable medulloblastoma). The "other" category includes 2 skin, 2 Bowen's, and 1 each of lymphoma, bronchopulmonary, renal, and Wilms' tumors.

To be noted separately is the fact that at least 4 patients (2 males and 2 females) developed tongue cancer following bone marrow transplantation; one had an earlier cheek cancer. The denominator for transplanted FA patients is not clear, and thus the true frequency cannot be stated, but it appears to be increased compared to non-transplanted FA. The possible contributions from immunosuppression with cyclophosphamide and irradiation cannot be ignored, although the reason for localization to the tongue is not obvious.

The liver is another site for tumors in FA. Twenty-nine patients were reported, of whom 20 had hepatocellular carcinomas, 7 adenomas, and 2 were not specified. One carcinoma and 1 adenoma had metastases. Two patients had both a carcinoma and an adenoma. All but one patient had received androgens, and thus the contribution of male hormones cannot be ignored. Nevertheless, none of the patients died directly from their liver tumor, and several were found at autopsy after death from another cause. Five patients had liver tumors plus leukemia, and 2 plus another cancer. In addition, peliosis hepatis was seen in 6 livers with tumors, and 7 without tumors. Focal nodular hyperplasia was also reported. We might speculate that the same types of cellular features which are interpreted as myelodysplasia in the marrow might also be present in the liver; certainly "dysplastic" morphology has been noted in the latter. When liver tumors are detected early in patients receiving androgens, the tumors may regress following discontinuation of treatment (alone or associated with marrow transplantation). Thus we recommend monitoring of patients on androgens with monthly liver function tests and 6 to 12 monthly abdominal ultrasound examinations.

The survival in FA has improved with time, although it is still low. The predicted probability of 50% survival in the entire group of FA patients in the literature is 19 years, while it is 30 years of age for those reported in the last 5 years. I can only speculate about whether this represents a real improvement, or a bias toward publication of older cases. Improved survival has resulted from bone marrow transplantation in a small number of patients, and from better supportive care in many. Patients who respond to androgens do slightly better overall than those with aplastic anemia who fail to respond.

The range of ages at which complications developed in FA is shown in *Figure 1*. The time line is such that the earliest complication is usually aplastic anemia. The next type of complication is leukemia, followed by liver disease, myelodysplasia, and then other tumors. Although these data represent literature reports, not a probability analysis, the general sense is that patients who do not succumb to complications from aplastic anemia are at risk of developing leukemia (or liver tumors if on androgens), and the risk after that is of oropharyngeal, gastrointestinal, or gynecological malignancies. We must keep in mind that bone marrow transplant, or gene therapy of hematopoietic stem cells, may cure aplastic anemia, and may prevent or cure leukemia, and reduce the risk of liver cancer related to androgen treatment, but will not impact (except perhaps negatively) on the occurrence of other cancers.

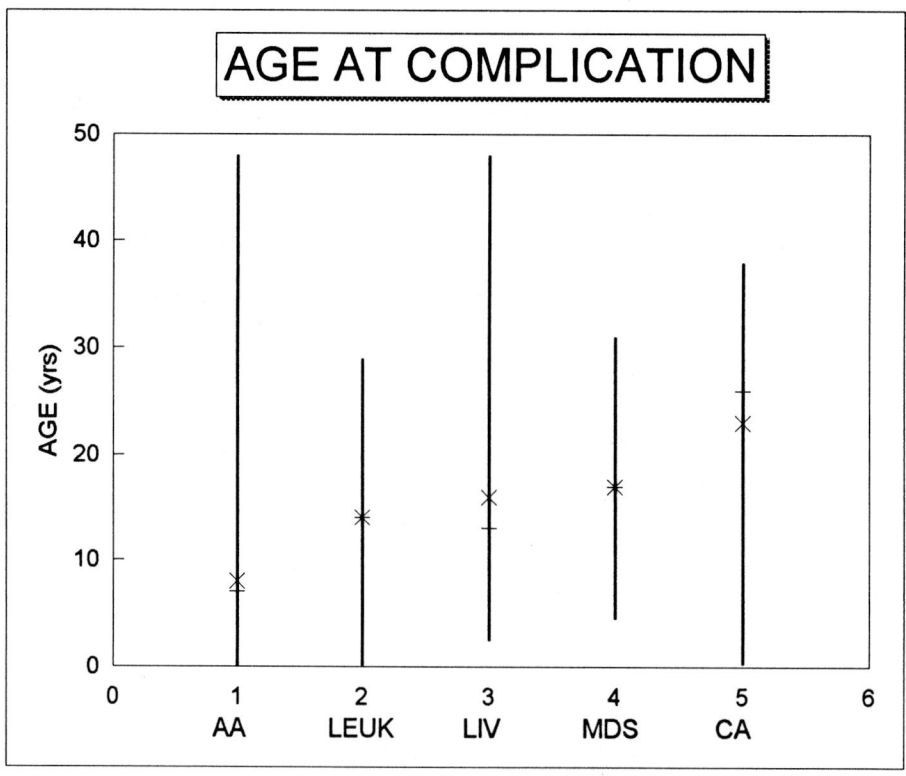

Figure 1. Schematic indicating the age range of FA patients at which complications developed. AA, aplastic anemia. Liv, liver. Leuk, leukemia. MDS, myelodysplasia (includes clonal anomalies). Ca, other cancers. — Range, X mean, – median.

References

1. Young NS, Alter BP. Aplastic Anemia: Acquired and Inherited. Philadelphia: WB Saunders Inc, 1994.
2. Alter BP, Young NS. The bone marrow failure syndromes. In: Nathan DG, Oski FA, eds. *Hematology of Infancy and Chilhood*. Philadelphia: WB Saunders Inc, 1993: 216-316.
3. Schroeder TM, Tilgen D, Kruger J, Vogel F. Formal genetics of Fanconi's anemia. *Hum Genet* 1976; 32: 257-288.
4. Rogatko A, Auerbach AD. Segregation analysis with uncertain ascertainment: Application to Fanconi anemia. *Am J Hum Genet* 1988; 42: 889-897.
5. Schroeder TM, Anschu"tz F, Knopp A. Spontane Chromosomenaberrationen bei familia"rer Panmyelopathie. *Humangenetik* 1964; 1: 194-196.
6. Sasaki MS, Tonomura A. A high susceptibility of Fanconi's anemia to chromosome breakage by DNA cross-linking agents. *Canc Res* 1973; 33: 1829-1836.
7. Auerbach AD, Wolman SR. Susceptibility of Fanconi's anaemia fibroblasts to chromosome damage by carcinogens. *Nature* 1976; 261: 494-496.
8. Berger R, Coniat ML, Gendron MC. Fanconi Anemia. Chromosome breakage and cell cycle studies. *Cancer Genet Cytogenet* 1993; 69: 13-16.
9. Arkin S, Brodtman D, Alter BP, Lipton JM. A screening test for Fanconi anemia using flow cytometry. *Blood* 1993; 82: 176a.
10. Strathdee CA, Duncan AMV, Buchwald M. Evidence for at least four Fanconi anaemia genes including FACC on chromosome 9. *Nature Genetics* 1992; 1: 196-198.
11. Gibson RA, Ford D, Jansen S, Savoia A, Havenga C, Milner RD, De Ravel TJ, Cohn RJ, Ball SE, Roberts I, Llerena JC, Vorechovsky I, Pearson T, Birjandi F, Hussein SS, Murer-Orlando M, Easton DF, Mathew CG. Genetic mapping of the FACC gene and linkage analysis in Fanconi anaemia families. *J Med Genet* 1994; 31: 868-871.
12. Whitney MA, Jakobs P, Kaback M, Moses RE, Grompe M. The Ashkenazi Jewish Fanconi anemia mutation: Incidence among patients and carrier frequency in the at-risk population. *Hum Mutat* 1994; 3: 339-341.
13. Verlander PC, Lin JD, Udono MU, Zhang Q, Gibson RA, Mathew CG, Auerbach AD. Mutation analysis of the Fanconi anemia gene FACC. *Am J Hum Genet* 1994; 54: 595-601.
14. Alter BP, Knobloch ME, Weinberg RS. Erythropoiesis in Fanconi's anemia. *Blood* 1991; 78: 602-608.
15. Alter BP, Knobloch ME, He L, Gillio AP, O'Reilly RJ, Reilly LK, Weinberg RS. Effect of stem cell factor on *in vitro* erythropoiesis in patients with bone marrow failure syndromes. *Blood* 1992; 80: 3000-3008.
16. Guinan EC, Lopez ED, Huhn RD, Felser JM, Nathan DG. Evaluation of granulocyte-macrophage colony-stimulating factor for treatment of pancytopenia in children with Fanconi anemia. *J Pediatr* 1994; 124: 144-150.
17. Rackoff WR, Orazi A, Robinson C, Cooper RJ, Alter BP, Freedman MH, Harris RE, Williams DA. Filgrastim (recombinant human granulocyte-colony stimulating factor, G-CSF) ameliorates neutropenia in patients with Fanconi anemia and stimulates multi-lineage hematopoiesis in some patients. *Blood* 1994; 84: 25a.
18. Alter BP, Scalise A, McCombs J, Najfeld V. Clonal chromosomal abnormalities in Fanconi's anemia: What do they really mean? *Br J Haematol* 1993; 85: 627-630.
19. Berger R, le Coniat M, Schaison G. Chromosome abnormalities in bone marrow of Fanconi anemia patients. *Cancer Genet Cytogenet* 1993; 65: 47-50.

Résumé

L'anémie de Fanconi est la forme la plus fréquente des syndromes d'aplasie médullaire héréditaire avec plus de 1 000 cas rapportés dans la littérature. Le diagnostic est fait par l'analyse des cassures chromosomiques ou l'étude de l'arrêt du cycle cellulaire; moins de 20% des patients aux USA sont de groupe C *in vitro*, les cultures de cellules souches hématopoïétiques comme le *stem cell factor* peuvent être stimulants en culture. *In vivo,* GM-CSF, IL-3 ou G-CSF augmentent la myélopoïèse alors que le G-CSF augmente parfois aussi, chez quelques patients, les plaquettes et l'hémoglobine. Les malades atteints de maladie de Fanconi ont une augmentation du risque de leucémie de plus de 10%, de syndrome myélodysplasique et ou de maladie clonale de 3%, de tumeur solide de 5%, de maladie hépatique de 4%. La leucémie est surtout myéloblastique et les anomalies chromosomiques dans les leucémies atteignent surtout les chromosomes 7 ou 5. Chez les malades non transformés en leucémie, nous avons trouvé que 30% d'entre eux avaient des anomalies cytogénétiques clonales variables dans le temps, sans spécifité pour un chromosome particulier. Les carcinomes squameux surviennent le plus souvent au niveau de l'oropharynx, du tube digestif ou de la sphère gynécologique avec une prédominance pour les malades du sexe féminin dans toutes les catégories. Le risque de cancer de la langue semble augmenté après greffe de moelle. Les tumeurs hépatiques sont plus souvent des hépatomes que des adénomes mais ne sont pas habituellement mortelles. Dans 10% des cas de tumeurs, plusieurs types étaient associés. Le temps d'âge d'apparition des complications était après 10 ans pour les leucémies, les maladies hépatiques et les anomalies clonales ou myélodysplasies et après 20 ans pour les tumeurs solides. La médiane de survie est de 19 ans; néanmoins, on observe une amélioration pour les malades plus récents.

Isolation and characterization of the Fanconi anemia genes

Manuel Buchwald[1], Ming Chen[1], Flora Krasnoshtein[1], Robert Cumming[1], Jeff Lightfoot[1], Linda Parker[1], Anna Savoia[2]

[1] Research Institute, Hospital for Sick Children, 555 University Avenue, Toronto, Ontario M5G 1X8, Canada and Department of Molecular and Medical Genetics, University of Toronto, tel.: (416) 813 63 50, fax: (416) 813 49 31 ; [2] Ospedale "Casa Sollievo della Sofferenza", San Giovanni Rotondo, Foggia, Italy

Abstract

Fanconi anemia (FA) is a genetically heterogeneous, autosomal recessive disorder characterized by pancytopaenia, a variety of congenital malformations and an increased susceptibility to the development of acute myelogenous leukemia. Cells from patients show an increased incidence of chromosomal aberrations and susceptibility to DNA cross-linking agents, in comparison to controls. We have exploited the sensitivity of FA cells to mitomycin C and diepoxybutane to isolate a set of cDNAs that complement the defect in FA(C) cells. The predicted protein shows no homology to known proteins nor does it show functional domains, thus requiring a more extensive approach to define its function. We have shown that the human FAC gene has two transcriptional start sites. The murine gene is expressed at low levels in mature tissues and at high levels in rapidly replicating cells of mesenchymal, epithelial, chondroblastic, osteoblastic and hematopoietic origin during embryonic development. Constitutive expression of FAC retards apoptosis in human and mouse cells deprived of growth factors. These results suggest that FAC may play a role in the protection of DNA during replication as well as in development. To test this hypothesis we have generated a mouse mutant in which the endogenous FAC locus has been inactivated.

Fanconi anemia (FA) is an autosomal recessive disorder, characterized by pancytopaenia, congenital malformations and an increased predisposition to the development of leukemia. FA patients have usually presented with aplastic anemia and one or more of a group of congenital malformations, especially radial ray defects in the arms and hands [1]. The clinical diagnosis of FA patients has been facilitated by assaying patients' cells for elevated chromosomal breakage, especially after treatment of cells with diepoxybutane (DEB) [2]. Some clinical variability is due to genetic heterogeneity. We first showed that FA patients could be classified into 2 complementation groups on the basis of somatic cell hybrid assays with FA cell lines, implying a minimum of two FA genes. We have extended the genetic analysis and shown that at least 4 genes, named *FAA* to *FAD*, are implicated in the disease [3]. Results submitted for publication indicate that there is a fifth gene, *FAE* [4]. At this time, insufficient data precludes correlation between complementation group and phenotype. *FAC* sequence alterations have been found in more than 30 FA patients. Mutations have been described that lead to polypeptide truncation (322ΔG, Q13X, R185X, R548X), aberrantly spliced transcripts (IVS4+4A-T) or base substitutions (L554P)(see [5]). The IVS4+4A-T mutation is present in the majority of FA patients of Ashkenazi Jewish descent and leads to a severe phenotype [6,7]. More precise relationships between genetic events and clinical outcomes will be possible after the other FA genes and their mutations are identified. However, other FA genes have yet to be found.

The basic defect in FA

Hypotheses to account for the pleiotropic FA phenotype postulate abnormalities in DNA repair, oxygen metabolism and growth factor homeostasis (see [5,8]). FA has been described as a DNA repair disorder in which the defect(s) lie in the repair of DNA cross-links, a view inferred from the increased sensitivity of FA cells to DNA crosslinking agents [9] and from their hypomutability [10]. Defects in DNA repair would cause abnormal cell replication in hematopoietic and osteogenic cells and lead to the developmental defects. However, biochemical studies of DNA repair defects in FA cells have been inconclusive or contradictory. This may represent the confounding effect of studying cells from different complementation groups or the fact that the repair defects may be secondary to the true basic defect. The most convincing evidence for a DNA repair defect is in FA(A), where cell extracts are defective in incising crosslinked DNA and have lower amounts of a protein that binds to interstrand cross-links [11].

The basic defect is also considered to arise from defects in oxygen metabolism. This would explain the sensitivity of the growth of FA cells to ambient oxygen, also reflected in increased chromosomal aberrations and as accumulation of cells in the G2 phase of the cell cycle [12]. The sensitivity to oxygen could be due either to increased production of toxic intermediates (*e.g.* free radicals) or to their decreased removal. The sensitivity of FA cells to DNA cross-linking agents is explained as resulting from aberrant handling of metabolites produced during their intracellular activation. The increased sensitivity to ambient oxygen could also affect the growth of FA cells *in vivo*, including those in the hematopoietic and osteogenic lineages.

The near universal bone marrow failure and the high incidence of congenital malformations in FA patients have led to suggestions that the FA genes function directly in cellular growth and/or differentiation [8]. Antisense nucleotides complementary to FAC mRNA inhibit the *in vitro* clonal growth of normal erythroid and granulocyte-macrophage progenitor cells, even in the presence of exogenous growth factors [13]. Similarly, peripheral blood $CD34^+$ cells isolated from a FA(C) patient and infected with a recombinant adeno-associated virus containing FAC cDNA, exhibit a 5-10 fold increase in the number of progenitor colonies formed *in vitro* compared to mock infected cells [14]. FA fibroblasts grow slower and senesce more rapidly than matched controls and demonstrate ultrastructural and physiological changes characteristic of cells from aged individuals. The FA gene products may play roles in the homeostasis of growth factors, many of which act in both hemopoiesis and osteogenesis. Addition of IL-6 to FA lymphoblast cultures reduces the sensitivity of these cells to mitomycin C (MMC) and DEB and decreases the number of chromosomal breaks [15]. Increased amounts of TNFα have been reported in FA cell cultures and in patient serum samples and anti-TNFα antibodies partially correct the chromosomal fragility of FA cells. If the basic defect in FA involves growth factor homeostasis, this might also be reflected in related processes, for example, apoptosis, or programmed cell death, implicated in the G2 arrest and death of cells treated with DNA crosslinking agents. A relationship between apoptosis and FA is also implied by the involvement of apoptosis in hemopoiesis and embryonic development, *i.e.* formation of the forelimb, which are abnormal in many FA patients.

Because of the above-mentioned interrelationships between cell growth, repair of DNA cross-links, oxygen metabolism, growth factor function and apoptosis, we do not know which, if any, is the primary defect caused by the mutations in the FA genes. Our approach has been to identify the defective genes by functional complementation, exploiting the increased sensitivity of FA cells to DNA cross-linking agents, and use the cloned genes as the vehicle to define the basic defect. We therefore expected that our identification of one of the FA genes [16] would identify at least one basic defect. However, the sequence of FAC shows no homology to known proteins nor known functional motifs and the function of FAC and the defective metabolic pathway(s) in FA still need to be defined.

Cloning and characterization of the *FAC* gene

We have reviewed the various attempts to clone the FA genes [5,17]. Failed attempts were based on the use of surrogate cell lines or animal models and on genomic or cDNA complementation of the MMC-sensitive phenotype of FA cells. We exploited an episomal vector (pREP4), based on the Epstein-Barr virus regulatory elements, to overcome the poor transfectability of human cells and cloned a set of cDNAs that specifically complemented the MMC- and DEB-sensitivity of FA(C) cells [16]. In the FA(C) cells used in the selection we identified a mutation predicted to produce an L554P substitution. We subsequently showed that this mutation led to an inactive cDNA [18]. *FAC* was mapped to 9q22.3 by *in situ* hybridization [3] and confirmed by genetic analysis of known FA(C) patients. A polymorphism within *FAC* has also been found. The complementing cDNAs contain three alternative 3' UTRs, each terminated by a consensus polyadenylation signal, in combination with one of two 5' UTRs. We hypothesized that the 5' UTRs reflected the presence of alternative transcriptional start sites that were spliced to a common downstream exon [16].

The *FAC* coding region contains 14 exons [19] and leads to a predicted protein of 558 amino acids [16,20]. The non-coding 5' exons, now called −1 and −1a, have suitable splice signals at their 3' ends but not at their 5' ends, consistent with the hypothesis of alternative transcriptional start sites [16]. The region upstream of exon −1 has promoter activity in transfection assays using a luciferase reporter gene. All 16 exons have been mapped to phages isolated from a genomic library. Because several introns are larger than 20 kb we have not yet been able to determine the complete genomic structure of *FAC*. The minimum size of *FAC* is 150 kb. The 3' terminal half of the mouse *FAC* gene was isolated during the development of a mouse model; the human and mouse genes are strikingly similar in this region. The mouse ORF shows 79% amino acid similarity to the human.

Studies of *FAC* expression

The analysis of gene expression can yield two essential pieces of information about gene function: the sites and levels where the gene functions and the mechanisms which mediate expression. In the case of *FAC*, the pleiotropic phenotype and the presence of two putative transcription start sites point to a complex regulation. We have pursued two parallel projects: to identify the promoter region of the gene [21] and to characterize the pattern of expression during development [22]. Both the human and mouse genes are ubiquitously expressed at low levels in adult tissues [16,19]. Analysis of *FAC* expression, using PCR-derived cDNA libraries from single hemopoietic cells, shows that higher levels of expression can be detected in less differentiated (multi-lineage progenitors) than in more differentiated cells (single lineage progenitors). We have tested the hypothesis that defects in FA alter apoptosis in two hematopoietic cell lines: MO7e, a human cell line derived from a megakaryocytic leukemia and dependent on either IL-3 or GM-CSF for survival and 32D, a murine myeloid progenitor cell line isolated from long term bone marrow cultures and dependent on IL-3. Both cell lines die by apoptosis upon factor withdrawal. We overexpressed *FAC* using a recombinant retroviral vector based on the Moloney Murine Leukemia Virus. MO7e and 32D cells overexpressing *FAC* showed a significant delay in cell death compared to the neomycin controls following IL-3 deprivation. FACS analysis confirmed that both MO7e and 32D cells infected with the FAC virus had significantly less (up to 50%) apoptotic cells, 2 and 3 days after IL-3 deprivation, compared to the *neo* infected controls. Thus, *FAC* appears to play a role in the apoptotic pathway of hemopoietic cells.

FAC expression during mouse embryogenesis is high in undifferentiated mesenchymal cells 8-10 days *p.c.* Starting at 13 days, expression becomes restricted to regions with rapidly replicating chondro- and osteoprogenitors (*e.g.* perichondrium), a pattern that persists to later stages (15-19.5 days), except in regions where differentiation has taken place (*e.g.* hypertrophic chondrocytes of the epiphyseal growth plate). As bone development proceeds, expression is seen in osteogenic and hematopoietic cells in the zone of calcification [22].

It is of interest to determine whether these changes in expression are mediated by transcriptional or posttranscriptional mechanisms. In the case of *FAC*, transcriptional regulation may involve either changes in the activity of one promoter or differential use of two promoters. The latter possibility is raised by the presence of alternative 5' UTRs in FAC messages [16]. Using RT-PCR, we have found that transcripts containing exon –1 are ubiquitous while those with exon –1a can be detected in lymphoblasts treated with DNA damaging agents and in human fetal tissues (*e.g.* bone at 12 weeks gestation). Similar transcription has not yet been determined in the mouse. The single murine *FAC* cDNA isolated from an adult liver library contained a 5' UTR region that resembled human exon –1. RACE-PCR on various mouse RNAs has identified an alternative 5' UTR.

Relating the function of *FAC* to its structure

Determination of the structure of FAC may provide clues to function through homology to proteins of known function. If the *FAC* structure is novel, this result will be of general interest in the protein structure field. The primary structure provides little information. The predicted ORF codes for a protein of 558 amino acids (63 kD) with a preponderance of hydrophobic amino acids (average hydrophobicity 0.17) but no predicted transmembrane domains [16]. *In vitro* transcription and translation of the cDNA produces a protein of 60 kD [18] and a protein of similar size is immunoprecipitated from lymphoblasts or transfected cells by anti-FAC antibodies [23,24]. The predicted protein has no obvious nuclear localization motifs and, as determined by immunofluorescence and subcellular fractionation, appears to be primarily cytoplasmic, though some is also present in the nucleus [23,24]. Comparison of the primary sequences of the human, mouse and bovine proteins does not reveal any obvious regions of higher homology, which could point to functional domains.

As a preliminary step towards purification of FAC, we have cloned the human FAC ORF into the pGEX-3X plasmid. When analyzed by SDS-PAGE, the fusion protein is approximately 82 kDa, yielding an estimated size of 55 kDa for FAC, somewhat smaller than that predicted. Since FAC with an epitope tag at the N terminus is fully functional in complementation assays, for purification of the mouse FAC protein, we cloned the mouse FAC ORF in the vector pTrcHisA, which allows high level expression of recombinant proteins with a 6-histidine tag at the N terminus. SDS-PAGE analysis of the mouse FAC protein shows a band of about 64 kDa, the expected size.

The function and structure of FAC can also be approached by cloning and analyzing orthologs of human *FAC*. Identification of the ortholog in "model organisms" such as the mouse, zebrafish or *Drosophila* can offer different or complementary experimental approaches to analyzing the biochemistry, regulation, development and disease progression in FA. Though mouse *FAC* has already been identified, and a *FAC* "knock-out" mouse has been produced and is being characterized, FA(C) models in organisms such as zebrafish and *Drosophila* offer further advantages. In addition to their value in developmental and genetic studies, the cloning of *FAC* orthologs should facilitate structure and function studies. Comparisons of sequences from distantly related species will allow the delineation of the minimal conserved functional domains. The human, mouse and bovine cDNAs share a 55% amino acid identity among them, suggesting that by comparing the sequences of more species, the important domains will be narrowed further. Using the mouse probe, hybridizing fragments have been seen in DNA from chicken, zebrafish and *Drosophila*, and perhaps in *Xenopus*.

Development of a mouse model for *FA(C)*

Availability of mouse (or other animal) models of human genetic diseases facilitates the genetic and developmental analysis of the disorder and serves as a tool to develop specific therapies. Because of the large reservoir of natural mouse mutants that have been collected over time, it is possible that a mouse model for a given genetic disease already exists. We have mapped mouse *FAC* to chromosome 13 [25]. This assignment indicates that the homology map between human chromosome 9 and mouse chromosome 4 is interrupted in the region of *FAC*. Mapping of the mouse *Fac* gene to chromosome 13 eliminates as a possible mouse model the mutant *an* (Hertwig's anemia), which is located in chromosome 4 [26]. However, the map location of the *f* (flexed-tail) mutant on chromosome 13 makes this a possible candidate. Homozygous *f* mutants are small at birth and have a transient hypochromic, microcytic anemia. Some affected animals have a flexed tail and a belly spot. While adults have normal blood values, they have a defective response to hemopoietic stress. Thus, *f* mutants may represent a mild form of FA, perhaps because they carry a leaky mutation. However, *f* mice show no hypersensitivity to MMC, suggesting they are not mouse equivalents to FA(C).

The alternative and more direct approach is to develop a mouse mutant by molecular and embryological methods. Two significant breakthroughs that allow this approach have been the development of pluripotent embryonic stem (ES) cell lines that can be manipulated *in vitro* and subsequently used to derive whole animals and the development of methods to identify homologous recombination in cell culture. Because in some instances the mouse model mimics the human disease (CF) while in other instances it does not (Lesch-Nyhan), the fidelity of disease replication in the animal model cannot be assumed in advance of the experiment.

The mouse *FAC* cDNA was used as a probe to screen a genomic library of mouse strain 129. More than twenty positive clones were isolated. Three of these were mapped and found to be overlapping, encompassing the genomic region from exon 8 to the end of the 3'UTR of the mouse cDNA. A targeting vector was constructed using the most 5' mouse genomic sequence available. The end result of the homologous recombination is that exon 8 is deleted and the *neo* gene is inserted. Based on data from our laboratory showing that the last exon, exon 14, is essential for the complementing function of the *FAC* gene product, the disruption in the middle of the murine *FAC* gene should render this locus biologically inactive. This targeting vector was linearized and electrophorated into R1 embryonic stem (ES) cells which were derived from the 129 mouse strain. The cells then underwent double selection using G418 and gangcyclovir. Of 102 clones screened, 18 positive cell lines were identified. To make sure that the homologous recombination took place in the expected manner, all of the 18 positive cell lines were analyzed on the second arm and confirmed to be correct recombinants [27]. Four targeted cell lines have been used to produce chimeric mice. 129-derived ES cells were aggregated *ex vivo* into the morulas derived from CD1 mice and then implanted into foster mothers. Twenty two chimeras were obtained; moderately and strongly chimeric mice were bred and those resulting in germline transmission bred to homozygosity. No apparent mortality has been observed among homozygous FAC^- mice. The oldest mice are now 5 months old; their phenotype is being characterized.

Acknowledgements

Work at HSC was supported by operating grants from the Medical Research Council of Canada and the National Cancer Institute of Canada. Support was also received from the Fanconi Anemia Research Fund, Inc (FARF) and from ChildCan. Work at San Giovanni Rotondo was supported by Telethon – Italy, Italian Ministry of Health, AIRFA and FARF. We also thank the families of FA patients for their continuing support.

References

1. Fanconi G. Familial constitutional panmyelocytopathy, Fanconi Anemia (FA). I. Clinical aspects. *Semin Hematol* 1967; 4: 233-240.
2. Auerbach AD, Adler B, Chaganti RSK. Prenatal and postnatal diagnosis and carrier detection of Fanconi anemia by a cytogenetic method. *Pediatrics* 1981; 67: 128-135.
3. Strathdee CA, Duncan AMV, Buchwald M. Evidence for at least four Fanconi anemia genes including *FACC* on chromosome 9. *Nature Genet* 1992; 1: 196-198.
4. Joenje H, Lo Ten Foe JR, Ostra AB, van Berkel CGM, Rooimans MA, Schroeder-Kurth T, Wegner R-D, Gille JJP, Buchwald M, Arwert F. Evidence for a new Fanconi anemia gene. (submitted for publication)
5. dos Santos CC, Gavish H, Buchwald M. Fanconi anemia revisited: old ideas and new advances. *Stem Cells* 1994; 12: 142-153.
6. Verlander PC, Lin JD, Udono MU, Zhang Q, Gibson RA, Mathew CG, Auerbach AD. Mutation analysis of the Fanconi anemia gene *FACC*. *Am J Human Genet* 1994; 54: 595-601.
7. Whitney MA, Saito H, Jakobs PM, Gibson RA, Moses RE, Grompe MA. A common mutation in the *FACC* gene causes Fanconi anaemia in Ashkenazi-Jewish individuals. *Nature Genet* 1993; 4: 202-205.
8. Liu JM, Buchwald M, Walsh CE, Young NS. Fanconi anemia and novel strategies for therapy. *Blood* 1994; 84: 3995-4007.
9. Ishida R, Buchwald M. Susceptibility of Fanconi's anemia lymphoblasts to DNA cross-linking and alkylating agents. *Cancer Res* 1982; 42: 4000-4006.

10. Papadopoulo D, Guillouf C, Mohnrenweiser H, Moustacchi E. Hypomutability in Fanconi anemia cells is associated with increased deletion frequency at the HPRT locus. *Proc Natl Acad Sci USA* 1990; 87: 8383-8387.
11. Lambert MW, Tsongalis GJ, Lambert WC, Hang B, Parrish DD. Defective DNA endonuclease activities in Fanconi's anemia, complementation group A, cells. *Mutation Res* 1992; 273: 57-71.
12. Joenje H, Arwert F, Eriksson AW, De Koning J, Oostra AB. Oxygen-dependence of chromosomal aberrations in Fanconi's anemia. *Nature* 1981; 290: 142-143.
13. Segal GM, Magenis RE, Brown M, Keeble W, Smith TD, Heinrich MC, Bagby GC. Repression of Fanconi anemia gene (FACC) inhibits growth of hematopoietic progenitor cells. *J Clin Invest* 1994; 94: 846-852.
14. Walsh CE, Nienhuis AW, Samuski RJ, Brown MG, Miller JL, Young NS, Liu JM. Phenotypic correction of Fanconi anemia in human hematopoietic cells with a recombinant adeno-associated virus vector. *J Clin Invest* 1994; 94: 1440-1448.
15. Rosselli F, Sanceau J, Gluckman E, Wietzerbin J, Moustacchi E. Abnormal lymphokine production: a novel feature of the genetic disease Fanconi anemia. II. *In vitro* and *in vivo* spontaneous production of tumor necrosis factor. *Blood* 1994; 84: 1216-1225.
16. Strathdee CA, Gavish H, Shannon W, Buchwald M. Cloning of cDNAs for Fanconi anaemia by functional complementation. *Nature* 1992; 356: 763-767.
17. Strathdee CA, Buchwald M. Molecular and cellular biology of Fanconi anemia. *Am J Pediat Hematol Oncol* 1992; 14: 177-185.
18. Gavish H, dos Santos CC, Buchwald M. Leu_{554}-Pro substitution completely abolishes complementing activity of the Fanconi anemia (FACC) protein. *Human Mol Genet* 1993; 2: 123-126.
19. Gibson R. Buchwald M, Roberts RG, Mathew CG. Characterization of the exon structure of the Fanconi anemia group C gene by vectorette PCR. *Human Mol Genet* 1993; 2: 35-38.
20. Wevrick R, Clarke CA, Buchwald M. Cloning and analysis of the murine Fanconi anemia group C cDNA. *Human Mol Genet* 1993; 2: 655-662.
21. Savoia A, Centra M, Lanzano L, de Cillis GP, Zelante L, Buchwald M. Characterization of the 5' region of the Fanconi anemia group C gene. *Hum Mol Genet* (in press).
22. Krasnoshtein F, Buchwald M. Analysis of the pattern of expression of the Fanconi anemia C (*Facc*) gene during murine development. *Am J Hum Genet* 1994; 55: A125
23. Youssoufian H. Localization of Fanconi anemia C protein to the cytoplasm of mammalian cells. *Proc Natl Acad Sci USA* 1994; 91:7975-7979.
24. Yamashita T, Barber DL, Zhu Y, Wu N, D'Andrea AD. The Fanconi anemia polypeptide FACC is localized to the cytoplasm. *Proc Natl Acad Sci USA* 1994; 91: 6712-6716.
25. Wevrick R, Barker, JE, Nadeau JH, Szpirer C, Buchwald M. Mapping of the murine and rat *Facc* genes and assessment of flexed-tail as a candidate mouse homolog of Fanconi anemia group C. *Mammalian Genome* 1993; 4: 440-444.
26. Lyon MF, Searle AG (eds) Genetic variants and strains of the laboratory mouse. Oxford: Oxford U Press, 1981.
27. Chen M, Auerbach W, Auerbach A, Joyner AL, Buchwald M. Targeted disruption of the murine *Facc* gene: towards the establishment of a mouse model for Fanconi anemia. *Am J Hum Genet* 1994; 55: A216.

Résumé

L'anémie de Fanconi est une maladie génétiquement hétérogène à transmission autosomale et récessive caractérisée par une pancytopénie, des malformations congénitales et une augmentation du risque de leucémie aiguë myéloblastique. Les cellules des malades ont une augmentation des aberrations chromosomiques ainsi qu'une sensibilité accrue aux agents pontants. Nous avons utilisé cette sensibilité des cellules de Fanconi à la mitomycine C et au Diepoxybutane pour isoler une série de cDNAs complémentant le défaut de *FA(C)*. La protéine ainsi prédite ne montre aucune analogie avec des protéines connues, ni de domaine fonctionnel, ce qui demande des études plus extensives pour connaître sa fonction. Nous avons démontré que le gène humain *FA(C)* a deux sites de transcription de départ. Le gène murin est exprimé en faible quantité sur les tissus matures et en grande quantité sur les cellules se divisant rapidement, mésenchimales, épithéliales, chondroblastiques, ostéoblastiques et hématopoïétiques pendant le développement embryonnaire. L'expression constitutive de *FA(C)* retarde l'apoptose dans les cellules humaines et murines en l'absence de facteurs de croissance. Ces résultats semblent démontrer que *FA(C)* pourrait jouer un rôle dans la protection du DNA pendant la réplication et pendant le développement. Pour tester cette hypothèse, nous avons développé un modèle de souris mutante dans lequel le locus *FA(C)* endogène a été inactivé.

Mutation analysis of the Fanconi anemia gene *FAC*

Arleen D. Auerbach and Peter C. Verlander

Laboratory of Human Genetics and Hematology, The Rockefeller University New York, New York, USA, tel.: (212) 327 7533, fax: (212) 327 8232

Abstract

Fanconi anemia (FA) is a genetically heterogeneous autosomal recessive disorder defined by hypersensitivity of cells to DNA cross-linking agents; FAC, the gene for complementation group C (FA-C), has been cloned. Two common mutations, IVS4 +4 A→T and 322delG, and several rare mutations have been reported in affected individuals. Results of our SSCP study of DNA samples from FA patients enrolled in the International Fanconi Anemia Registry (IFAR), maintained at The Rockefeller University since 1982, indicate that approximately 15% of patients exhibited pathogenic mutations in FAC. IVS4 is found exclusively in individuals of Jewish ancestry; the ancestry of carriers of 322delG is primarily northern European. Our analysis showed a correlation between genetic and clinical features in FA-C individuals; all patients with IVS4 exhibited a severe phenotype with multiple birth defects and early onset of hematologic abnormalities, while 322delG was associated with a mild form of the syndrome. We have developed amplification refractory mutation system (ARMS) assays for the five pathogenic mutations found in our SSCP study of the IFAR population. These assays provide a means for rapid, non-radioactive testing and we have applied these assays to screen a healthy Jewish population. In addition, we have applied these ARMS assays to (1) assign newly diagnosed FA patients to group C, (2) provide rapid carrier testing for FA-C families, and (3) provide prenatal diagnosis for FA-C families. Thirty-five IVS4 carriers were identified in a screen of genomic DNA samples from 3104 Jewish individuals, primarily of Ashkenazi descent, for a carrier frequency of >1%; no 322delG carriers were found. No carriers for IVS4 were detected in DNA samples from 563 Iraqi Jews ascertained in Israel. With a carrier frequency greater than 1% and simple testing available, the IVS4 mutation merits inclusion in the battery of carrier tests routinely provided to the Ashkenazi Jewish population.

Fanconi anemia (FA) is an autosomal recessive disorder characterized clinically by diverse congenital abnormalities and a predisposition to bone marrow failure and malignancy, particularly acute myelogenous leukemia (AML) [1-3]. FA patients display a wide range of clinical features: patients may be severely affected, with multiple congenital malformations, or may have a mild phenotype with no major malformations. The considerable overlap of the FA phenotype with that of a variety of genetic and non-genetic diseases makes diagnosis on the basis of clinical manifestations alone difficult [1]. FA cells exhibit an abnormally high level of baseline chromosomal breakage and are hypersensitive to both the cytotoxic and clastogenic effects of DNA cross-linking agents such as diepoxybutane (DEB) and mitomycin C (MMC) [4]. The relationship of this DNA instability to the cancer susceptibility of FA patients is unknown. Diagnosis of FA is now facilitated by the study of chromosomal breakage induced by DNA cross-linking agents such as DEB [5], which provides a unique marker for the FA genotype. This cellular characteristic can be utilized as a diagnostic test to identify the preanemic patient as well as the patient with aplastic anemia or leukemia who may or may not have the classic physical stigmata associated with FA. Heterozygotes for FA cannot be detected by the DEB test.

FA is found in all races and ethnic groups and has been reported to have a carrier frequency of 1:300 [6]. The true gene frequency may be considerably higher than this; a low estimate would result from a lack of ascertainment of cases due to the occurrence of extreme phenotypic heterogeneity in the syndrome, leading to difficulty in establishing the clinical diagnosis of FA.

In addition to the clinical heterogeneity seen in FA, extensive genetic heterogeneity has been reported [7,8]. At least five different complementation groups have been defined [7,9]; the relationship between complementation groups detected by different laboratories as well as the full extent of heterogeneity in FA remain to be determined. Only one of these genes, *FAC*, which maps to chromosome 9q22.3 [7], has been cloned [10]. This gene corrects the DNA cross-link hypersensitivity of a complementation group C (FA-C) cell line. Study of genomic DNA revealed that *FAC* contains 14 exons ranging in size from 53 to 204 bp [11]. The DNA sequence of this gene has no substantial similarity to any known gene family. The *FAC* cDNA is predicted to encode a polypeptide of 558 amino acids with a molecular mass of ~60 kDa. The function of the *FAC* gene product is still unknown. The protein has been shown to bind to several other proteins to form a complex which localizes exclusively to the cytoplasmic compartment to the cell [12-14]. This would seem to exclude a direct role for *FAC* and *FAC*-related proteins in DNA repair, as had been widely assumed on the basis of the cellular phenotype of hypersensitivity to DNA damage. In this paper we review our *FAC* mutation studies performed on DNA samples from FA patients enrolled in the International Fanconi Anemia Registry (IFAR), and our analysis of genotype-phenotype correlations in these patients.

Mutation analysis of *FAC*

SSCP analysis

FA patients have been screened for mutations in *FAC* by SSCP analysis [15] and by chemical mismatch cleavage analysis. [16-18] Results of our SSCP study of DNA samples from FA patients enrolled in the IFAR, maintained at The Rockefeller University since 1982, indicate that approximately 15% of patients exhibited pathogenic mutations in *FAC*. These patients can be classified as FA-C on this basis. The specific mutations detected in our study are shown in *Table I*. In addition to the disease causing mutations, two variants were found that did not segregate with the disease allele in multiplex families, indicating that they represent polymorphisms. One of the presumptive pathogenic mutations was found in only one family with one affected individual; the possibility that this mutation represents a normal variant cannot be ruled out. The distribution of alleles in IFAR families with mutations in *FAC* is seen in *Table II*. The most frequent mutations in this gene are IVS4 + 4 → AT (IVS4), an A to T transversion four bases into

Table I. *FAC* mutations and variants.

	Location	Base	Base change	Amino acid	Reference
Mutations					
Q13X	exon 1	292	C→T	Gln→Stop	Verlander *et al* 1994
322delG	exon 1	322	deletion	frameshift	Strathdee *et al* 1992
IVS4 +4 A→T	intron 4	712+4	A→T	splice site	Whitney *et al* 1993
R185X	exon 6	808	C→T	Arg→Stop	Gibson *et al* 1993
R548X	exon 14	1897	C→T	Arg→Stop	Murer-Orlando *et al* 1993
L554P	exon 14	1916	T→C	Leu→Pro	Strathdee *et al* 1992
Variants					
D195V	exon 6	839	A→T	Asp→Val	Verlander *et al* 1994
S26F	exon 1	332	C→T	Ser→Phe	Verlander *et al* 1994
G139E	exon 4	671	G→A	Gly→Glu	Whitney *et al* 1993

Table II. Distribution of *FAC* alleles.

	Allele 1				
Allele 2	Q13X	322delG	IVS4	R185X	L554P
Q13X	1	2			
322delG		1			
IVS4			20		
R185X		2		1	
unknown	1	6			1

the intron 4 donor splice site, and 322delG, a deletion in exon 1 resulting in a frameshift and a premature stop codon. These two mutations were present in 84% of FA-C families. IVS4 is found exclusively in individuals of Jewish ancestry while the ancestry of carriers of 322delG is primarily northern European.

ARMS assays

We have recently developed amplification refractory mutation system (ARMS) assays for the five pathogenic mutations found in the SSCP study of the IFAR population [19]. These assays provide a means for rapid, non-radioactive testing and we have applied these assays to screen a healthy Jewish population for IVS4 and 322delG, the two most common FA alleles. In addition, we have applied these ARMS assays to [1] assign newly diagnosed FA patients to group C, [2] provide rapid carrier testing for FA-C families, and [3] provide prenatal diagnosis for FA-C families.

All mutation-specific primers anneal to the plus strand, and were designed so that the 3' base matched the point of the mutation. The second primer for each assay was the forward primer for the exon containing the mutation [11]. Primers were designed to have a predicted annealing temperature of 56°C. In order to reduce background, a second mismatch was introduced at the third base from the 3' end in some primers, so that two of the last three nucleotides would be mismatched in an individual lacking the mutation. The ARMS assays can be combined in two multiplex reactions as shown in *Table III*. Assay A includes primers for the two common mutations, IVS4 and 322delG, while Assay B includes primers for Q13X, R185X, and L554P. Each assay includes a set primers for *FAC* exon 13 as a positive control for the PCR reaction.

In order to determine the frequency of IVS4 carriers in the Jewish population, genomic DNA samples ascertained anonymously from 3104 Jewish individuals, primarily of Ashkenazi descent, were obtained from Dor Yeshorim, an organization that provides genetic testing services to the religious Jewish community in New York. DNA samples from 563 Iraqi Jews from Israel were supplied by Dr. Uri Seligsohn, in order to determine if the IVS4 mutation is present in the Sephardic Jewish population as well. Thirty-five IVS4 carriers were identified in the Dor Yeshorim population, for a carrier frequency of >1%; no 322delG carriers were found. No carriers for IVS4 were detected in the Iraqi Jewish sample *(Table IV)* [19].

Twenty-one probands from the IFAR, for whom both parents have Ashkenazi Jewish ancestry, were screened for *FAC* mutations, and twenty were homozygous for IVS4; the one remaining patient had no detectable *FAC* mutation. Four additional probands with Ashkenazi ancestry on only one side of their family were also been tested, and none carry IVS4. The fact that 100% of FA-C chromosomes of Jewish origin carry the IVS4 mutation is strong evidence for a founder effect.

Table III. ARMS assay primers.

Mutation	Primers	Product
Assay A		
322delG	5'-ACCATTTCCTTCAGTGCTGG-3' 5'-AAAGTGGAAGCCTGATA**CA**-3'	147 bp
IVS4 +4 A→T	5'-GTAGGCATTGTACATAAAAG-3' 5'-AAACATTTCAAAAGTGATAAATATTAAAT**TC**<u>A</u>-3'	220 bp
control	5'-CCTAGAAGTATGTCTGTCCTG-3' 5'-CTCTCCTTGACTAGGATGCTG-3'	303 bp
Assay B		
Q13X	5'-ACCATTTCCTTCAGTGCTGG-3' 5'-AGCTTCTGCATCCAAAACT<u>A</u>-3'	121 bp
R185X	5'-GTCCTTAATTATGCATGGCTC-3' 5'-AATAAGTGGGACACAAAC**GC**<u>A</u>-3'	111 bp
L554P	5'-GGATAGGGCTTCTTTCAGGG-3' 5'-CTTCTAGACTTGAGTTCA**C**<u>G</u>-3'	258 bp
control	5'-CCTAGAAGTATGTCTGTCCTG-3' 5'-CTCTCCTTGACTAGGATGCTG-3'	303 bp

Bold indicates a base that is mismatched when annealed to the wild-type sequence.
Underline indicates a base that matches a mutation.

Table IV. IVS4 carrier frequency in Jews.

	Carriers	Non-carriers	Total	Frequency
Ashkenazi	35	3069	3104	1.1%
Iraqi	0	563	563	0%

Genotype-phenotype correlation for FA-C patients

Our studies have shown a correlation between genetic and clinical features in FA-C individuals [15]. All our patients with IVS4 exhibited a severe phenotype with multiple birth defects and early onset of hematologic abnormalities, while 322delG was associated with a mild form of the syndrome. Another exon 1 mutation found in our population, Q13X, is carried only by individuals of Southern Italian ancestry. Like 322delG, Q13X is associated with a mild phenotype. In a recent study in which we examined the correlation between height, endocrinopathy and mutations in *FAC*, we found that patients with the IVS4 mutation (8 individuals) had significantly shorter stature than the mean for age (mean height standard deviation score -4.30 ± 0.73, $p=0.002$) [20]. Hypothyroidism also occurred more frequently in the IVS4 patients. While fifty-seven percent of IVS4 patients exhibited growth hormone (GH) insufficiency, 45% of patients without this mutation (mostly non-FA-C patients) also had GH insufficiency in this study. In another example of a possible genotype-phenotype correlation, we found that the two patients who developed moyamoya syndrome, in the IFAR database comprised of 434 patients, were compound heterozygotes for the 322delG and R185X mutations in the *FAC* gene [21].

Affected sib-pair analysis of patients in the international Fanconi anemia registry (IFAR)

In order to better understand the correlation between genotype and phenotype in FA patients, we have recently performed an analysis of congenital malformations exhibited by 434 patients reported to the IFAR between 1982 and 1994 [22]. At least one major malformation was reported in 284 patients (65%). This data set included 53 families with two or more affected siblings, and was comprised of 120 siblings affected with FA. Sixty-seven of these individuals (56%) had at least one congenital malformation. Our study indicates that there is both interfamilial and intrafamilial phenotypic variation in the specific types of congenital malformations among affected siblings in these 53 sibships; even two sets of monozygotic (MZ) twins showed phenotypic discordancy. One set of MZ twins was diagnosed prenatally as affected with FA, and the pregnancy was terminated. Postmortem evaluation of both stillborn male fetuses revealed that twin fetus A had a duplicated distal phalanx of the right thumb while twin fetus B had no physical stigmata of FA [23]. The second MZ twin pair comprised 7 year old females with FA. One had unilateral absence of the radius, bilateral absent thumbs and an absent right clavicle. The other had a bifid right thumb, hypoplastic left thumb and absent left clavicle. Although these twins had congenital malformations involving the same organ systems, they were discordant for specific congenital malformations [22]. The sib-pair analysis of the 53 multiplex families, which included complementation group C and non-C families, also showed that the intrafamilial variation for the presence or absence of any congenital malformation, as well as the type of malformation exhibited, is non-random. To explain this non-random occurrence of malformations among FA siblings, we postulate that the phenotypic features of an affected individual depend on the specific FA mutation, somatic DNA instability, other genes and environmental factors.

Conclusion

The source of the phenotypic heterogeneity found in FA patients has been an open question; the relative contributions of complementation group, specific mutations, and random factors has remained unknown. Sibship analysis of multiplex FA families indicates that FA has both random and non-random components: while the specific manifestation of the disease is random, the severity of the disease is non-random. In addition, genotype-phenotype analysis of FA-C patients demonstrats that the variation in the severity of the disease is more likely to be a function of the specific mutation than of the complementation group.
The high carrier frequency of the IVS4 mutation in Ashkenazi Jews places FA-C in the group of so-called "Jewish" diseases that include Tay-Sachs, Gaucher, and Canavan disease, among others [24]. Carrier screening programs have been implemented for the Ashkenazi population for several of the diseases which occur at high frequency in this population. With a carrier frequency greater than 1% and simple testing available, the IVS4 mutation merits inclusion in the battery of tests routinely provided to the Jewish population.

Acknowledgments

The authors thank the many physicians who referred patients to the International Fanconi Anemia Registry (IFAR). This work was supported in part by grant R01 HL32987 from the National Institutes of Health.

References

1. Giampietro PF, Adler-Brecher B, Verlander PC, Pavlakis SG, Davis JG, Auerbach AD. The need for more accurate and timely diagnosis in Fanconi anemia. A report from the International Fanconi Anemia Registry. *Pediatrics* 1993; 91: 1116-1120.
2. Butturini A, Gale RP, Verlander PC, Adler-Brecher B, Gillio AP, Auerbach AD. Hematologic abnormalities in Fanconi anemia. An International Fanconi Anemia Registry study. *Blood* 1994; 84: 1650-1655.
3. Auerbach AD, Allen RG. Leukemia and preleukemia in Fanconi anemia patients: a review of the literature and report of the International Fanconi Anemia Registry. *Cancer Genet Cytogenet* 1991; 51: 1-12.
4. Auerbach AD, Rogatko A, Schroeder-Kurth TM. International Fanconi Anemia Registry: relation of clinical symptoms to diepoxybutane sensitivity. *Blood* 1989; 73: 391-396.
5. Auerbach AD. Fanconi anemia diagnosis and the diepoxybutane (DEB) test. *Exp Hematol* 1993; 21: 731-733.
6. Swift M. Fanconi's anaemia in the genetics of neoplasia. *Nature* 1971; 230: 370-373.
7. Strathdee CA, Duncan AMV, Buchwald M. Evidence for at least four Fanconi anaemia genes including FACC on chromosome 9. *Nature Genet* 1992; 1: 196-198.

8. Mann WR, Venkatraj VS, Allen RG, Liu Q, Olsen DA, Adler-Brecher B, Mao J, Weiffenbach B, Sherman SL, Auerbach AD. Fanconi anemia: evidence for linkage heterogeneity on chromosome 20q. *Genomics* 1991; 9: 329-337.
9. Joenje H, Lo Ten Foe JR, Oostra AB, van Berkel CGM, Rooimans MA, Schroeder-Kurth TM, Wegner R-D, Gille JJP, Buchwald M, Arwert F. Classification of Fanconi anemia patients by complementation analysis: evidence for a fifth gentic subtype. *Blood* 1995; in press.
10. Strathdee CA, Gavish H, Shannon WR, Buchwald M. Cloning of cDNAs for Fanconi's anaemia by functional complementation. *Nature* 1992; 356: 763-767.
11. Gibson RA, Buchwald M, Roberts RG, Mathew CG. Characterisation of the exon structure of the Fanconi anaemia group C gene by vectorette PCR. Hum *Molec Genet* 1993; 2: 35-38.
12. Yamashita T, Barber DL, Zhy Y, Wu N, D'Andrea AD. The Fanconi anemia polypeptide FACC is localized to the cytoplasm. *Proc Natl Acad Sci USA* 1994; 91: 6712-6716.
13. Youssoufian H. Localization of Fanconi anemia C protein to the cytoplasm of mammalian cells. *Proc Natl Acad Sci, USA* 1994; 91: 7975-7979.
14. Youssoufian H, Auerbach AD, Verlander PC, Steimle V, Mach B. Identification of cytosolic proteins that bind to the Fanconi anemia polypeptide (FACC) *in vitro*: evidence for a myltimeric complex. *J Biol Chem* 1995; in press.
15. Verlander PC, Lin JD, Udono MU, Zhang Q, Gibson RA, Mathew CG, Auerbach AD. Mutation analysis of the Fanconi anemia gene FACC. *Am J Hum Genet* 1994; 54: 595-601.
16. Gibson RA, Hajianpour A, Murer-Orlando M, Buchwald M, Mathew CG. A nonsense mutation and exon skipping in the Fanconi anaemia group C gene. *Hum Molec Genet* 1993; 2: 797-799.
17. Whitney MA, Saito H, Jakobs PM, Gibson RA, Moses RE, Grompe M. A common mutation in the FACC gene causes Fanconi anaemia in Ashkenazi Jews. *Nature Genet* 1993; 4: 202-205.
18. Murer-Orlando M, Llerena JC, Birjandi F, Gibson RA, Mathew CG. FACC gene mutations and early prenatal diagnosis of Fanconi's anemia. *Lancet* 1993; 342: 686.
19. Verlander PC, Kaporis AG, Liu Q, Zhang Q, Seligsohn U, Auerbach AD. Carrier frequency of the IVS4 +4 AT mutation of the Fanconi anemia gene *FAC* in the Ashkenazi Jewish population: evidence for a founder effect. *Am J Hum Genet* 1994; submitted.
20. Huma Z, Auerbach AD, Verlander PC, Giampietro PF, Gertner JM. Endocrinological outcome of children with Fanconi anemia. *J Pediatr* 1995; submitted.
21. Pavlakis SG, Verlander P, Gould RJ, Strimling BC, Auerbach AD. Fanconi anemia and moyamoya: evidence for an association. *Neurology* 1995; in press.
22. Giampietro PF, Verlander PC, Maschan A, Davis JG, Auerbach AD. Fanconi anemia: a model for somatic gene mutation during development. *Am J Med Genet* 1994; 52: 36-37.
23. Adler-Brecher B, Zhang Q, Flit Y, Gray DL, Beaver HA, Reid JE, Auerbach AD. Prenatal diagnosis of Fanconi anemia in monozygotic twin boys with discordant phenotype. *Am J Hum Genet* 1992; 51(suppl): A251.
24. Motulsky AG. Jewish diseases and origins. *Nature Genet* 1995; 9:99-101.

Résumé

La maladie de Fanconi est une maladie génétique hétérogène à transmission autosomale récessive définie par une hypersensibilité aux agents pontants du DNA; le gène du groupe de complémentation C a été cloné. Deux mutations fréquentes, IVS4+4 T et 322delG, et quelques mutations plus rares ont été décrites. Notre étude en SSCP des échantillons de DNA des patients inclus depuis 1982 dans le registre international des maladies de Fanconi établi au Rockefeller University montre qu'approximativement 15% des patients ont une mutation de *FAC*. IVS4 est retrouvée exclusivement chez les malades d'origine juive alors que 322delG se retrouve chez les sujets originaires d'Europe du Nord. Notre analyse a montré l'existence d'une corrélation entre les aspects génétiques et cliniques; tous les malades avec la mutation IVS4 ont une forme sévère avec de nombreuses malformations et une aplasie précoce alors que la mutation 322delG est associée à une forme de gravité modérée. Nous avons développé un test ARMS *(amplification refractory mutation system)* pour les 5 mutations trouvées dans l'étude par SSCP. Ce test permet une identification rapide, par un test non radioactif des principales mutations. Il est appliqué pour le dépistage dans la population juive normale. De plus nous avons appliqué l'ARMS 1) pour le diagnostic de mutation C chez les malades nouvellement diagnostiqués, 2) pour détecter les porteurs dans les familles atteintes, 3) faire le diagnostic prénatal. Trente-cinq porteurs de IVS4 ont été identifiés sur 3104 juifs ashkénases testés avec une fréquence de >1%; aucune mutation 322delG n'a été trouvée; Aucune mutation IVS4 n'été trouvée chez les juifs d'origine irakienne. Avec une fréquence de >1% et un test simple, la mutation IVS4 devrait être systématiquement introduite dans la batterie des tests à la recherche d'anomalies génétiques chez les juifs ashkénases.

Classification of Fanconi anemia patients by complementation analysis

Hans Joenje, for EUFAR*

Department of Human Genetics, Free University, Van der Boechorststraat 7, NL-1081 BT Amsterdam, The Netherlands, tel.: (31 20) 548 27 64, fax: (31 20) 548 33 29

Summary

Currently four genetic subtypes or 'complementation groups' (FA-A through FA-D) have been distinguished among 7 unrelated FA patients. We used genetically marked Fanconi anemia (FA) lymphoblastoid cell lines representing each of the 4 presently known complementation groups to carry out classification of additional FA patients through cell fusion and complementation analysis. Additional patients were identified belonging to groups A, C and D. Assignment of patients to the FA-C group was confirmed by mutations detected in the FAC gene. One cell line complemented all 4 reference cell lines and therefore represented a fifth complementation group, designated FA-E. These results suggest that at least 5 genes are involved in a pathway that, when defective, causes bone marrow failure in FA patients.

Fanconi anemia (FA) is a recessive disease featuring diverse clinical symptoms including progressive panmyelopathy and a markedly increased risk of acute myeloid leukemia. FA cells exhibit an increased spontaneous chromosomal instability and are hypersensitive to the clastogenic and cytotoxic effects of crosslinking agents, such as mitomycin C (MMC), diepoxybutane (DEB), cyclophosphamide and cisplatinum [1, 2]. FA is genetically heterogeneous: 4 com-

---

* EUFAR (European Fanconi Anemia Research) is a concerted action sponsored by the Commission of the European Union. Participants *EU countries:* E Gluckman, E Moustacchi (France); M Digweed, H Hoehn, T Schroeder-Kurth, W Friedrich, W Ebell (Germany); F Arwert, H Joenje, ML Kwee, LP ten Kate, A Westerveld, MZ Zdzienicka (The Netherlands); A Savoia, D del Principe, L Zanisco, V Poggi, B Rotoli (Italy); JJ Ortega (Spain); C Mathew, EC Gordon-Smith, J Burn (United Kingdom); M Siimes (Finland); N Clausen (Denmark); A Békássy (Sweden). *Non-EU countries:* S Temtamy (Egypt); M Alikasifoglu, C. Altay, H Kayserili (Turkey); D Schuler (Hungary); M Karwacki (Poland). Additional support: The European Cancer Centre Amsterdam, the Fanconi Anemia Research Fund Inc, Eugene, Oregon. This investigation was carried out in collaboration with Dr M Buchwald (Hospital for Sick Children, Toronto, Canada), with support from the Medical Research Council of Canada.
A full account of this study will appear elsewhere (Joenje H, Lo Ten Foe JR, Oostra AB, Van Berkel CGM, Rooimans M, Schroeder-Kurth T, Wegner R-D, Gille JJP, Buchwald M, Arwert F. Classification of Fanconi anemia patients by complementation analysis: evidence for a fifth genetic subtype. *Blood,* in press.

plementation groups (FA-A through FA-D) have been distinguished based on somatic cell hybridization studies [3], implying that at least 4 genes cooperate to support normal hematopoiesis in non-affected individuals. The gene for group C (*FAC*) (see [4], for nomenclature) is the only FA gene cloned thus far [5]. *FAC* codes for a cytoplasmically localized [6, 7] protein with unknown function.

Complementation analysis has been limited to only 7 patients sofar. The analysis critically depended on the use of a HAT-sensitive (hprt⁻), ouabain-resistant derivative of a FA lymphoblastoid cell line (HSC72OT) as a fusion donor, which permitted selective outgrowth of hybrids by HAT + ouabain selection. MMC sensitivity of the hybrid cell lines obtained upon fusion with 6 FA lymphoblast lines indicated that 3 were identical to HSC72OT (defined as group A) whereas the remaining 3 were 'non-A' [8]. Strathdee *et al* [3] recently succeeded in introducing drug resistance markers into each of these 3 non-A cell lines by transfection with pSV2neo (conferring G418 resistance) or pSV2hph (for hygromycin resistance), which allowed hybrid selection in the presence of G418 plus HAT. All possible combinations of the 3 non-A lines resulted in MMC-resistant hybrid cell lines, implying that each cell line represented a separate complementation group, designated FA-B, FA-C and FA-D (ref 3).

To extend the analysis to a larger number of patients we prepared new genetically marked derivatives (G418 resistant/HAT sensitive) of the original FA-B, FA-C and FA-D cell lines to be used as 'universal fusion donors' in the genetic classification of FA patients.

Methods

Patients and cell lines

Epstein-Barr virus-immortalized cell lines were established from blood samples obtained from patients diagnosed as having FA on the basis of clinical symptoms in combination with hypersensitivity to mitomycin C or diepoxybutane, as determined in a standard chromosomal breakage test.

Cell culture and complementation analysis

Culture medium was RPMI 1640 plus 1 mM glutamine (Gibco) supplemented with 1 mM sodium pyruvate and 10% fetal calf serum (Gibco). Complementation analysis was carried out by polyethylene-induced fusion of lymphoblasts derived from an unclassified patient with each of the four genetically marked cell lines representing the four known FA subtypes, i.e. HSC72OT (FA-A), HSC230NT-sp1 (FA-B), HSC536NT-E6 (FA-C) and HSC62NT-sp8 (FA-D). "OT" refers to ouabain-resistance and thioguanine resistance (=HAT sensitivity); "NT" refers to G418 and thioguanine resistance. Selection of hybrids was done with medium containing HAT plus ouabain (fusions with HSC72OT) or HAT plus G418 (fusions with the FA-B, -C and -D reference cell lines). Crosslinker sensitivity of cell lines and hybrids was assessed in a standard growth inhibition assay [9].

Results and discussion

Figure 1 illustrates the classification of patient 1 as belonging to group FA-C, based on the persistence of the FA phenotype (MMC sensitivity) when fused with the reference FA-C cell line.

Complete correction of the sensitive phenotype was observed when the cells were fused with the FA-A, -B and -D reference cell lines (not shown). As summarized in *Table I*, 12 out of the 13 cell lines analyzed behaved similarly in that persistence of the FA phenotype was observed in combination with only one reference cell line, while the other combinations resulted in a resistant phenotype. In this way 7 patients were classified as FA-A, 4 as FA-C and one as FA-D; none could be assigned to the B group. Independent validation of the FA-C assignments was obtained by the finding that all 4 FA-C cell lines apparently had pathogenic sequence variations in both alleles of the *FAC* gene (JR Lo Ten Foe *et al*, submitted for publication). One cell line, from patient 8, was complemented by all four reference cell lines and thus represented a fifth complementation group (E, *Table I*). Two additional experiments confirmed this conclusion. First, the results obtained on MMC cytotoxicity were confirmed with two other crosslinking agents for which FA cells are known to be hypersensitive [9], namely diepoxybutane (DEB) and cisplatinum. Second, MMC-induced chromosomal breakage was complemented in all hybrid cell lines obtained after fusion with the cells from patient 8 (results not shown). Thus, these results strongly suggest that patient 8 represents a new complementation group, FA-E.

Our data together with those on the 7 patients typed earlier [3, 8] indicate that FA-A is the most prevalent group among ethnically and clinically unselected FA patients from North-America/Canada and Europe (55%; 95% confidence interval: 32-77%). The numbers for the other groups are still too small to derive a reliable estimate of their prevalences. We are cur-

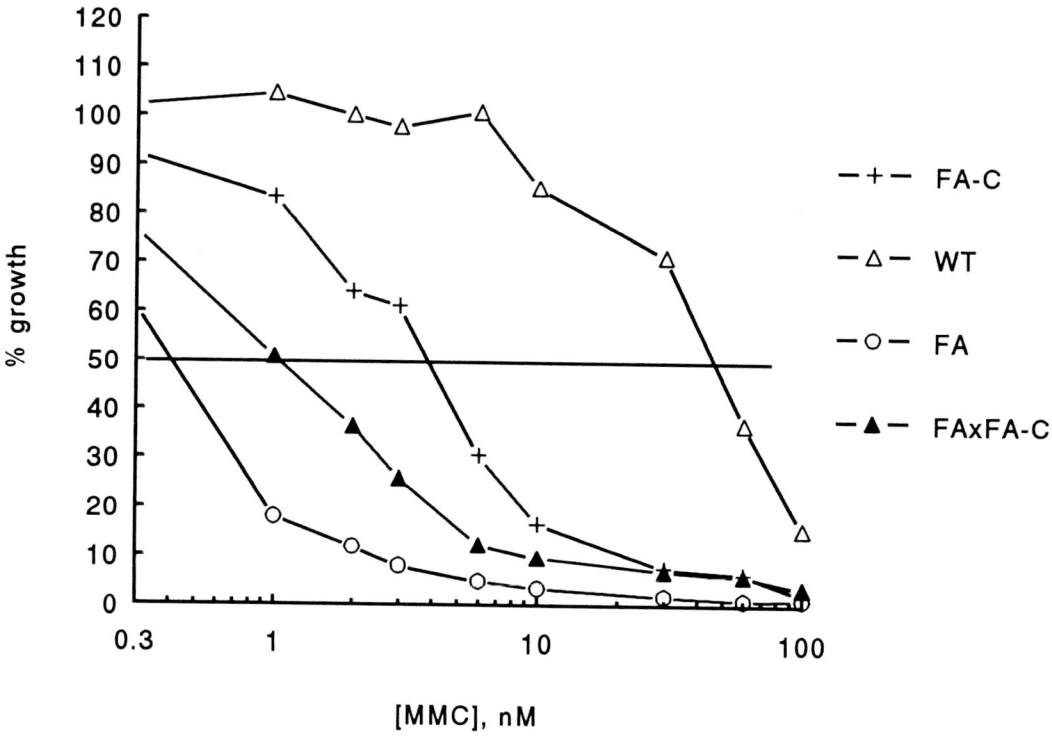

Figure 1. Example of a complementation test. The results allow assignment of a patient (FA) to complementation group C, based on the persistence of MMC sensitivity (lack of complementation) in a hybrid with the cell line representing group C (FA-C). The horizontal line indicates MMC concentrations causing 50% inhibition of growth in the various cell lines.

Table I. Complementation analysis of 13 FA patients[1].

	Fusion hybrids with reference cell line				
Patient:	A	B	C	D	**Diagnosis**
1	+	+	−	+	C
2	−	+	+	+	A
3	+	+	−	+	C
4	−	+	+	+	A
5	−	+	+	ND	A
6	−	+	+	+	A
7	−	+	+	+	A
8	+	+	+	+	E
9	−	+	+	+	A
10	+	+	−	+	C
11	+	+	−	+	C
12	−	+	+	+	A
13	+	+	+	−	D

[1] +: IC_{50} value for MMC-induced growth inhibition was greater than 20 nM (indicative of complementation); −: no complementation (IC_{50} less than 5 nM). Wildtype lymphoblasts typically have an IC_{50} value of 20-40 nM MMC. FA reference cell lines had IC_{50} values of 2-10 nM. ND, not done.

rently extending our analysis to FA patients in Europe, which would allow a more accurate estimate of the distribution of patients in the various complementation groups and potentially identify new groups. When linked to the clinical phenotype, such data might reveal distinct associations of complementation group with specific clinical symptoms and prognosis of individual patients.

References

1. Liu JM, Buchwald M, Walsh CE, Young NS. Fanconi anemia and novel strategies for therapy. *Blood* 1994; 84: 3995.
2. Joenje H, Mathew C, Gluckman E. Fanconi anemia research: current status and prospects. *Eur J Cancer* 1995; 31A(2): 268-272.
3. Strathdee CA, Duncan AMV, Buchwald M: Evidence for at least 4 Fanconi anaemia genes including FACC on chromosome 9. *Nature Genet* 1992; 1: 196.
4. Lehmann AR, Bootsma D, Clarkson SG, Cleaver JE, McAlpine PJ, Tanaka K, Thompson LH, Wood RD. Nomenclature of human DNA repair genes. *Mutation Res* 1994; 315: 41.
5. Strathdee CA, Gavish H, Shannon WR, Buchwald M. Cloning of cDNAs for Fanconi's anaemia by functional complementation. *Nature* 1992; 356: 763. Correction: 1992; 358: 434.
6. Yamashita T, Barber DL, Zhu Y, Wu N, D'Andrea AD. The Fanconi anemia polypeptide FACC is localized to the cytoplasm. *Proc Natl Acad Sci USA* 1994; 91: 6712.
7. Youssoufian H. Localization of Fanconi anemia C protein to the cytoplasm of mammalian cells. *Proc Natl Acad Sci USA* 1994; 91: 7975.
8. Duckworth-Rysiecki G, Cornish K, Clarke CA, Buchwald M. Identification of two complementation groups in Fanconi anemia. *Som Cell Mol Genet* 1985; 11: 35.
9. Ishida R, Buchwald M. Susceptibility of Fanconi's anemia lymphoblasts to DNA-crosslinking and alkylating agents. *Cancer Res* 1982; 42: 4000.

Résumé

Actuellement quatre sous-groupes génétiques ou groupes de complémentation ont été décrits (FA-A à FA-D). Nous avons utilisé des lignées lymphoblastoïdes représentant chacun des groupes de complémentation connu pour classer les patients par fusion cellulaire et analyse de complémentation. Des patients ont ainsi pu être classés. Pour le groupe C, la classification a pu être confirmée par l'étude de la mutation du gène *FAC*. Une lignée cellulaire était complémentaire des 4 lignées de référence et représente donc un cinquième groupe désigné FA-E. Ces résultats indiquent qu'au moins 5 gènes sont impliqués dans le mécanisme de l'aplasie médullaire liée à l'anémie de Fanconi.

Mechanisms of mutagenesis in Fanconi anemia. Possible relation with predisposition to AML

D. Papadopoulo, A. Laquerbe and E. Moustacchi

URA 1292 CNRS, Institut Curie, Section de Biologie, 26, rue d'Ulm, 75231 Paris Cedex 05, France, tel.: (33 1) 40 51 67 10, fax: (33 1) 46 33 30 16

Summary

Fanconi anemia (FA) is a cancer prone disorder characterized by increased chromosomal instability. In normal human lymphoblasts, base substitutions were the most frequent type among the spontaneous or the psoralen photoinduced mutations. In contrast in FA lymphoblasts, more than 60% of spontaneously arised or psoralen photoinduced mutants at the chromosomally located hypoxanthine phosphoribosyl transferase (HPRT) gene result in deletions. The patterns of psoralen photoinduced HPRT deletions in FA suggest that the action of a site-specific mechanism may take place.

With xeroderma pigmentosum and ataxia telangiectasia, Fanconi anemia (FA) belongs to a group of rare inherited human autosomal recessive diseases designated as "DNA repair disorders". Since their principal cellular feature is the hypersensitivity to specific DNA damaging agent(s), it is thought that each of these diseases reflects a defect in a more or less specific repair pathway (for review see [1]) which will confere predisposition to malignancy. Therefore the characterization of the involved genes and of their function may help our understanding of the complex cellular response to a DNA injury and may provide informations on whether the inaccurate processing of DNA lesions is implicated in the cancer proneness.
FA is characterized by progressive bone marrow failure and an increased incidence of acute myeloid leukemia (AML) [2, 3]. Cells derived from FA patients show chromosomal instability and are abnormally sensitive to the cytotoxic and clastogenic effects of DNA cross-linking agents. Although the underlying molecular defect is still unknown, there is evidence that DNA repair is affected. Indeed, using the well defined FA cell lines, belonging to the genetic complementation groups "A" and "D", we and others have previously shown that the repair of psoralen photolesions is to some extent impaired in FA cells [4-9].
Exposure of repair proficient human cells to psoralens photoadditions (PUVA) is mutagenic with the majority of the mutations being base-substitutions [10-13]. In contrast in FA cells, a very high frequency of deletions has been observed among the induced mutants (14-15), although FA cells were found to be hypomutable after PUVA when the endogenous loci, *HPRT* and Na^+/K^+ *ATPase*, were considered [16].

Southern blot hybridization analysis of $HPRT^-$ mutants revealed an increased deletion frequency in FA cells [14]. In order to obtain more information on the mutagenic pathways operating on psoralen photolesions in human cells, sequence analysis has been performed on induced $HPRT^-$ mutants derived from normal and FA lymphoblasts. Our analysis showed that the mutagenic processing of lesions in normal cells leads essentially to targeted base substitutions whereas, in FA "D" cells, the same lesions lead predominantly to intragenic deletions. However, the recovered base substitutions in FA cells were similar to those observed in normal cells according to type, sequence and strand distribution. In order to obtain information on the mechanism(s) of deletion mutagenesis operating in FA cells, the analysis of breakpoint junctions in deletion FA mutants was undertaken and indicated that the molecular mechanism underlying formation of deletions may involve a site-specific recombination process.

Material and methods

Cell lines, photosensitizing treatment and mutant isolation as well as structural analysis of genomic DNA and sequence analysis of breakpoint junctions were as previously described [11, 12, 14, 17].

Results

FA cells are highly deletion prone

As can be seen in *Figure 1,* in normal human lymphoblasts base substitutions were the most frequent type among the spontaneous (82%) or the psoralen photoinduced mutations (90%). In contrast, in FA lymphoblasts, more than 60% of spontaneously arised or psoralen photoinduced $HPRT^-$ mutants were due to deletions of the *HPRT* coding sequences [11, 12, 14]. The deletions were detected and mapped by Southern blotting techniques and/or by multiplex PCR analysis. They were of various sizes, from loss of individual exons or clusters of exons representing relatively small regions to loss of the entire gene or of a major part of the gene. Among the $HPRT^-$ clones isolated from FA "D" lymphoblasts, the intragenic deletions predominate. It is of interest to note that, in spontaneously arised FA mutants, more than half of the deletions involved exon 4. In contrast to spontaneous $HPRT^-$ mutants, among the psoralen photoinduced deletions, those involving exon 3 were the most frequent [17].

Two different – size deletions in FA cells have the same breakpoint

In order to gain information about the mechanism involved in the deletion formation, we have sequenced the breakpoint junctions in several deletion mutants derived from FA lymphoblasts (group D). To localize such breakpoint junctions, we used PCR amplification of genomic DNA in combination with several oligonucleotide primer pairs located in introns flanking the missing exon(s). The PCR amplification procedure was carried out in parallel in deletion mutants and in a wild type *HPRT* clone. The PCR product yielded a single fragment with the expected size in both clones if the amplified fragment is not included in the deletion. Failure to see a PCR product only in mutant clones indicated either that the amplified region was deleted in the

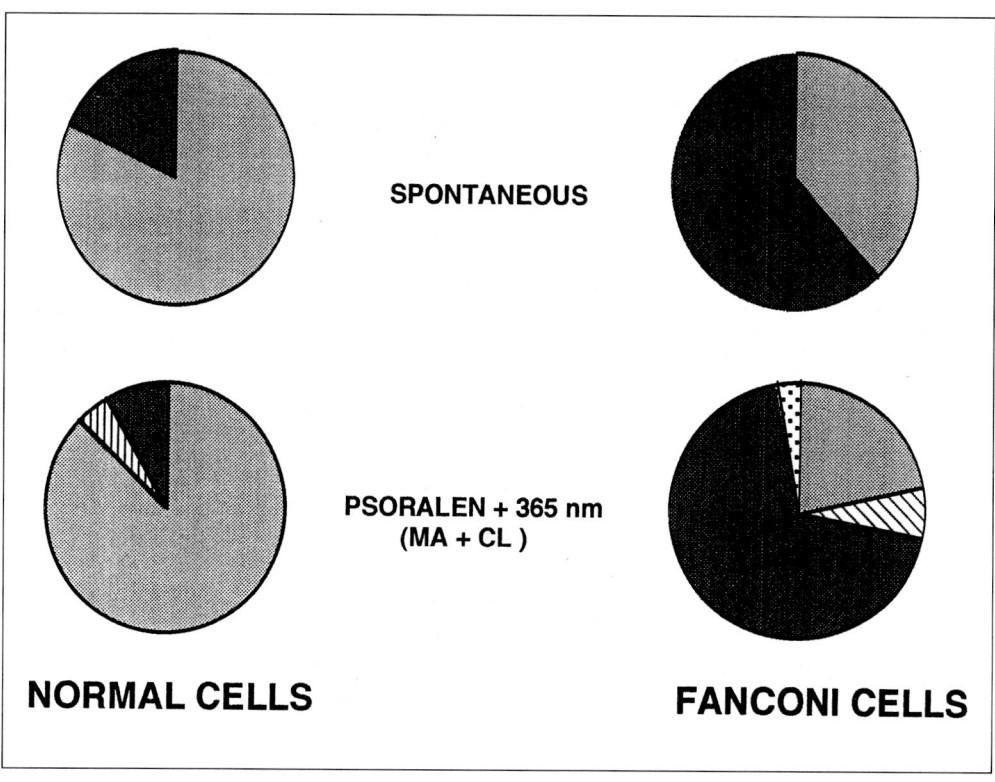

Figure 1. Relative proportions of different types of *HPRT⁻* mutants observed among spontaneous or psoralen photoinduced mutants in normal and in Fanconi anemia lymphoblasts.

▒▒▒ base substitution   ███ deletions   \\\\\ frameshift (–1)   ∷∷∷ insertions

mutant analysed or that the deletion was extended into the primer's site(s). Attempts were then made with alternative primers pairs. Primers flanking the junctions were designed to yield a PCR product for direct sequencing.

Among all FA deleted mutants (> 50 *HPRT⁻* clones), spontaneous or psoralen photoinduced, only one was due to a deletion of exons 2 and 3. The sequence analysis showed a deletion of 4988 bp. The deleted fragment is flanked in the wild-type sequence by TGGTA at the 5'-end and by TGGAT at the 3'-end of the deletion. Intriguingly the analysis of the size of PCR products from 5 mutants missing exon 3 suggested that the deletions involved were similar. The sequence analysis revealed that the deletions in all 5 mutants were identical and the deletion encompassed 586 bp of the *HPRT* sequence including 39 bp from the 3'-end of exon 3. The deletion has a 4 bp direct repeat (CATT) at the breakpoints, one copy of which being preserved in the novel junction. As can be seen in *Figure 2*, the breakpoint at the 3'-end of the deletion involved in these mutants was located only at 12 bp upstream of the breakpoint of the deletion involved in mutant missing exons 2 and 3.

The analysis of the sequences at the junctions of these two different size deletions recovered in FA lymphoblasts revealed that the same sequence motif CACTGTG was present at both 3' break-sites. This motif is identical to the highly conserved heptamer which plays an essen-

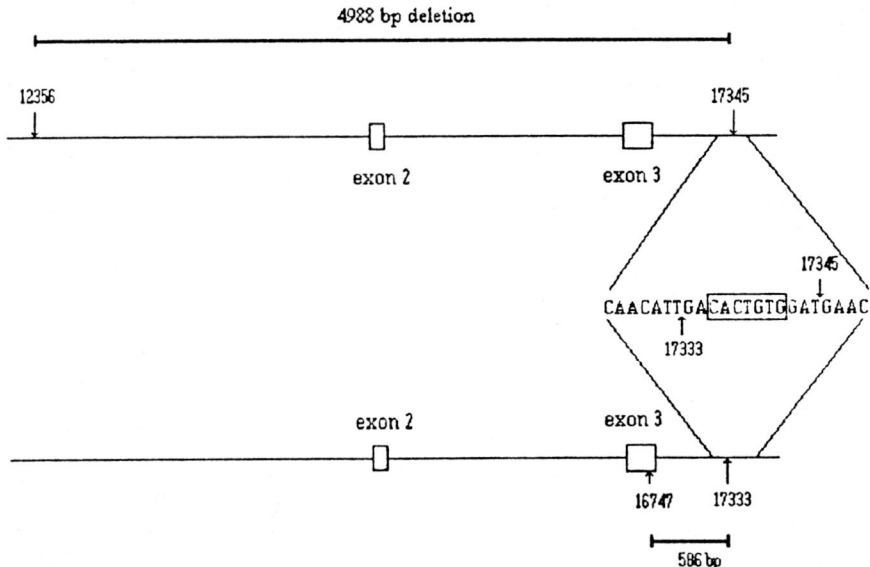

Figure 2. Schematic representation of a site of deletion in the human *HPRT* gene. In mutants FTA 37, FTA 40, FTA 41, FTB 15 and FTB 18, exon 3 was deleted and in FTA 32, exons 2 and 3 were deleted (17). At or close to the 3' breakpoint junctions represented by the arrows, there is a perfect V(D)J recombinase type heptamer (CACTGTG) in these 6 FA-derived psoralen photoinduced mutants.

tial role in recombination signals sequences in the V(D)J cleavage and joining, the site specific recombination system known to assemble seven different loci in developing B and T lymphocytes. The minimum sequence requirements for V(D)J joining has been extensively studied. It has been reported [18, 19] that a nonamer-less signal allowed recombination at detectable level but a heptamer-less signal did not. This suggests that the heptamer is the more essential element of the two. Within the heptamer, only four base pairs appear to be critical in initiating and completing the reaction, but as expected, mutations in the heptamer region adjacent to the joining site reduced the recombination drastically. With regard to these findings, the perfect heptamer found at the 3' breakpoint in *HPRT*⁻ deleted mutants involving exon 3, combined with the role that psoralen photolesions probably play and the presence of the 4-6 bp repeat at the break-sites might explain the relatively high occurence (25%) of this type of break among the induced mutants. At the *HPRT* locus, there are 11 perfect V(D)J heptamer motifs [20]. The heptamer at the 3' breakpoint in mutants missing exon 3 and 2,3 is one of them.

Discussion

Mutational response and high frequency of deletions in FA

Using the *HPRT* locus as a target gene, we have shown that, while the mutagenic processing of photolesions results essentially in base substitutions in normal cells, in FA cells among the *HPRT*⁻ mutants, intragenic deletions predominates [11, 12, 14]. The substantial increase in the frequency of deletions after induction of DNA damage in a gene coding for a non-essential enzyme suggests that such an event may also take place in essential genes in FA, leading to cell death. Several cellular divisions are required for the *in vitro* detection of *HPRT*⁻ clones and proneness to deletion may result in loss of potential mutants. The observed depressed levels of induced *HPRT*⁻ and ouabain resistant mutants in FA lymphoblasts, as opposed to normal cells [16], can be interpreted on this basis.

In vivo the *HPRT*⁻ spontaneous frequency was the same in lymphocytes from FA patients and from age matched healthy donors whereas the variant frequency at the glycophorin A (*GPA*) locus was significantly increased in erythrocytes from the FA patients [21]. The variant cell frequency for the *GPA* marker measures the amount of somatic cell genotoxicity that has occured at the *GPA* locus in bone marrow erythroïd precursor cells. The variants are not likely to be selected against *in vivo* since individuals totally lacking the *GPA* cell surface glycoprotein show no clinical symptoms. Also the life span and function of the erythrocytes are not affected by such loss [22]. In the case of MN blood type, NO variants originate from mutation, deletion or loss of the chromosome bearing the M marker, whereas NN variants result from chromosome loss plus duplication or mitotic recombination. The frequency of both classes is elevated in FA patients. It may be questioned if this increase in *GPA* variant frequencies in FA is related to a more rapid cycling of the remaining precursor stem cells or to a genuine increase in the spontaneous mutation rates. We tend to favor this last possibility since compared to healthy donors with no exception all the FA children demonstrated higher frequencies of NO and NN variants although their hematological condition ranged from severe to mild depression in red blood cell counts.

Such a hypermutability at the *GPA* locus would reflect a bias towards mutational events leading to deletions (or chromosome loss) rather than point mutations. In accord with this, it should be noted that xeroderma pigmentosum cells which are particularly prone to point mutation induction demonstrate a hypermutability at the *HPRT* locus and a normal response at the *GPA* locus [23]. Deletions appear to be fundamental in the FA pathology. It may be then asked why such deletion events, when taking place in essential genes, may be tolerated in red blood cells precursors but not in lymphoïd cells, as suggested above. The simplest explanation would be that, in the *in vivo* context, such potentially lethal events are not expressed in lymphocytes and erythrocytes precursors because of the presence of growth factors and possible metabolic cooperation. In contrast, when cells have to undergo multiple cell cycles *in vitro*, as necessary for the *HPRT*⁻ assay, these deleterious events may be expressed and lead to an apparent hypomutability for this locus.

The results reported for FA suggest that chromosomal instability, deletion proneness and high levels of *GPA* variants are closely related. Since loss of heterozygosity events in a number of genes, including proto-oncogenes and their suppressors, is an important event in multistep carcinogenesis, the ability of cells to produce high frequencies of deletions may explain the predisposition to cancer in certain genetic syndromes including FA. The intrinsic defect of hematopoïetic stem cells, the specific predisposition to myelogenous leukemia, the high frequencies of chromosomal aberrations and of chromosome loss as well as of gene deletion appear to be closely related characteristics of the FA pathology.

DNA sequence analysis and site-specific deletion breakpoint patterns at the chromosomally located HPRT locus

The comprehension of the mechanisms underlying the genomic rearrangements in human pathological states is important as chromosomal translocations, intrachromosomal duplications, large or intragenic deletions, are at the basis of important biological processes and constitute a major class of disease-related genetic events. Several mechanisms have been suggested to account for deletion formation in mammalian cells: homologous recombination between repetitive sequences [24-26], nonhomologous recombination between regions with short blocks of junctional homology [27-30]; stretches of alternating purines and pyrimidines [31]; homopurines and homopyrimidines tracts [32].

Characterization of the sequences at and near the breakpoints of deletions in FA cells provided informations on the mechanism(s) underlying the genomic rearrangements in this disorder. In the present study the analysis of the breakpoint junctions in several internal deletions produced at the *HPRT* gene in FA mutants showed that the rearrangements involving a given exon were identical even when the FA mutants derived from different psoralen phototreatments. Moreover the analysis of the sequences at the deletion junctions suggests that the rearrangements might be generated by a cleavage at the heptamer sequence that normally plays a role in immunoglobulin and TCR gene rearrangement. This reminds the observations of Fuscoe *et al* [20, 33] concerning an aberrant V(D)J recombination activity at the human *HPRT* locus in fetal T-cells as opposed to adult cells in which point mutations become predominant.

The breakpoint junctions in all FA mutants analysed so far suggest the action of a site-specific mechanism which shares features with a V(D)J recombinase-mediated events. These include essentially perfect or closely matched heptamer motifs at the, or close to, the 3'-termini of all deletions, in the case of the psoralen photoinduced mutants or of the spontaneous mutants [17]. It can be noted that in all induced mutants a short (2-4 bp) sequence homology at each breakpoint is present, one copy of which is retained in the novel junctions. Moreover, in mutants isolated after psoralen phototreatment, the prefered sites for psoralen photoadditions (ATT, ATTTT, TAT, TATA) can be observed immediately before the consensus heptamer. Consequently an obvious explanation for the precision of deletions observed in $HPRT^-$ mutants photoinduced by psoralen treatments in FA cells might be the association of: *1)* the presence of the specific sequences close to the sequences modified by psoralen photoadditions which should then serve as signals for an illegitimate V(D)J type cleavage; *2)* searching of short homology which would direct and define the subsequent end joining. Knowing that the average mutation frequency for doses used for isolation of psoralen photoinduced $HPRT^-$ mutants was 12-16 x 10^{-6} and that 66% of FA mutants are due to deletions, it can be expected that the frequency of V(D)J mediated mutations in FA lymphoblasts is between 7 x 10^{-6} and 9 x 10^{-6}.

In normal human lymphoblasts the frequency of deletions was low, less than 20% among the spontaneous and between 0% and 10% among the psoralen photoinduced mutants. Moreover, among the few deleted mutants deriving from normal cells there is no evidence for site-specific events. The sequencing of psoralen photoinduced mutants indicated that the mutagenic mechanism(s) leading to targeted base substitutions is(are) the major pathway(s) operating in normal human lymphoblasts [11, 12].

The role of V(D)J recombinase in the production of chromosomal abnormalities in B- and T-cell tumor pathogenesis is crucial. There are a number of examples where the recombinase is involved in the creation of chromosome aberrations via specific recognition of signal-like sequences. V(D)J recombinase-mediated translocations have been implicated as contributing factors in leukemogenesis [35, 36]. Most of these translocations involve an Ig or a TCR gene, normal substrate for V(D)J activity and a presumed or known oncogene on a different chromosome arm [37-39]. Whether an aberrant action of the V(D)J machinery in FA cells may be related to chromosomal instability and to the higher predisposition to leukemia caracteristic for this disorder is an appealing suggestion which remains to be consolidated.

Acknowledgements

We are grateful to J Fuscoe for discussion. This research was supported by grants from CNRS, ARC, LNFC and GREG (France).

References

1. Hanawalt PC, Sarasin A. Cancer prone hereditary diseases with DNA processing abnormalities. *Trends in Genetics* 1986; 2: 124-9.
2. Schroeder TM, Anschultz F, Knopp A. Spontane chromosomen-aberrationen bei familiarer Panmyelopathie. *Humangenetik* 1964; 1: 194-6.
3. Auerbach AD, Wolman SR. (1976) Susceptibility of Fanconi's anemia fibroblasts to chromosome damage by carcinogens. *Nature* 1976; 261: 494-6.
4. Papadopoulo D, Averbeck D, Moustacchi E. The fate of 8-methoxypsoralen photoinduced DNA interstrand cross-links in Fanconi's anemia cells of defined genetic complementation groups. *Mutation Res* 1987; 184: 271-80.
5. Averbeck D, Papadopoulo D, Moustacchi E. Repair of 4,5',8-trimethylpsoralen plus light-induced DNA damage in normal and Fanconi's anemia cell lines. *Cancer Res* 1988; 48: 2015-20.
6. Matsumoto A, Vos JMH, Hanawalt PC. Repair analysis of mitomycin C-induced DNA crosslinking in ribosomal RNA genes in lymphoblastoid cells from Fanconi's anemia patients. *Mutation Res* 1989; 217: 185-92.
7. Rousset S, Nocentini S, Revet B, Moustacchi E. Molecular analysis by electron microscopy of the removal of psoralen-photoinduced DNA cross-links in normal and Fanconi's anemia fibroblasts. *Cancer Res* 1990; 50: 2443-8.
8. Rousset S, Nocentini S, Santella R, Gasparro F, Moustacchi, E. Immunological probing of induction and repair of 8-methoxypsoralen photoadducts in DNA from Fanconi anemia and normal human fibroblasts: Quantitative analysis by electron microscopy. *J Photochem Photobiol, Part B* 1992; 18: 27-34.
9. Hang B, Yeung AT, Lambert MW. A damage-recognition protein which binds to DNA containing interstrand cross-links is absent or defective in Fanconi anemia, complementation group A, cells. *Nucleic Acids Res* 1993; 21: 4187-92.
10. Bredberg A, Nachmansson N. Psoralen adducts in a shuttle vector plasmid propagated in primate cells: high mutagenicity of DNA cross-links. *Carcinogenesis* 1987; 8: 1923-7.
11. Guillouf C, Laquerbe A, Moustacchi E, Papadopoulo D. Mutagenic processing of specific monoadducts differ in normal and Fanconi anemia cells at human *HPRT* locus. *Mutagenesis* 1993; 8: 355-61.
12. Papadopoulo D, Laquerbe A, Guillouf C, Moustacchi E. Molecular spectrum of mutations induced at the *HPRT* locus by a cross-linking agent in human cell lines with different repair capacities. *Mutation Res* 1993; 294: 167-77.
13. Yang SC, Lin JG, Chion CC, Chen LY AND Yang JL. Mutation specificity of 8-methoxypsoralen plus two doses of UVA irradiation in the HPRT gene in diploid human fibroblasts. *Carcinogenesis* 1994; 15: 201-207.
14. Papadopoulo D, Guillouf C, Mohrenweiser H, Moustacchi E. Hypomutability in Fanconi anemia cells is associated with increased deletion frequency at the *HPRT* locus. *Proc Natl Acad Sci USA* 1990; 87: 8383-7.
15. Bredberg A, Sandor Z, Brant M. Mutational response of Fanconi anaemia cells to shuttle vector site-specific psoralen cross-links. *Carcinogenesis* 1995; 16: 555-61.
16. Papadopoulo D, Porfirio B, Moustacchi E. Mutagenic response of Fanconi's anemia cells from a defined complementation group after treatment with photoactivated bifunctional psoralens. *Cancer Res* 1990; 50: 3289-94.
17. Laquerbe A, Moustacchi E, Fuscoe JC, Papadopoulo D. The molecular mechanism underlying formation of deletions in Fanconi anemia cells may involve a site specific recombination. *Proc Natl Acad Sci USA* 1995; 92: 831-5.
18. Akira S, Okazahi K, Sakano H. Two pairs of recombination signals are sufficient to cause immunoglobulin V(D)J joining. *Science* 1987; 238: 1134-8.
19. Hesse JE, Lieber K, Mizuuchi K, Gellert M. V(D)J recombination: a functional definition of the joining signals. *Genes Develop* 1989; 3: 1053-61.
20. Fuscoe JC, Zimmermann LJ, Lippert MJ, Nicklas JA, O'Neill JP, Albertini RJ. V(D)J recombinase-like activity mediates hprt gene deletion in human fetal T-lymphocytes. *Cancer Res* 1991; 51: 6001-5.
21. Sala-Trepat M, Boyse J, Richard P, Papadopoulo D, Moustacchi E. Frequencies of *HPRT*$^-$ lymphocytes and glycophorin A variants erytrocytes in Fanconi anemia patients, their parents and control donors. *Mutation Res* 1993; 289: 115-26.
22. Furthmayr H. Structural comparison of glycophorins and immunochemical analysis of genetic variants. *Nature* 1978; 271: 519-24.

23. Langlois RG, Nisbet BA, Bigbee WL, Ridinger DN, Jensen RH. An improved flow cytometry assay for somatic mutations at the glycophorin A locus in humans. *Cytometry* 1990; 11: 513-21.
24. Lehrman MA, Schneider WJ, Suedhof TF, Brown MS, Goldstein JL, Russell DW. Mutation in LDL receptor Alu-Alu recombination deletes exon encoding transmembrane and cytoplasmic domains. *Science* 1985; 227:140-6.
25. Chen SJ, Chen Z, Font MP, d'Auriol L, Larsen CJ, Berger R. Structural alterations of the BCR and ABL genes in Ph1 positive acute leukemias with rearrangements in the BCR gene first intron: further evidence implicating Alu sequences in the chromosome translocation. *Nucleic Acids Res* 1989; 17: 7631-42.
26. Stoppa-Lyonnet D, Carter PE, Meo T, Tosi M. Clusters of intragenic Alu repeats predispose the human C1 inhibitor locus to deleterious rearrangements. *Proc Natl Acad Sci USA* 1990; 87: 1551-5.
27. Canning S, Dryja TP. Short, direct repeats at the breakpoints of deletions of the retinoblastoma gene. *Proc Natl Acad Sci USA* 1989; 86: 5044-8.
28. Hentborn PS, Smithies O, Mager DL. Molecular analysis of deletions in the human (-globin gene cluster: deletion junctions and locations of breakpoints. *Genomics* 1990; 6: 226-37.
29. Love DR, England SB, Speer A, Marsden RF, Bloomfield JF, Roche AL, Cross GS, Mountford RC, Smith TJ, Davies KE. Sequences of junction fragments in the deletion-prone region of the dystrophin gene. *Genomics* 1991; 10: 57-67.
30. Morris T, Thacker J. Formation of large deletions by illegitimate recombination in the *HPRT* gene of primary human fibroblasts. *Proc Natl Acad Sci USA* 1993; 90: 1392-6.
31. Boehm T, Mengle-Gaw L, Kees UR, Spurr N, Lavenir I, Forster A, Rabbits TH. Alternating purine-pyrimidine tracts may promote chromosomal translocations seen in a variety of human lymphoid tumours. *EMBO J* 1989; 8: 2621-31.
32. Weinreb A, Collier DA, Birshtein BK, Wells RD. Left-handed Z-DNA and intramolecular triplex formation at the site of an unequal sister chromatid exchange. *J Biol Chem* 1990; 265: 1352-9.
33. Fuscoe JC, Zimmerman LJ, Harrington-Brock K, Burnette L, Moore MM, Nicklas JA, O'Neill JP, Albertini RJ.V(D)J recombinase-mediated deletion of the *hprt* gene in T-lymphocytes from adult humans. *Mutation Res* 1992; 283: 13-20.
34. Lieber MR. The mechanism of V(D)J recombination: A balance of diversity, specificity, and stability. *Cell* 1992; 70: 873-6.
35. Tsujimoto Y, Jaffe E, Cossman J, Gorham J, Nowell PC, Croce CM. Clustering of breakpoints on chromosome 11 in human B-cell neoplasms with the t(11;14) chromosome translocation. *Nature* 1985; 315: 340-3.
36. Boehm T, Rabbits TH. The human T cell receptor genes are targets for chromosomal abnormalities in T cell tumors. *FASEB J* 1989; 3: 2344-59.
37. Finger LR, Harvey RC, Moore RCA, Showe LC, Croce CM. A common mechanism of chromosomal translocation in T- and B-cell neoplasia. *Science* 1986; 234: 982-5.
38. Gu Y, Cimino G, Adler H, Nakamura T, Prasad R, Canaani O, Mois DT, Jones C, Nowell PC, Croce CM *et al.* The (4;11)q (q21;q23) chromosome translocation in acute leukemia involve the V(D)J recombinase. *Proc Natl Acad Sci USA* 1992; 89: 10464-8.
39. Brown L, Cheng JT, Chen Q, Siciliano MJ, Crist W, Buchanon G, Baer R. Site-specific recombination of the *tal-1* gene is a common occurrence in human T-cell leukemia. *EMBO J* 1990; 9: 3343-51.

Résumé

La maladie de Fanconi est une maladie prédisposant au cancer, caractérisée par une instabilité chromosomique. Dans les lymphoblastes humains normaux, des substitutions de bases sont les plus fréquentes parmi les mutations spontanées ou photoinduites par le psoralène. Dans les lymphoblastes de maladie de Fanconi, plus de 60% des mutants spontanés ou photoinduits par le psoralène provoquent des délétions chromosomiques situées au gène hypoxanthine phosphoribosyl transférase *(HPRT)*. Les aspects des délétions de *HPRT* photoinduites par le psoralène dans la maladie de Fanconi suggèrent que l'activité d'un mécanisme spécifique de site peut survenir.

4) Epidemiology

4) *Epidémiologie*

Preliminary results on epidemiology of aplastic anemia in Thailand

S. Issaragrisil, for the Thai Aplastic Anemia Study Group

Division of Hematology, Department of Medicine, Faculty of Medicine, Siriraj Hospital, Mahidol University, Bangkok 10700, Thailand, tel.: (662) 411 2012, fax: (662) 412 9783

Summary

A population based case-control study of aplastic anemia has been conducted in Thailand since 1989. The objectives are to document the incidence of the disease, and to study the etiologies in a case-control analysis. An overall incidence in Bangkok was 3.9 per million per year; which is twice as high as in Western countries. The incidence appears to be higher in Khonkaen, the northeast of Thailand and lower in Songkla, the south of Thailand. There is a difference in the age pattern between Bangkok and the two rural areas, with double incidence peaks at ages 15-24 and over 60 in Bangkok, and a more steady increase in incidence with increasing age in the rural areas.

Among the substantive results of case-control analysis, there is a strong inverse association with socioeconomic status as measured by total family income. There are also significant positive associations with occupational exposure to solvents, especially thinners and glues, and with grain farming. In Khonkaen, the latter association has been estimated to account for 30% of cases. Given this very high etiologic fraction, it is important to determine which specific exposure is increasing the risk. The association does not appear to be due to pesticide use. While some drugs are associated (e.g., sulfonamide), the overall drug attributability of aplastic anemia appears to be low in Thailand. It is noteworthy that there continues to be no evidence of association with chloramphenicol. Household pesticide use appears to be relatively safe.

There is a belief that aplastic anemia is more common in the Far East than in the West [1,2]. This belief is based on the number of patients seen annually in Asian hospitals compared with Western hospitals [3]. In Thailand the prevalence of aplastic anemia appears to be high. At Siriraj Hospital, 60-70 new cases of aplastic anemia are seen annually and more than 1,500 cases have been diagnosed. However, the high number of patients may reflect selective referral from other hospitals in Bangkok and the rural areas.

The population-based case control study of aplastic anemia has been conducted in Thailand since 1989. The objectives are to document the incidence of aplastic anemia in Thailand and to study the etiologies in a case-control analysis. The methods employed are similar to those used in the International Agranulocytosis and Aplastic Anemia Study (IAAAS)[4]. Briefly, all cases of aplastic anemia that occur in the region of Bangkok, Khonkaen in the northeast, and Songkla in the South are identified by regular contact with all hospitals with more than 100 beds. Possible cases are reviewed to confirm the diagnosis. For each case, four hospital controls of the same sex and a similar age are enrolled. Information on demographic variables, relevant medical history, and history of exposure to drugs, pesticides, other chemicals and various other factors are obtained from cases and controls by interview. Standard case-control methods are used to analyze the data. In addition, census data are used to estimate the overall incidence of aplastic anemia in the study region.

Incidence

The annual incidence of aplastic anemia in the three study region is shown in *Table I*. In Bangkok, the incidence over six years of data collection was 3.9 per million. The incidence in Songkla was lower, at 3.0 per million, and it was higher in Khonkaen, at 5.0 per million. There was a striking variation in the incidence rates in Bangkok proper and surrounding suburbs, with groupings of low, intermediate, and high incidence. In Nakornpathom and Pathumthani, the rates were 2.5 and 2.4 per million; in metropolitan Bangkok the rate was 3.6 per million; and in Nonthaburi, Samutprakan, and Samutsakorn, the rates were 5.7, 6.6, and 6.7 per million. The pattern is sufficiently consistent that is unlikely to be a chance phenomenon. Two of the high incidence suburbs are contiguous, suggesting that there may be some common environmental exposure there. Other possibilities that were considered included different patterns of migration from rural areas into the city, and common occupational exposures in the high incidence suburbs. Further exploration of these issues was not revealing, and at present the incidence pattern cannot be explained, although it still seems most likely to be due to environmental factors that vary considerably in their distribution in the Bangkok region.

Table II shows the incidence in Bangkok according to age and sex. Consistently throughout the study there has been a peak in the 15-24 year age group, and in recent analyses, another peak among those aged at least 60 years. The pattern continued among both men and women, with rates of 7.6 and 6.0 per million at age 15-24, and 9.3 and 6.3 per million at age ≥60. The overall incidence was somewhat higher in men than in women, at 4.2 and 3.7 per million.

As shown in *Table III* the pattern of incidence according to age was different in the rural areas, with a consistent increase in incidence with increasing age, rising to 15 per million in Khonkaen and 25 per million in Songkla. In Khonkaen, the incidence was marginally higher among men, whereas in Songkla, it was higher among women.

There is no explanation at present for the different age patterns in the incidence among the three study regions, but as the numbers are now reasonably stable in the rural areas, the differences are not likely to be due to chance. The pattern in the rural areas is more conventional than the double peak observed in Bangkok. There may be etiologic clues in the regional variations, although there is no explanation in the case-control comparison.

The overall incidence rate of 3.9 per million in Bangkok, 3.0 in Songkla , and 5.0 in Khonkaen are higher than those from studies conducted in Western countries. In the IAAAS, with diagnostic criteria that were identical to those used in the present study, there was an average incidence of 2.0 per million in six European regions and Israel with a range from 0.6 to 3.0 [4]. Subsequent studies in France (1984-1987) and the United Kingdom (1985) yielded annual incidence rates of 1.4 and 2.3 per million, respectively [5,6]. The incidence in Thailand was higher than any of these.

Table I. Incidence of aplastic anemia in Thailand according to region.

Region	Population	Number of Cases	Rate per Million
Bangkok (1989-1994)	8,754,000	207	3.9
Songkla (11/91-12/94)	4,994,000	48	3.0
Khonkaen (11/91-12/94)	7,644,000	119	5.0

Table II. Annual incidence of aplastic anemia in greater Bangkok, 1989-1994 according to age and sex.

Age interval	Annual rate per million (no. of cases)		
	Male	Female	Total
0-14	2.0 (16)	2.2 (16)	2.1 (32)
15-24	7.6 (38)	6.0 (30)	6.8 (68)
25-39	4.1 (32)	1.8 (14)	2.9 (46)
40-59	2.9 (12)	6.2 (26)	4.6 (38)
≥60	9.3 (12)	6.3 (10)	7.7 (22)
Total	4.2 (110)	3.7 (97)	3.9 (207)

Table III. Annual incidence of aplastic anemia in Khonkaen and Songkla, 11/91-12/94, according to age, and sex.

Age Interval	Annual rate per Million (No. of Cases)					
	Khonkaen			Songkla		
	Male	Female	Total	Male	Female	Total
0-14	0.5 (2)	0.2 (1)	0.4 (3)	1.0 (3)	0 (0)	0.5 (3)
15-24	4.8 (14)	2.1 (6)	3.5 (20)	0.6 (1)	3.1 (5)	1.8 (6)
25-39	8.4 (22)	4.7 (12)	6.6 (34)	1.8 (3)	0.6 (1)	1.2 (4)
40-59	7.2 (13)	15.5 (29)	11.4 (42)	4.5 (5)	5.3 (6)	4.9 (11)
≥ 60	19.7 (12)	11.2 (8)	15.1 (20)	20.3 (9)	30.0 (15)	25.4 (24)
Total	5.2 (63)	4.7 (56)	5.0 (119)	2.7 (21)	3.4 (27)	3.0 (48)

Case-control analysis

An analysis of the data for aplastic anemia was conducted based on 284 cases and 1174 controls. Multiple logistic regression was used to estimate the relative risks for selected factors when the confounding effects of other factors were simultaneously taken into account. Factors included in the model were age, sex, region, year of hospital admission, years of education, total household income, history of hookworm and tuberculosis, truck driving, farming, occupational exposure to various drugs and pesticides. Exposure to drugs and pesticides was defined as any use in the five-month period beginning four weeks before admission, because we judged that more recent use was likely to have taken place after the onset of aplastic anemia for many cases.

The results for various demographic factors are shown in *Table IV*. Among cases and controls who were at least 15 years of age, the relative risk estimate was modestly elevated for those whose height was less than 150 cm compared to those whose height was at least 170 cm, but there were very few subjects in the lowest height category (<140), and the data could not be considered to indicate a trend. There was no association with body mass index. There was a strong inverse association with both years of education and household income adjusted for inflation. With regard to birthplace, cases tended more often than controls to have been born outside of Bangkok.

There was no association for dengue fever, and somewhat elevated but not significant multivariate relative risk estimates for history of hookworm (2.4) and tuberculosis (2.1).

There was no evidence of association with employment in the textile metal and wood industries. Grain farming and occupational exposure to solvents were strongly associated, with relative risks of 3.0 (95% confidence interval, 1.8-5.2) for grain farming and 3.6 (2.1-6.3) for solvents. There were also a significant association for truck driving, with a relative risk of 3.3 (1.2-9.4), and an elevated relative risk estimate for occupational pesticide exposure (1.8) that approached statistical significance.

The association with grain farming was largely confined to Khonkaen. As shown in *Table V*, 46% of the cases there were grain farmers, and the multivariate relative risk estimate was 2.9 (1.6-5.3). Many of the grain farmers were not exposed to pesticides, and for this group the association was similar to the overall result (crude relative risk, 3.8), indicating that it is not explained by pesticide exposure. There was also an elevated relative risk estimate for other farming employment (2.4), but it was not statistically significant. In contrast with grain farmers, many of the latter subjects were exposed to agricultural pesticides (63% of the cases and 21% of the controls).

With regard to agricultural pesticide exposure, there was a borderline overall association, with a multivariate relative risk estimate of 2.3 (1.0-5.6). Most exposures were to organophosphates; the crude relative risk (3.1) was similar to the overall result, but the multivariate estimate was considerably lower at 1.6 (0.5-5.0).

Details of solvent exposure are given in *Table VI*. There was no evidence of association in Songkla or Khonkaen, with similar or lower prevalence of exposure in cases than in controls. In Bangkok, there were relatively few exposures to benzene, but the crude relative risk estimate was elevated, at 2.2. There were significant associations for glues (multivariate estimate, 5.5; 95% confidence interval, 1.4-21), thinners (4.0; 1.6-10), and other solvents (6.7; 2.8-16).

Exposure to specific drugs in days 29-180 before hospital admission is shown in *Table VII*. There was no association with chloramphenicol, with 1% of both cases and controls exposed. However, the upper 95% confidence limit of 3.2 did not exclude a modest association. There were significant elevations in the multivariate relative risk estimates for sulfonamides, at 4.1 (1.2-13), thiazides, at 5.7 (1.2-27), and corticosteroids, at 3.4 (1.5-8.0), and borderline elevations for tetracyclines, at 2.8 (1.0-7.9) and mebendazole, at 4.8 (0.9-24). There was no association

Table IV. Demographic factors among 284 cases of aplastic anemia and 1174 controls.

Factors	Cases		Controls		Crude relative risk	95% confidence interval
	No	(%)	No	(%)		
Height*						
≥ 170	44	(18)	189	(18)	1.0**	–
160-169	86	(34)	421	(39)	0.9	(0.6–1.3)
150-159	87	(35)	370	(34)	1.0	(0.7–1.5)
140-149	20	(8)	68	(6)	1.3	(0.7–2.3)
< 140	2	(1)	5	(0.5)	1.7	(0.3–9.0)
Unknown	10	(4)	23	(2)	–	–
Years of education						
≥ 7	64	(23)	416	(35)	1.0**	–
4-6	174	(61)	618	(53)	1.8	(1.3–2.5)
< 4	41	(14)	138	(12)	1.9	(1.3–3.0)
Unknown	5	(2)	2	(0.2)	–	–
Household income (baht/month) †						
≥ 5000	86	(30)	531	(45)	1.0**	–
1500-4999	130	(46)	494	(42)	1.6	(1.2–2.2)
< 1500	64	(23)	130	(11)	3.0	(2.1–4.4)
Unknown	4	(1)	19	(2)	–	–

* Confined to 249 cases and 1076 controls with age ≥15 years.
** Reference category.
† Income adjusted for inflation to 1989 baht. The inflation rates were:
1990, 6%; 1991, 5.7%; 1992, 4.1%; 1993, 4.6%; 1994, 5%. Test for trend, p = 0007.

Table V. Farming and exposure to occupational pesticides among cases of aplastic anemia and controls in Khonkaen.

	Cases		Controls		Crude relative risk	Multivariate relative risk (95% confidence interval)
	No	(%)	No	(%)		
Grain Farming	37	(46)	57	(19)	4.1	2.9 (1.6–5.3)
No occupational Pesticide Exposure	31	(46)	52	(19)	3.8	–
Other Farming*	9	(11)	19	(6)	3.0	2.5 (0.8–7.9)
Occupational Pesticide Exposure	13	(16)	17	(6)	3.1	2.8 (1.1–7.5)
Organophosphates	10	(12)	13	(4)	3.1	1.6 (0.4–5.8)
Carbamates	4	(5)	7	(2)	2.1	1.6 (0.2–11)
Organochlorines	3	(4)	3	(1)	3.7	1.6 (0.1–24)
Paraquat	3	(4)	2	(0.7)	5.6	–
Other	3	(4)	1	(0.3)	11	–

* Fruit (3 cases, 4 controls), Vegetable (3, 3), Cotton (1,0), Tobacco (1, 0), Truck Driver (1, 1), Laborer (0, 3), Cowpuncher (0, 2), Gardener (0, 2), Dairy (0, 1), Agricultural Scientist (0, 1), Security Guard (0, 1), Unknown (0, 1).

Table VI. Details of solvent exposure among 160 cases of aplastic anemia and 698 controls in Bangkok.

Solvent	Cases		Controls		Crude relative risk	Multivariate relative risk (95% confidence interval)
	No	(%)	No	(%)		
Benzene	2	(1)	4	(0.6)	2.2	–
Glues	6	(4)	5	(1)	5.4	5.5 (1.4-21)
Thinners	10	(6)	14	(2)	3.3	4.0 (1.6-10)
Other solvents	12	(8)	12	(2)	4.6	6.7 (2.8-16)
Any solvents	27	(17)	34	(5)	4.0	4.6 (2.5-8.7)

Table VII. Exposure to drugs in days 29-180 before admission among 284 cases of aplastic anemia and 1174 controls.

Drug	Cases		Controls		Crude relative risk	Multivariate relative risk (95% confidence interval)
	No	(%)	No	(%)		
Chlorampenicol	4	(1)	12	(1)	1.4	0.8 (0.2-3.2)
Sulfonamides	6	(2)	8	(1)	3.2	4.1 (1.2-13)
Tetracyclines	7	(3)	13	(1)	2.3	2.8 (1.0-7.9)
Thiazides	6	(2)	5	(0.4)	5.1	5.7 (1.2-27)
Corticosteroids	15	(5)	14	(1)	4.6	3.4 (1.5-8.0)
Mebendazole	5	(2)	3	(0.3)	7.0	4.8 (0.9-24)
Benzodiazepines	10	(4)	18	(2)	2.3	1.3 (0.5-3.6)
Beta Blockers	4	(1)	5	(0.4)	3.3	1.0 (0.1-7.3)
Salicylates						
< 4 days/week	23	(8)	124	(11)	0.8	0.6 (0.4–1.6)
≥ 4 days/week	37	(13)	122	(10)	1.3	1.1 (0.7–1.7)
≥ 4 days/week for ³ 4 weeks	10	(4)	26	(2)	1.6	1.3 (0.6–3.1)
Paracetamol						
< 4 days/week	51	(18)	247	(21)	0.8	0.9 (0.6–1.4)
≥ 4 days/week	72	(25)	265	(23)	1.1	1.1 (0.7–1.6)
Pyrazolones	5	(2)	29	(3)	0.7	0.5 (0.2-1.5)
NSAIDs	5	(2)	11	(1)	1.9	1.9 (0.5-6.5)

with benzodiazepines, beta blockers, salicylates, paracetamol, and pyrazolones. There were few users of nonsteroidal anti-inflammatory drugs. The upper confidence limits for the three groups of analgesics excluded increases in risk of as low 80%, indicating the relative safety of these drugs with regard to aplastic anemia. Of particular interest is the lack of association observed for salicylates taken at least four days a week, and at least four days a week for at least four weeks, because significant elevations in risk were reported for these categories in the IAAAS [4]. In terms of other comparisons with the latter study, a borderline association had been reported for sulfonamides, and a significant increase in risk for corticosteroids [4].

Results for exposure to various groups of household pesticides are given in *Table VIII*. Organophosphates and carbamates were very commonly used, with overall prevalence of exposure in controls of 30% and 47%, respectively. For organophosphates, carbamates, and pyrethrines, the relative risk estimates for exposure less than four days a week and at least four days a week were all close to or below 1.0, with upper confidence limits below 2.0, suggesting that these compounds are relatively safe in household use in Thailand. For organochlorines, which were less commonly used, the relative risk estimate for at least four days a week was 4.1, with a lower confidence limit of 1.0; there was no evidence of association for less frequent use. There was no overall evidence of association with other household pesticides.

Table VIII. Exposure to household pesticides in days 29-180 before admission among 284 cases of aplastic anemia and 1174 controls.

Pesticide	Cases No	Cases (%)	Controls No	Controls (%)	Crude relative risk	Multivariate relative risk (95% confidence interval)
Organophosphates						
< 4 days/wk	62	(22)	283	(24)	0.9	1.0 (0.6–1.6)
≥ 4 days/wk	11	(4)	68	(6)	0.6	0.7 (0.2–1.9)
Carbamates						
< 4 days/wk	68	(24)	260	(22)	1.0	1.1 (0.8–1.7)
≥ 4 days/wk	50	(18)	289	(25)	0.7	0.6 (0.4–0.9)
Organochlorines						
< 4 days/wk	9	(3)	31	(3)	1.2	1.4 (0.5–3.4)
≥ 4 days/wk	5	(2)	13	(1)	1.6	4.1 (1.0–16)
Pyrethrines						
< 4 days/wk	19	(7)	86	(7)	0.9	1.0 (0.5–1.9)
≥ 4 days/wk	4	(1)	35	(3)	0.5	0.5 (0.1–1.9)
Other	5	(2)	50	(4)	0.4	0.4 (0.2–1.2)

Hepatitis study

The analysis included 177 cases and 183 controls who had been tested for hepatitis A, B and C. The overall results for hepatitis A, B, and C are shown in *Table IX*. For hepatitis A, as determined by anti HAV IgG, the multivariate relative risk estimate was 2.9 (1.2-6.7). There was no

Table IX. Results of serological testing among 177 cases of aplastic anemia and 183 controls.

Test result	Cases No	(%)	Controls No	(%)	Crude relative risk	Multivariate relative risk (95% confidence interval)
Hepatitis A	166	(94)	148	(81)	3.6	2.9 (1.2-6.7)
Hepatitis B	111	(63)	109	(60)	1.1	1.2 (0.7–2.0)
Core only	18	(10)	17	(9)	1.1	1.0 (0.4–2.3)
Antibody	77	(44)	84	(46)	1.0	1.1 (0.6–1.9)
Antigen	16	(9)	8	(4)	2.2	2.2 (0.8–6.1)
Hepatitis C	12	(7)	10	(6)	1.3	1.2 (0.5-3.3)
Hepatitis A only	59	(33)	52	(28)	3.6	2.5 (0.9-7.2)
Hepatitis B only	4	(2)	13	(7)	1.0	0.9 (0.2-4.0)
Hepatitis A + B	107	(61)	96	(53)	3.5	3.0 (1.1-8.4)
Hepatitis A + B Antigen	16	(9)	8	(4)	6.3	5.2 (1.4-20)

evidence of association for hepatitis B, as measured by various tests, except for an elevated but not statistically significant relative risk estimate (2.2) for positive surface antigen. The overall relative risk for hepatitis B was 1.2 (0.7-2.0). There was no association with hepatitis C, with a low positivity rate. The separate and combined effects of hepatitis A and B were also evaluated; there was a significant positive association with infection by both viruses, with an estimate of 3.0 (1.1-8.4), and an elevated point estimate that approached statistical significance for hepatitis A only (2.5). For positivity to hepatitis A and hepatitis B surface antigen, the relative risk estimate was 5.2 (1.4-20). It is interesting to note that all of the subjects who were positive to B surface antigen were also positive for hepatitis A.

The analysis was repeated for subjects under the age of 25 years (data not shown). The pattern was similar to the overall data; the crude relative risk estimate for hepatitis A was 4.0 (1.6-9.7); for A only it was 3.6 (1.2-11); and for A and B combined it was 4.0 (1.3-12). Again, there was no association with hepatitis C.

There appears to be an association only with hepatitis A, and not with the other types. Since the transmission of hepatitis A is related mostly to poor sanitation, it is possible that the association reflects and underlying factor that is also related. It seems unlikely that the virus itself is related to the risk of aplastic anemia.

Etiologic fractions for selected factors

Etiologic fractions were calculated based on the overall relative risks for the two salient associations, grain farming in Khonkaen and solvent exposure in Bangkok, and for associated drugs overall in relation to aplastic anemia. Etiologic fractions were based on the 30% of the incidence of aplastic anemia in Khonkaen can be explained by grain farming, due to the high prevalence of exposure there. This etiologic fraction is higher than anything reported for aplastic anemia in the IAAAS [4]. In Bangkok, solvent exposure can account for 13% of the incidence, and in all regions combined, associated drugs for 10%. The latter figure is to be contrasted with the 25% reported in the IAAAS [4]. It demonstrates that the etiology of aplastic anemia is less well understood, although factors have been identified in the present study that contribute substantially to what is known.

Conclusion

This series of 284 cases of aplastic anemia is the largest from a single epidemiologic study. The major findings are: a complete description of the incidence in Bangkok and two rural regions of Thailand, including interesting patterns by age, with a double peak in Bangkok; a strong inverse association with socioeconomic status, present in all three areas; and association with occupational exposure to solvents in the Bangkok area, accounting for about 13% of the incidence there; a strong association with grain farming in the two rural areas that does not appear to be explained by pesticides, and which accounts for as much as 30% of the incidence in Khonkaen; a possible association with agricultural pesticide exposure in Khonkaen; and association with truck driving, which is not elucidated further; relatively low drug attributability, with associated drugs explaining only about 10% of the incidence, and an interesting lack of association with chloramphenicol; the relative safety of household pesticides, which are very commonly used in Thailand; and a positive association with hepatitis A seropositivity.

References

1. Aoki K, Ohtani M, Shimizu H. Epidemiological approach to the etiology of aplastic anemia. In: Hibino S, Takaku F, Shahidi T, eds. Aplastic anemia. Baltimore: University Park Press, 1978: 155-70.
2. Young NS, Issaragrisil S, Chieh CW, Takaku F. Aplastic anaemia in the Orient. *Br J Haematol* 1986; 62: 1-6.
3. Whang KS. Aplastic anemia in Korea: a clinical study of 309 cases. In: Hibino S, Takaku F, Shahidi T, eds. Aplastic anmia. Baltimore; University Park Press 1978: 225-42.
4. Kaufman DW, Kelly JP, Levy M, Shapiro S. The drug etiology of agranulocytosis and aplastic anemia. New York: Oxford University Press, 1991.
5. Mary JY, Baumelou E, Guiguet M and the French Cooperative Group for Epidemiological study of Aplastic Anemia. Epidemiology of aplastic anemia in France. A prospective multicentric study. *Blood* 1990; 75: 1646-53.
6. Cartwright RA, McKinney PA, Williams L, *et al*. Aplastic anemia incidence in parts of the United Kingdom in 1985. *Leuk Res* 1988; 6: 459-63.

Résumé

Une étude de population cas-contrôle des aplasies médullaires a été faite en Thaïlande depuis 1989. Les objectifs sont d'étudier l'incidence et l'étiologie de la maladie. L'incidence globale à Bangkok est de 3,9 par million par an, ce qui est deux fois plus élevé que dans les pays occidentaux. L'incidence semble plus élevée dans la région de Khonkaen, au nord-est de la Thaïlande et plus basse au Songkla, au sud de la Thaïlande. Il y a une différence d'âge entre Bangkok et les deux régions rurales, avec deux pics d'âge à Bangkok à 15-24 ans et au-dessus de 60 ans, et une augmentation progressive avec l'âge dans les populations rurales.

Parmi les résultats de l'étude cas-contrôle, il y a une association significative entre la maladie et une diminution du statut socio-économique mesuré par les revenus familiaux. Il existe également une corrélation positive avec les solvants, particulièrement les colles et vernis et les graines pour l'agriculture. A Khonkaen, cette dernière association est retrouvée dans 30% des cas. En raison de cette grande fréquence de risque retrouvé, il est important de rechercher quelle exposition augmente spécifiquement le risque. L'association ne semble pas liée à l'utilisation de pesticides. Les pesticides domestiques ne semblent pas incriminés. Certains médicaments comme le sulfonamide sont associés, mais les causes médicamenteuses en particulier le Chloramphenicol semblent rarement la cause des aplasies médullaires en Thaïlande.

Epidemiology of aplastic anemia: the French experience

J.-Y. Mary, M. Guiguet, E. Baumelou and the French cooperative group for epidemiological study of aplastic anemia

INSERM U 263, Centre de Bioinformatique, Université Paris 7 (Case 7113), 2, place Jussieu, 75251 Paris Cedex 05, France, tel.: (33 1) 44 27 78 86, fax: (33 1) 44 27 69 12

Abstract

Between May 1984 and December 93, a cooperative group, including 83 University medical centers throughout metropolitan France, prospectively recorded new cases of aplastic anemia (AA) defined as: at least 2 depressed blood cell lineages (hemoglobin $\leq$ 10g/100ml and reticulocytes $\leq$ 50 10^9/l, granulocytes $\leq$ 1.5 10^9/l, platelets $\leq$ 100 10^9/l) and a bone marrow biopsy compatible with the disease. Analysis of the three first years of the register indicates that France is a zone of moderate incidence (1.5/year/million inhabitants) with an excess of cases after 60 years, specially in females. Two of every three cases had a severe disease with a fatality rate of 34% one year after diagnosis. Suspected etiology was unknown in about 3 cases out of 4. Careful analysis of available data on AA incidence in the literature demonstrates its overestimation in three situations: absence of confirmation of the diagnosis by a biopsy, use of death certificates for case recruitment, retrospective ascertainment of cases.

In parallel to this register, a case control study was conducted between 1985 and 1988 to investigate possible etiologic factor of AA. Using a standardized questionnaire, trained investigators interviewed one case and three controls, matched for age, sex and interviewer: two hospitalized patients and one neighbor of the case. 147 cases, 287 hospitalized controls and 108 neighbors were interviewed. The part of the study dedicated to occupational exposure was limited to cases and controls aged 18 to 70 years, leading to 98 cases, 181 hospitalized controls and 72 neighbors. The occurrence of aplastic anemia was analyzed by matched design with relation to medical history, to drug use during the last five years and specifically during the last year, to 15 year occupational history, grouped into exposure categories by jobs done for one year or more. Three times more cases reported having suffered from clinical hepatitis during the last six months than either type of control. Similarly, a higher proportion of cases reported a history of chronic immune disorder, mainly rheumatoid arthritis, and a previous use of gold salts and of D-Penicillamine. An excess of Colchicine and of Allo-thiopurinol intake was observed among the cases. A moderate risk was associated with any use of Acetaminophen or salicylates, but the therapeutic intake of salicylates within the last year was associated with an elevated risk of aplastic anemia. No differences appeared between the cases and both groups of controls relative to any group of occupations investigated. A positive relationship between exposure to glues and AA was observed, as well as a trend towards an increased risk after exposure to paints. Although borderline not significant, a small excess of exposure to pesticides was observed among the cases when compared to hospitalized controls. This large spectrum case-control study confirmed the vanishing role of previously known toxics in the etiology of aplastic anemia. Moreover, differences observed with recently published studies suggest that targeted studies on each category of drugs according to the treated pathologies should be initiated. Moreover, the association with glues and paints which came out from several recent studies needs further investigation because of the large heterogeneity of compounds included in these products.

Aplastic anemia (AA) is known to be a rare but severe disease. Until recently, descriptive epidemiology of this disease was limited, based mainly on death statistics [1-3]. Although drugs have been considered as etiological factors in about one third of the cases [4-6], the implication of most drugs in the etiology of AA has been suspected in the past decades from national drug side effects surveillance data or case-history reports [5-8]. Some effects concerning the relationship between occupational exposure and the occurrence of aplastic anemia have been well documented, such as benzene [9] or radiation exposure [10], but they are now disapppearing as a result of either replacement of the toxic substance, or increase in protection and control of the exposure level. Conversely, other toxic effects due to the lack of consistency of published results are still being debated. In France, a prospective multicentric survey has been carried out from May, 1984 to derive information concerning the descriptive epidemiology of the disease in a well defined population [11]. In parallel, a case-control study has been undertaken to analyse risk factors associated with the disease, the patient's medical history [12], drug intake [12] and occupational exposure [13].

Incidence

Material and methods

This population based study was performed between May, 1984 and December, 1993 with the active cooperation of 83 medical centers covering the whole of France. Recruitment of new cases was performed in two steps. First, new cases were recorded by the responsible clinician in each center using a standardized registration form, excluding patients with neoplastic or granulomatous disease involving the bone marrow, cases following chemotherapy or radiotherapy, and patients with spleno-megaly, systemic lupus erythematosus or other conditions masquerading as AA. This form was sent to the coordinating center to allow careful verification and data validation. A follow-up form was sent by the coordinating center to the clinician 1 month after the diagnosis, and then every 6 months, in order to update patient status. Finally, information about suspected etiology of the disease was requested of the clinician, who was not aware of any information obtained during the case-control study. In a second step, patients coming from abroad for disease treatment and those with constitutional disease were excluded. Registered cases were then identified for analysis according to the following criteria: at least two depressed blood cell lineages at the time of diagnosis prior to blood product transfusion; *i.e.*, (1) hemoglobin value ≤ 10 g/100 ml with a reticulocyte count $\leq 50 \times 10^9$/l, (2) polymorphonuclear count $\leq 1.5 \times 10^9$/l, (3) platelet count $\leq 100 \times 10^9$/l, and a bone marrow biopsy specimen with decreased cellularity compatible with the disease, showing no significant fibrosis or neoplastic infiltration. Severity of the disease at diagnosis was assessed using Camitta's criteria [14]. The population under study was drawn from the French National Census of 1982 adjusted for the increase of the population during the study period. Crude and stratum specific incidence rates were calculated from these projections by age, sex, place of residence. Data were expressed according to sex, age and place of residence through the ratio of the observed number of cases to the corresponding expected number, assuming no influence of the stratum on the incidence, ratio referred to as stratum specific incidence rate (stratum SIR).

Results

During the three first years of the registry, 250 new cases had their initial diagnosis confirmed out of 284 registered cases. Among the 34 excluded patients, 13 and 20 failed criteria in relation to biopsy and to blood evaluation, respectively. Only one record had insufficient data to confirm patient's diagnosis. Annual incidence rate was 1.51 per million inhabitants (95% confidence interval: 1.32 – 1.70), stable over the three year period. The main characteristics of the descriptive epidemiology are shown in *Table I*. Among females there was a sharp incidence peak above the age of 60, with twice as many cases as expected ($P < .001$). In males, two incidence peaks were observed; in the 15 to 29 ($P < .01$) and in the above 60-year-old ($P < .05$) age groups. The peaks over 60 in males and females appeared to the stable over the three year period, whereas the peak in young adult males was restricted to the first year of the study. No excess was observed in rural areas (less then 2 000 inhabitants), but it was noted in small cities (2 000 – 20 000 inhabitants) ($P < .001$), a fact which was constant throughout the observation period.

Table I. Aplastic anemia incidence according to sex, age and place of residence.

	Standardized incidence ratio (per year)
• Sex ratio close to 1	
- males	1.03 (0.99 - 1.09 - 1.03)
• Excess of cases in:	
- females above the age of 60	1.98 (1.98 - 2.08 - 1.90)
- males above the age of 60	1.40 (0.85 - 1.55 - 1.69)
- males aged 15 to 29	1.53 (2.30 - 1.27 - 1.10)
• Excess of cases in:	
- small cities (2 000 to 20 000 inhabitants)	1.52 (1.57 - 1.50 - 1.48)
• No excess in:	
- rural areas (less than 2 000 inhabitants)	0.87 (0.71 - 0.85 - 0.93)

Fatality rate was 34% during the year following the diagnosis. About two thirds of the confirmed cases were diagnosed as severe AA. In males, there was an excess of severe cases (87%) in young patients (less than 15 years of age) ($P < .05$). In females, the same trend was observed. The time elapsed since the evidence of the first symptoms until diagnosis was significantly shorter for younger patients ($P < .02$) and for severe cases ($P < .02$). Suspected etiology of the disease was reported by the clinicians in 243 cases. About 74% of these cases of AA were declared as idiopathic, and 13 cases were associated with hepatitis. Among the 32 cases in which a drug association was suspected, 6 were attributed to gold compounds and 1 to chloramphenicol. Twelve cases were declared to be related to a possible toxic exposure.

Discussion

Table II summarizes the previously published results for incidence rates of AA [11, 15-23]. Although these rates are not strictly comparable due to the absence of age and sex standardization in most studies, a rough examination of incidence levels could be envisioned due to the

Table II. Descriptive epidemiology of aplastic anemia according to existing literature: incidence rate ($/10^6$/year)

Study period	Ref.	Region	Population studied	Type of survey	Source of cases	Standard population	Number of cases	Combined incidence	Incidence Male	Female
61-65	15	Israel	–	?	MR	no	93	7.8	7.1	8.7
70-78	16	Baltimore area	whites	Ret	MR/DC	local	94		7.0	6.1
					MR		62		4.8	3.8
70-81	17	3 counties in South Carolina	whites	Ret	MR/DC	local	20		11.7	5.4
80-84	21	7 European regions and Israel	–	Pros	MR	local	168	2.2		
		Ulm area					56	2.9		
		Israel					21	1.6		
71-78	18	Northern region of England	–	Ret	MR	no	174	6.8		
85	19	Parts of United Kingdom	–	Pros	?	no	49	2.3	1.4	3.2
66-77	20	Southern area of Buenos Aires	–	Ret	MR	no	35	6.0		
84-87	11	Metropolitan France	–	Pros	MR	world	250	1.4	1.6	1.3
89-94	22-23	Bangkok	–	Pros	MR	no	207	3.9	4.2	3.7
91-94	23	Songkla					48	3.0	2.7	3.4
		Khonkaen					119	5.0	5.2	4.7

MR = medical record; DC = death certificate; Ret = retrospective; Pros = prospective; Ref.= reference absence of large differences in age/sex structure of the populations studied, except for the Thai study [22-23]. These differences should be interpreted with caution, taking into account the number of registered cases in the different studies, which varied from 27 to up to 250. For instance, data published by Szklo et al for males [16] led to a 95% confidence interval of 3.2 to 6.5 for cases identified by medical records. This large interval stressed the importance of sample size on the accuracy of estimates.

Some of these discrepancies could be accounted for by differences in diagnosis criteria. We applied different criteria for diagnosis of aplastic anemia recently published in the literature [21, 24] to our data. Among the evaluable cases identified in our registry as AA, 98 and 94% were selected according to Camitta's and IAAAS criteria, respectively. Among our rejected patients, those who did not fullfil our criteria or whose diagnosis was changed during the follow-up, 10 and 4, among the 28, were selected using the same criteria, respectively. This indicates that rather similar results would have been obtained when using these different criteria.

In the older studies [15,25], no bone marrow cellularity was required for case definition, AA being, solely, defined as pancytopenia. In a recent study, a retrospective examination of 213 consecutive cases of pancytopenia observed in an hematology laboratory of a large hospital that includes most of the medical and surgical specialities, was conducted. Only 10% of these pancytopenias could be ascribed to AA [26]. This rough estimate applied to data, where the sole diagnostic criterium was pancytopenia, results in an incidence rate of 1.3 for Sweden and of 0.8 for Israel, figures of the same order of magnitude than our own incidence rate [11] and the incidence published by the IAAAS for Israël [21].

The high mortality rates published for AA in Japan [1] and in the United States and Canada [2] raise the problem of the proportion of those deaths attributed to AA which were actually due to AA. Wallerstein et al [3] reported that only 60 cases could be confirmed among the 290 cases with death certificates. In the study conducted in the Baltimore area [16], among 111 death certificates designated as aplastic anemia or pancytopenia, only 55% met the criteria of AA, when case notes were used. The use of death certificates clearly overestimates the incidence estimate. Finally, prospective identification of cases, with confirmation by follow-up of registered cases, is clearly more accurate than a retrospective search of cases through medical records and/or death certificates. Clearly, some methodological problems arise from using retrospective studies, which lead to much higher incidence rates than prospective ones. It has been claimed for a long time that AA was more frequent in the Orient that in western countries [27]. The only prospective study performed in Thailand following a strict methodology gave an annual incidence rate between 3 and 5 per million, a figure lower than incidence rates observed in the United States from retrospective studies. Consequently, in our opinion results obtained from retrospective studies and/or from death certificates should be ignored in favor of prospective studies.

Case-control study

Material and methods

The case source was the AA national register. The investigators, each in charge of a center, were trained and met regularly at the coordinating center to report problems that arose and to define uniform solutions. When a patient was reported to the coordinating center and, as soon as the diagnosis of AA was confirmed by bone marrow biopsy, the secretary at this center contacted the corresponding investigator to refer the case. Among 326 registered AA cases, 147 were included in our study. For the occupational part of the study restricted to 18 to 70 years of age, 98 out of 222 were included. In both parts of the study, there were no significant differences between their distributions as to any characteristic reported in the register. For each case, two different kinds of controls were required. The first two controls matching the case's sex and age (± 5 years) were identified on the admission board in the same hospital as the case after exclusion of patients with malignant disease or those treated in an intensive care unit. The third control had to be named by the case himself among his/her neighbors of the same sex and age (± 5 years). Two hundred and eighty seven hospitalized controls and 108 neighbors were interviewed. The corresponding figures were 181 and 72 for the occupational part of the case-control study.

All interviews were conducted through a standardized questionnaire covering personal and familial medical history, drug use (exposure to a known myelotoxic treatment in the five last years, drugs taken by brand name in an open-ended question with dosage, time, and duration of administration, during the five previous years for the well suspected myelotoxic drugs, and only the last year for the other drugs), occupational exposures over the last fifteen years (with data about the description of the tasks exposure, environmental conditions and protections for each occupation done for one year or more). Information concerning drug use, and the conversion from brand names to pharmacological names, were coded blindly by the same medical doctor who was unaware of the subject's status (case or control). For the drugs investigated over five years, the intakes were classified as therapeutic or not according to the total dosage. Information about occupation was examined blindly by a single toxicologist to determine if an exposure should be attributed or not to each component using a predefined checklist. The exposure was graded by the toxicologist as 'large' or not according to both intensity and frequency.

Statistical analysis was conducted according to the matching design with a variable number of controls [28]. Each group of controls – hospitalized or neighbors – was separately considered. When no difference in exposure was observed between the hospitalized control patients and the neighbors, and if the same trend was obtained in the comparisons between cases and each category of controls, a global analysis was performed by combining both types of controls. When dealing with several factors together, logistic regression was employed using a conditional regression model [28]. Comparative results were expressed by the corresponding odds ratio (OR) and its 95% confidence interval (95% CI). The etiologic fraction was calculated and, as the national register provided an estimate of the annual incidence of AA in France, an estimate of the excess of risk associated with drug use over the preceding year was calculated [29]. Assuming that the proportion exposed among the controls would be 0.1, an odds ratio greater than 3.5, 2.5 and 2.0 could be detected with a power of 90% in the case-neighbor, case-hospitalized control, case-any control comparisons, respectively. With a proportion of exposed controls expected at 0.3, odds ratios likely to be detected were 2.5, 2.3 and 1.9 in the same conditions [30].

Results

All factors significantly related to AA occurrence are described in *Table III*. A personal medical history of immunological disease, specially rheumatoid arthritis, was more frequently observed among the cases than among both types of controls. The known association between the use of gold salts and AA was evidenced both for any use during the 5 last years as well as during the last year. Very similar risks were observed for gold salt and D-Penicillamine intakes. However, the use of these two drugs was largely confounded by a medical history of rheumatoid arthritis and their relative contributions could not be separated.

Table III. Association of aplastic anemia occurrence with medical history, drug use and occupational exposures.

Risk factor	Type of factor	Period	Conditions	Controls Type	% exposed	Odds ratio Mean	95 % CI
Immunologic disease	Medical history	any	–	both	3.1	3.2	1.4 - 7.2
Rheumatoid arthritis	Medical history	any	–	both	1.0	6.8	1.8 - 25.
Gold salts	Drug use	one year	any or therapeutic	both	0.3	11.7	1.3 - 108.
D-Penicillamine	Drug use	one year	any or therapeutic	both	0.3	11.3	1.2 - 109.
Clinical hepatitis	Medical history	six months	–	both	2.5	2.8	1.2 - 7.0
Infectious episode	Medical history	six months	viral origin	neighbor	7.5	3.8	1.3 - 11.3
Sulfonamides	Drug use	one year	any	neighbor	1.9	6.0	0.7 - 50.
Non phenicol antibiotics	Drug use	one year	any	neighbor	17.8	2.9	1.4 - 6.4
Chloramphenicol	Drug use	one year	any or therapeutic	both	0.3	6.0	0.5 - 66.
Colchicine	Drug use	one year	any	both	0.5	7.5	1.5 - 39.
			therapeutic		0.3	15.0	1.8 - 128.
Allo-Thiopurinol	Drug use	one year	any	both	1.3	3.3	1.0 - 11.
			therapeutic		0.8	5.9	1.5 - 23.7
Salicylates	Drug use	one year	any	both	16.7	1.9	1.1 - 3.2
			therapeutic		4.5	5.1	2.3 - 11.0
Acetaminophen	Drug use	one year	any	both	7.9	2.0	1.0 - 3.8
			therapeutic		3.0	2.0	0.8 - 5.1
Fenamates	Drug use	one year	any	both	3.1	2.1	0.8 - 5.4
			therapeutic		2.6	2.0	0.7 - 5.8
Indolic derivatives	Drug use	one year	any	neighbor	1.9	5.0	0.6 - 43.
			therapeutic		0.0	ne	0.9 - ne
Glues	Occupational	15 years	any	both	17.0	2.7	1.5 - 5.0
			large		7.5	2.8	1.3 - 6.2
Paints	Occupational	15 years	any	both	19.4	1.8	1.0 - 3.4
			large		9.1	1.8	0.8 - 4.2
Pesticides	Occupational	15 years	any, all types	hospitalized	13.3	1.6	0.8 - 3.0
			large, insecticides		6.1	2.3	0.9 - 5.8
			large, fungicides		6.1	2.5	1.0 - 6.2
			large, weed killers		5.5	2.0	0.8 - 5.3

In the preceding six months, clinical symptoms of hepatitis, with or without any serological marker, were associated with a higher risk of AA. Other recent infectious episodes, as well as sulfonamide and other non phenicol antibiotic intakes, were significantly more frequent among hospitalized controls than among neighbors. In the case-neighbor control comparison, when events with a viral suspicion, like influenza, and events that often have a bacterial origin, like bronchitis, were analysed separately, the excess in cases relative to neighbor controls was only observed for "viral" infections. There were an elevated non significant and a significant odds ratios for the previous year use of sulfonamide and non-phenicol antibiotics, respectively. These intakes were associated with a recent history of an infectious episode and their respective roles could not be distinguished. Due to a low number of exposed subjects, the risk associated with the use of Chloramphenicol and Thiamphenicol cannot be accurately evaluated.

A significant association was found with any use of Colchicine or Allo-Thiopurinol during the last year. This association was more pronounced when analysing therapeutic use. When using the conditional regression model, for therapeutic use during the last year, the association was limited to Colchicine use with a corresponding odds ratio of 13.2 (95% CI: 1.5 – 115).

In the NSAID group of drugs, the results varied according to the pharmacological subtypes. Any use of salicylates in the last year was significantly associated with an increased risk of AA, as was any use of Acetaminophen. When only therapeutic use was considered, the association was significant only for salicylate intake. When using the conditional regression model for therapeutic use of salicylates and Acetaminophen in the last year, the association remained only for salicylates with an odds ratio of 4.3 (95% CI: 1.9 – 9.4). For indolic derivatives, when comparing cases to neighbor controls, and fenamates, the significant association observed during the last five years became non significant for any use or use at a therapeutic level during the last year.

None of the major groups of occupations tested was found to be associated with an increase of aplastic anemia. In particular, no excess risk was observed for the group "agricultural, animal husbandry, and forestry workers, fishermen and hunters" which, in our sample, included only farmers. There was a borderline non significant difference in history of occupational exposure to pesticides when comparing cases to hospitalized controls only. Cases were at least twice as likely as both groups of controls to have been exposed to glues or paints, a relationship still present after restriction to the 'large' level of exposure. When using the conditional regression model, the association with AA remained only for glues with an OR of 2.8 (95% CI, 1.3 to 5.8) and 3.2 (95%CI, 1.0 to 10.2) for any and 'large' exposure, respectively.

No excess of cases was associated with personal history of hematologic or allergic disease, recent vaccination, parental consanguinity, familial history of genetic or hematologic disease. No differences appeared between cases and both groups of controls relative to any intake of the propionic and carboxylic acids (among which is diclofenac), the oxicams, the pyrazolics (phenbutazone and oxyphenbutazone), the dipyron-dipyrin derivatives. There was no evidence of an increased risk for those exposed to any of the investigated categories of solvent.

Discussion

Cases were drawn solely from the National Register of AA. All cases identified during the study period could not be interviewed. However, a comparison of the cases included with those not included in the study, showed no differences.

In a case-control study, selection of controls is crucial. In the present study, two groups of controls were investigated. The first group was composed of patients admitted to the same hospital as the cases. A selection bias for these controls could not be excluded, even if a systematic selection was performed from the admission board to minimize the occurrence of this bias.

Among these hospitalized controls no specific disease was overrepresented, and this diversity prevented any potential bias due to hospitalisation for specific diseases which could be related to some drug intake or occupational exposure. However, a potential referral bias could not be excluded, cases and hospitalized controls reflecting a population from different areas. The second group of controls, taken from the general population, was personally named by the cases, leading to a possible geographic overmatching. Clearly, neither of these two control groups were perfect. Nevertheless, careful analysis of differences in exposure levels between the two groups of controls and in the association with AA according to control group, before eventually mixing them, emphasizes the importance of having these two groups, the ideal control group being somewhere in between according to each factor studied. For instance, when analyzing the possible role of farmer occupations, the proportion of farmers among hospitalized controls (6%) was similar to the one in the whole population (8%), which differed from that among neighbor controls (17%). Similarly, when investigating exposure to pesticides, the very small number of concordant pairs among cases and neighbors opposed to the high proportion of exposed in both groups was indicative of a likely overmatching of cases and neighbor controls, leading to a comparison of cases with hospitalized controls, only. In the IAAA study [31], the controls were hospitalized, but chosen as having pathological "conditions unrelated to drug use". As already stated by other authors [32], this selection could lead to an underexposure of the controls, as the ideal non-case controls, should be possibly exposed to the studied drugs.

The IAAAS group used an analysis of non matched data stratified on sex and age [33]. In addition to sex and age, our study matched for the investigator. By using the matching design, we eliminated the confounding effect of the demographic factors and we attempted to minimize the influence of interviewer variation as the same investigator interviewed a matched set of case and controls. This type of analysis appears to be valuable, even if it is responsible for a loss of numerous subjects (concordant sets) and, thereby, rendering more difficult the evaluation of the respective roles of different factors.

Table IV presents in a standardized way the main results obtained in the different case-control studies [12-13, 23, 33-38] which have investigated the role of either medical history, drug intake, or ocupational exposure. Recent studies show some fair agreement about an association with an history of clinical hepatitis [12, 38] or hepatitis A [23], indomethacin intake [12, 33], a borderline association with the use of Allo-Thiopurinol [12, 37], salicylates [12, 33, 38], sulfonamides [12, 23, 35], an absence of association with pyrazolones [12, 23, 33, 38]. The limited use of Chloramphenicol [12,23,35,38] renders the estimation of its association out of the scope of case-control studies. Some contradictory results have been published for carboxilic acids, specially diclofenac sodium [12-33], butazones [12, 33, 38]. The differences observed between some results of these reports could be due to differences in investigated delays for exposure time, in the extent or conditions of drug utilization according to countries and periods, and in the choice of controls with a possible linkage between the latter two. Concerning occupational exposures, no excess of farmers was observed, as already observed in a cohort study after 1960 [39] and in a case-control study [40]. Several studies agreed on the possible role of exposure to glues or paints [13, 23, 38]. The vanishing role of radiation exposure [13, 38] confirmed previous published results [41]. The role of Benzene exposure, at least in the present conditions, appears to be doubtful [42, 43], as well as solvent exposure.

Conclusion

In conclusion, a large case-control study on the etiological factors of AA was conducted in metropolitan France. According to this study and several reports, further studies are necessary

Table IV. Association of aplastic anemia with possible etiologic factors according to the literature.

Risk factors	Association* reported in the different case-control studies (percentage of exposed controls / particular conditions)			
Medical History	Linet's et al [38] any time before	IAAAS [33-37] —	French [12-13] any time before	Thai [23] 1 to 6 months before
Immunologic disease	0	0	+ (3)	0
Rheumatoid arthritis	0 (no case, no control)	0	+ (1)	0
			6 months before	
Hepatitis	+ (2/clinical)	0	+ (2.5/clinical)	+ (81/serology A)
Drug use	any time before	1 to 6 months before	1 year before	1 to 6 months before
Gold salts	0 (no case, no control)	0	+ (0.3)	0
D-Penicillamine	0	0	+ (0.3)	0
Sulfonamides	0	(+) (4)	(+) (2/any)	+ (1/any)
Non sulfonamides antibiotics	0	0	+ (18/any)	0
Chloramphenicol	0 (1 case, no control)	0 (0 case, 1 control)	(+) (0.3)	– (1 any)
Colchicine	0	0	+ (0.5/any ; 0.3/frequent)	0
Allo/Thiopurinol	(+) (19/any)	+ (1/any; 0.1/frequent)	+ (1/any; 0.8/frequent)	0
Salicylates	0	–; + (38/any; 2/frequent)	+ (17/any; 4/frequent)	– (21/any; 2/frequent)
Acetaminophen	0	(+) (17/any; 1/frequent)	+; (+) (8/any; 3/frequent)	– (44/any; 23/frequent)
Diclofenac sodium	0	+ (1/any)	– (5/any; 4/frequent)	0
Butazones	0 (1 case, 1 control)	+ (2/any; 0.2/frequent)	– (6/any; 2/frequent)	0
Pyrazolones	0	– (24/any; 1/frequent)	– (8/any; 2/frequent)	– (3 any)
Indomethacin	0	+ (1/any; 0.2/frequent)	(+) (2/any; 0/frequent)	0
Antithyroid	0	+ (0.2/any)	0	0
Furosemide	0	+ (4/any; 2/frequent)	0	0
Occupational exposure	any time before	—	1 year in the last 15 years	1 to 6 months before
Glues	0	0	+ (17/any; 8/large)	+ (1/any, Bangkok)
Paints	+ (4/any)	0	(+) (19/any; 9/large)	0
Pesticides	– (13/any)	0	(+) (13/any; 6/large)	(+) (6/any, Khonkaen)
Virus	(+) (2/any)	0	0	0
Solvents	– (21/any)	0	– (53/any; 28-34/large)	+ (5/any, Bangkok)
Benzene	+ (11/any)	0	0	– (1/any, Bangkok)
Radiation	– (16/any)	0	– (4/any; 1/large)	0

* +: significant; (+): trend; –:absence; 0: not tested.

to investigate the association of hepatitis with AA in relation to serological markers and viral DNA detection. This study also provided evidence of an association of AA with a history of immunological disease, particularly rheumatoid arthritis, whose responsibility should be analyzed apart from that of the anti-inflammatory treatments, especially gold salts and D-Penicillamine. The toxicity of the indolic derivatives is confirmed. The myelotoxicity of salicylates is highly suspect in several recent reports, especially for regular use, and requires further evaluation according to their wide use, as well as the debatable association with Allo-Thiopurinol intake. These results stress the importance of new epidemiological studies focused on the toxicity of these drugs, taken successively or contemporarily by assessing risk conditional on patients medical history and treatment indications. The association of AA with exposure to either paints or glues requires further specific investigations, taking into account the various compounds of these products.

Supported by a grant from the Ministère des Affaires Sociales et de la Solidarité Nationale, Direction Générale de la Santé and by grants 850017 and 489018 from Institut National de la Santé Et de la Recherche Medicale (INSERM).
Address reprint requests to JY Mary, Centre de Bioinformatique, INSERM U263, Université Paris 7, Case 7113, 2 place Jussieu, 75251 Paris Cedex 05, France.

References

1. Aoki K, Fujiki N, Shimizu H, Ohno Y. Geographic and ethnic differences of aplastic anemias in humans. In Najean Y (ed). Medullary aplasia. New York: Masson, 1980: 79-88.
2. Smick KM, Condit PK, Proctor RL, Sutcher V. Fatal aplastic anemia: an epidemiological study of its relationship to the drug chloramphenicol. *J Chron Dis* 1984; 17: 899-914.
3. Wallerstein RO, Condit PK, Kasper CK, Brown JW, Morrison FR. Statewide study of chloramphenicol therapy and fatal aplastic anemia. *JAMA* 1969; 208: 2045-50.
4. Bottiger LE and Bottiger B. Incidence and cause of aplastic anemia, agranulocytosis and thrombocytopenia. *Acta Med Scand* 1981; 210: 475-9.
5. Williams DM, Lynch RE, Cartwright GE. Drug induced aplastic anemia. *Semin Haemat* 1973; 10: 195-223.
6. Alter BP, Potter NU, Li FP. Classification and aetiology of the aplastic anemias. *Clin Haematol* 1978; 7: 431-65.
7. Heimpel H, Heit W. Drug induced aplastic anemia: clinical aspect. *Clinics in Haemat* 1980; 9: 641-62.
8. Vincent PC. Drug-induced aplastic anemia and agranulocytosis. Incidence and mechanisms. *Drugs* 1986; 31: 52-63.
9. Brief RS, Lynch J, Bernath T, Scala RA. Benzene in the workplace. *Am Ind Hyg Assoc* 1980; 41: 616-23.
10. Lewis EB. Leukemia, multiple myeloma and aplastic anemia in American radiologists. *Science* 1963; 142: 1492-4.
11. Mary JY, Baumelou E, Guiguet M. Epidemiology of aplastic anemia in France: a prospective multicentric study. *Blood* 1990; 75: 1646-53.
12. Baumelou E, Guiguet M, Mary JY and the French Cooperative Group for Study of Aplastic Anemia. Epidemiology of aplastic anemia in France: a case-control study. I: medical history and medication use. *Blood* 1993; 81: 1471-8.
13. Guiguet M, Baumelou E, Mary JY and the French Cooperative Group for Study of Aplastic Anemia. A case-control study of aplastic anemia. II. occupational exposures. *Int J Epidemiol* 1995 (in press).
14. Camitta BM, Thomas ED, Nathan DG, Gale RP, Kopecky KJ, Rappeport JM, Santos G, Gordon-Smith EG, Storb R. A prospective study of androgens and bone marrow transplantation for treatment of severe aplastic anemia. *Blood* 1979; 53: 504-14.
15. Modan B, Segal S, Shani M, Sheba C. Aplastic anemia in Israël: evaluation of the etiological role of chloramphenicol on a community-wide-basis. *Am J Med Sci* 1975; 270: 441-5.
16. Szklo M, Sensenbrenner L, Markowitz J, Weida S, Warm S, Linet M. Incidence of aplastic anemia in metropolitan Baltimore: a population-based study. *Blood* 1985; 66: 115-9.

17. Linet MS, McCaffrey LD, Morgan WF, Bearden JD, Szklo M, Sensenbrenner LL, Markowitz JA, Tielsch JM, Warm SG. Incidence of aplastic anemia in a three county area in South-Carolina. *Cancer Res* 1986; 46: 426-9.
18. Davies SM, Walker DJ. Aplastic anemia in the northern region 1971-1978 and follow-up of long term survivors. *Clin Lab Haemat* 1986; 8: 307-13.
19. Cartwright RA, McKinney PA, Williams L, Miller JG, Evans DIK, Bentley DP, Bhavnani M. Aplastic anemia incidence in parts of the United Kingdom in 1985. *Leukemia Research* 1988; 12: 459-63.
20. Aggio MC, Alvarez RV, Bartomioli MA, Maguitman O. Incidence and etiology of aplastic anemia in a defined population of Argentina (1966-1977). *Medicina (Buenos Aires)* 1988; 48: 231-33.
21. International Agranulocytosis and Aplastic Anemia Study. Incidence of aplastic anemia: the relevance of diagnostic criteria. *Blood* 1987; 70: 1718-21.
22. Issaragrisil S, Sritanasatavom C, Piankijagum A, Vaunasaeng S, Porapakkham Y, Leaverton PE, Kaufman DW, Anderson TE, Shapiro S, Young NS and the aplastic anemia study group. Incidence of aplastic anemia in Bangkok. *Blood* 1991; 77: 2166-8.
23. Issaragrisil S for the Thai aplastic anemia study group. Preliminary results on epidemiology of aplastic anemia in Thailand. In: Gluckman E, Coulombel L. Ontogeny of hematopoiesis. Aplastic anemia. Paris: INSERM, John Libbey Eurotext, 1995, vol. 235: 281-290.
24. Camitta BM, Rappeport JM, Parkmann R, Nathan DG. Selection of patients for bone marrow transplantation in severe aplastic anemia. *Blood* 1975; 45: 355-63.
25. Böttiger LE, Westerholm B. Aplastic anemia. I incidence and aetiology. *Acta Med Scand* 1972; 192: 315-8.
26. Imbert M, Scoazec JY, Mary JY, Jouault H, Rochant H, Sultan C. Adult patients with pancytopenia: a reappraisal of underlying pathology and diagnostic procedures in 213 cases. *Hematologic Pathol* 1990; 3: 159-67.
27. Young NS, Issaragrisil S, Chieh CW, Takaku F. Aplastic anemia in the Orient. *Br J Haematol* 1986; 62: 1-6.
28 Breslow NE, Day NE. Statistical methods in cancer research. vol I: The analysis of case-control studies. Lyon, International Agency for Research on cancer, 1980.
29 Kleinbaum DG, Kupper LL, Morgenstern H. Epidemiologic research. New York: Van Nostrand Reinhold Company, 1982.
30. Breslow NE, Day NE. Statistical methods in cancer research. Vol II: The design and analysis of cohort studies. Lyon: IARC, 1987.
31. International Agranulocytosis and Aplastic Anemia Study. The design of a study of the drug etiology of agranulocytosis and aplastic anemia. *Eur J Clin Pharmacol* 1983; 24: 833-36.
32. Kramer MS, Lane DA, Hutcinson TA. Analgesic use, blood dyscrasias, and case-control pharmacoepidemiology. A critique of the international agranulocytosis and aplastic anemia study. *J Chron Dis* 1987; 40: 1073-85.
33. The International Agranulocytosis and Aplastic anemia Study. Risks of agranulocytosis and aplastic anemia. A first report of their relation to drug use with special reference to analgesics. *JAMA* 1986; 256: 1749-57.
34. International Agranulocytosis and Aplastic Anemia Study. Risk of agranulocytosis and aplastic anaemia in relation to use of antithyroid drugs. *Br Med J* 1988; 297: 262-5.
35. International Agranulocytosis and Aplastic Anemia Study. Anti-infective drug use in relation to the risk of agranulocytosis and aplastic anemia. *Arch Intern Med* 1989; 149: 1036-40.
36. Kelly JP, Kaufman DW, Shapiro S. Risks of agranulocytosis and aplastic anemia in relation to the use of cardiovascular drugs: The international Agranulocytosis and Aplastic Anemia study. *Clin Pharmacol Ther* 1991; 49: 330-41.
37. Kaufman DW, Kelly JP, Levy M, Shapiro S. The drug etiology of agranulocytosis and aplastic anemia. New York: Oxford University Press, 1991.
38. Linet MS, Markowitz JA, Sensenbrenner LL, Warm SG, Weida S, van Natta M L, Szklo M. A case-control study of aplastic anemia. *Leukemia Research* 1989; 13: 3-11.
39 Gallagher RP, Threlfall WJ, Jeffries E, Band PR, Spinell J, Coldman AJ. Cancer and aplastic anemia in British Columbia farmers. *JNCI* 1984; 72: 1311-5.
40 Wang HH, Grufferman S. Aplastic anemia and occupational pesticide exposure: a case-control study. *J Occup Med* 1981; 23: 364-6.
41 Matanoski GM, Seltser R, Sartwell PE, Diamond EL, Elliott EA. The current moratlity rates of radiologists and other physician specialists: specific causes of death. *Am J Epidemiol* 1975; 101: 199-210.

42 Ott MG, Townsend JC, Fishbeck WA, Langner RA. Mortality among individuals occupationally exposed to benzene. *Arch Environ Health* 1978; 33: 3-10.
43 Yin SN, Li Q, Tian F, Du C, Jin C. Occupational exposure to benzene in China. *Br J Ind Med* 1987; 44: 192-5.

Résumé

Un groupe collaboratif, réunissant 83 services hospitaliers universitaires couvrant tout le territoire métropolitain, a enregistré prospectivement entre mai 1984 et décembre 1993 les cas incidents d'aplasie médullaire (AM) définis par : au moins 2 lignées sanguines atteintes (taux d'hémoglobine $\leq$ 10g/100ml et nombre de réticulocytes < 50 10^9/l, taux de polynucléaires neutrophiles $\leq$ 1,5 10^9/l, taux de plaquettes $\leq$ 100 10^9/l) et une biopsie médullaire compatible avec le diagnostic. L'analyse des 3 premières années de recueil montre que la France est une zone d'incidence modérée (1,5 cas/an/million d'habitants) avec un excès de cas chez les personnes âgées de plus de 60 ans, particulièrement chez les femmes. Deux cas sur trois étaient atteints d'aplasie sévère et le taux de survie était de 66 % un an après le diagnostic. L'étiologie suspectée était inconnue pour 74 % des cas. L'analyse des données de la littérature montre la surestimation des taux d'incidence en l'absence de biopsie pour confirmer le diagnostic, lorsque des certificats de décès sont utilisés pour identifier les cas, lorsque les cas sont recherchés rétrospectivement.

Parallèlement à ce registre, une étude cas-témoin a été menée entre 1985 et 1988 dans un but étiologique. Des enquêteurs, formés et utilisant un questionnaire standard, ont interviewé chaque cas et trois témoins appariés au cas sur l'âge, le sexe et l'enquêteur : 2 témoins hospitalisés et un témoin voisin du cas. Les questionnaires de 147 cas, 287 témoins hospitalisés et 108 voisins ont été obtenus. La partie expositions professionnelles de cette enquête a été limitée aux individus âgés de 18 à 70 ans, avec 98 cas, 181 témoins hospitalisés et 72 voisins enquêtés. L'association entre AM et les antécédents médicaux, les prises médicamenteuses dans les 5 années précédentes, et particulièrement au cours de la dernière année, et les expositions professionnelles dans les 15 années précédentes a été analysée en tenant compte de l'appariement entre cas et témoins. Un excès d'antécédents récents d'hépatite clinique a été observé chez les cas par rapport à chaque groupe de témoins. Les cas ont rapporté plus fréquemment que les témoins des antécédents de maladie immunologique, en particulier de polyarthrite rhumatoïde, ainsi que des prises de sels d'or et de D-penicillamine. Un excès de prise de colchicine et d'Allo-thiopurinol a été observé chez les cas. Un risque modéré a été associé à toute prise de salicylés ou de paracétamol, un risque plus élevé n'existant que pour les salicylés dans les cas d'utilisation à dose thérapeutique au cours de la dernière année. La répartition des différentes professions analysées était identique chez les cas et les témoins. Une association entre AM et l'exposition aux colles a été observée, ainsi qu'une tendance à la surexposition des cas aux peintures. Une tendance, bien que non significative, à la surexposition aux pesticides a été observée chez les cas par rapport aux témoins hospitaliers. Cette enquête à large spectre confirme la diminution des risques d'AM associés aux produits toxiques précédemment mis en évidence. Les différences observées entre cette étude et d'autres récemment publiées suggèrent la nécessité de mise en place d'enquêtes spécifiques sur le rôle de certains médicaments conjointement aux pathologies traitées. De plus, le rôle des expositions professionnelles aux colles et aux peintures, souligné par plusieurs enquêtes récentes, devrait être étudié de façon détaillée du fait de l'hétérogénéité des composants de ces produits.

5) Treatment of aplastic anemia

5) Traitement des aplasies médullaires

Transplant and nontransplant therapy for patients with severe aplastic anemia: an update of the Seattle experience

H.J. Deeg, K. Doney, C. Anasetti and R. Storb

Clinical Research Division, Fred Hutchinson Cancer Research Center, and the Department of Medicine, University of Washington School of Medicine, 1124 Columbia Street, M 318, Seattle, WA 98104, USA, tel.: (206) 667 5985, fax: (206) 667 6124

Summary

For nearly all patients with severe aplastic anemia up to approximately 50 years of age who do have an HLA genotypically- or phenotypically-identical related donor, marrow transplantation is the treatment of choice. With currently used conditioning and GVHD prophylactic regimens, disease-free survival in excess of 90% is achieved. In patients without a matched related donor, transplant results are generally inferior, and immunosuppressive therapy with ATG, CSP, glucocorticoids with or without the addition of hematopoietic growth factors is currently seen as the preferred treatment. However, patients failing this therapy are high risk candidates for subsequent transplants from alternative donors. With transplants from an HLA-nonidentical related donor, approximately 50% of patients are currently surviving. With transplants from a phenotypically matched or a single-locus mismatched unrelated donor, 30% of patients are surviving. Engraftment is achieved in most patients. However, the incidence of GVHD remains high and its complications, in particular infections, frequently prove fatal.

Allogeneic bone marrow transplantation for the treatment of severe aplastic anemia was pioneered in the early 1970's. The major problem in initial studies was graft rejection observed in 30%-60% of patients even with an HLA-identical sibling donor. Failure of sustained engraftment appeared to be related to allosensitization, generally secondary to transfusions given pretransplant [reviewed in 1]. Indeed, in previously untransfused patients, graft rejection was infrequent and survival was superior [2]. The majority of patients, however, continued to present for transplantation after having been transfused. The problem of graft rejection in these patients was overcome by modifying the conditioning regimens, in Seattle by including infusion of viable donor buffy coat cells after the marrow, and at other institutions by incorporating total body irradiation (TBI), total lymphoid irradiation (TLI) or a modification of TLI, thoracoabdominal irradiation (TAI) [1]. More recently, a combination of antithymocyte globulin (ATG) and cyclophosphamide (Cy) has been used successfully [3]. In addition, transfusion policies, the quality of transfusion products, and other prophylactic and therapeutic measures changed over time, leading to a decline in graft rejection [4]. Experimental data from canine models suggest that the risk of allosensitization can be further reduced by exposing the transfusion products to ultraviolet [5] or gamma irradiation [6].

Other problems included graft-versus-host disease (GVHD), both acute and chronic, and infections. The incidence of GVHD has been reduced substantially by the use of drug combinations, in particular methotrexate (MTX) plus cyclosporine (CSP) [7], a regimen originally developed in canine models [8, 9]. T-cell depletion has been used by some investigators [10]. Improved infection prophylaxis, particularly against viral infections, has reduced the morbidity and mortality rates related to these problems [11]. Late complications such as secondary malignancies are rare but severe; irradiation as part of the conditioning regimen, and GVHD and its therapy have been identified as risk factors [12-14].

Immunosuppressive therapy has been used in patients without a suitable donor or those who were not transplant candidates for other reasons. ATG was given either alone or in combination with androgens or glucocorticoids (with or without the infusion of HLA-incompatible marrow), with the addition of CSP or hematopoietic growth factors [15-17]. However, even though many patients respond to treatment, hematopoiesis generally does not return to normal. Furthermore, late complications including paroxysmal nocturnal hemoglobinuria (PNH), myelodysplastic syndromes (MDS), or acute myeloid leukemias have been reported with frequencies ranging from 15%-45% [18].

Here we present an update of treatment results obtained in Seattle.

Results with bone marrow transplantation

Syngeneic transplants

It is infrequent that patients with aplastic anemia, an infrequent disease, have a syngeneic donor. Nine such transplants have been carried out in Seattle. These transplants have generally been uncomplicated. However, as observed by others, some of these patients do not achieve sustained engraftment with marrow infusion only; despite the absence of a histocompatibility barrier, these require conditioning, either with cyclophosphamide, or in some instances with TBI before achieving sustained engraftment [19]. Three Seattle patients have died, one after three transplants and disease recurrence, one with multiorgan failure 7 years posttransplant, and one died with acute leukemia 10 years posttransplant at the age of 75 years. Six patients are surviving 3–21 (median 7) years posttransplant.

Allogeneic transplants

HLA-identical transplants. The problem of graft rejection is largely avoided by transplanting untransfused patients [2]. In patients who have received transfusions, sensitization is overcome by adding to the conditioning regimen of Cy, 50 mg/kg for four doses, the infusion of viable donor buffy coat cells after the marrow infusion [20]. With this approach, the probability of rejection has declined to 10% or less. However, there was a higher incidence of chronic GVHD even though the incidence of acute GVHD was not increased [21].

In the 1980's, based on encouraging results in canine models [8, 9], we investigated the efficacy of combination regimens for GVHD prophylaxis. A combination of MTX given on days 1, 3, 6, and 11 plus CSP given on days −1 to 180 reduced the incidence of acute GVHD (grades II-

IV) to 18% compared to 60% among patients given intermittent MTX only on days 1 to 102 [7]. Concurrently, survival improved to approximately 70%. In these patients, the prevalence of chronic GVHD still was 40%-50% at 1-2 years posttransplant. However, most patients could eventually be taken off therapy and only 10% had evidence of chronic GVHD by 10 years posttransplant [22].

Encouraged by the success of a regimen which combined Cy, 50 mg/kg for 4 days, and ATG, 30 mg/kg for three doses, in patients conditioned for second transplants after rejecting their initial grafts, the same regimen was then given to patients with aplastic anemia for initial conditioning. Results have recently been reported [3]. Thirty-nine patients were transplanted, 38 with marrow from an HLA-identical sibling and one from a phenotypically-matched father. Patients were 2-52 (median 24.5) years of age, 87% had been transfused, and 41% had received immunosuppressive therapy. All were given MTX and CSP as GVHD prophylaxis. Two patients (5%) rejected their grafts but were successfully retransplanted. Acute GVHD grades II or III occurred in 15% of patients and chronic GVHD in 34%. Survival was 92% at 3 years. It appears, therefore, that this is currently the regimen of choice for patients up to approximately 50 years of age with an HLA-matched related donor.

Transplants from related donors other than HLA genotypically-identical siblings. Ten patients have been transplanted from phenotypically-matched related donors after conditioning with Cy at 50 mg/kg for four doses. All patients had sustained engraftment and except for one patient who died in an accident all are surviving more than 3 years. Various GVHD prophylactic regimens were used; the incidence of acute GVHD grades II-IV was 35% [23 and unpublished].

Fifteen patients were conditioned with Cy at 50 mg/kg for four doses and transplanted from a related donor mismatched for at least one HLA antigen in either the HVG or GVH direction, or one or two antigens in both directions. Nine of 14 evaluable patients failed to achieve sustained engraftment. None are currently surviving. Causes of death were graft failure, infection, and GVHD [23].

A group of 16 patients was then conditioned with Cy, 60 mg/kg for two doses, and TBI, 6 x 200 cGy. Only two patients failed to achieve sustained engraftment and eight are currently surviving 2 years or longer after transplantation. All evaluable patients in this group developed grades II-IV acute GVHD. Causes of death generally were infections [23 and unpublished].

Transplants from unrelated volunteer donors. Thirty-four patients have been transplanted since 1985. Similar to patients given transplants from HLA-nonidentical related donors, all had previously received two or more courses of immunosuppressive therapy [26]. Patients were 4-47 (median 20.5) years of age. The donor was phenotypically HLA-identical (including molecular typing for DRB_1) in 26 cases, and mismatched for one class I or class II antigen in eight patients. Conditioning regimens consisted of Cy 60 mg/kg x 2 plus TBI 6 x 200 cGy without ATG (n=17), or with 6 doses of ATG (n=4); Cy 50 mg/kg for 4 doses plus ATG 30 mg/kg for 3 doses (n=5); Cy 50 mg/kg x 4 plus ATG x 3 plus TBI 3 x 200 or 2 x 200 cGy (n=6); Cy 60 mg/kg x 2 plus TBI 11 x 120 cGy and selectively T-cell depleted marrow (n=1); or Cy 60 mg/kg x 2 plus TBI 3 x 200 cGy (n=1). Some of these data have been presented previously [1, 24, 25]. Three patients died early (hemorrhage, infection). Of 31 evaluable patients, 25 had sustained engraftment. Of these, 18 developed acute GVHD grades II-IV. Among 23 who were at risk, 13 developed chronic GVHD. Currently, 10 patients are surviving 3 to 88 months posttransplant.

Thus, overall results are significantly inferior to those obtained with transplants from HLA-identical siblings. In particular, a Cy plus ATG regimen, very successful with related transplants [3], proved disappointing [25]. A protocol combining Cy plus ATG plus low-dose fractionated TBI is currently still active as a multi-institutional study. Additional studies are required to further reduce conditioning-related toxicities and the incidence of GVHD.

Results with immunosuppressive therapy

These results will be described in detail elsewhere (K. Doney et al. unpublished). Briefly, 288 patients who did not have a suitable donor were treated. Immunosuppressive therapy consisted of ATG alone (n=223) or ATG plus HLA-mismatched marrow (n=50), ATG plus recombinant GM-CSF (n=13) or other regimens (n=2) [15-17]. Overall, 15% showed complete, 16% partial, and 10% minimal responses; 42% of patients are surviving. Currently active protocols involve the use of ATG, CSP, and hematopoietic growth factors.

Acknowledgments

This work was supported in part by grants HL36444, CA15704, and CA18221 awarded by the National Institutes of Health, DHHS; by the Josef Steiner Krebsstiftung; and by the National Marrow Donor Program/Baxter Health Care Division. We thank Deborah Monroe and Katherine Newton for data tracking and Bonnie Larson and her colleagues for typing the manuscript.

References

1. Storb R. Bone marrow transplantation for aplastic anemia. In: Forman SJ, Blume KG, Thomas ED, eds. *Bone Marrow Transplantation.* Boston, MA: Blackwell Scientific Publications, 1994: 583-594.
2. Storb R, Thomas ED, Buckner CD, Clift RA, Deeg HJ, Fefer A, Goodell BW, Sale GE, Sanders JE, Singer J, Stewart P, Weiden PL. Marrow transplantation in thirty "untransfused" patients with severe aplastic anemia. *Ann Intern Med* 1980; 92: 30-36.
3. Storb R, Etzioni R, Anasetti C, Appelbaum FR, Buckner CD, Bensinger W, Bryant E, Clift R, Deeg HJ, Doney K, Hansen H, Martin P, Pepe M, Sale G, Sanders J, Singer J, Sullivan KM, Thomas ED, Witherspoon RP. Cyclophosphamide combined with antithymocyte globulin in preparation for allogeneic marrow transplants in patients with aplastic anemia. *Blood* 1994, 84: 941-949.
4. Deeg HJ, Self S, Storb R, Doney K, Appelbaum FR, Witherspoon RP, Sullivan KM, Sheehan K, Sanders J, Mickelson E, Thomas ED. Decreased incidence of marrow graft rejection in patients with severe aplastic anemia: Changing impact of risk factors. *Blood* 1986; 68: 1363-1368.
5. Deeg HJ, Aprile J, Graham TC, Appelbaum FR, Storb R. Ultraviolet irradiation of blood prevents transfusion-induced sensitization and marrow graft rejection in dogs. Concise Report. *Blood* 1986; 67: 537-539.
6. Bean MA, Storb R, Graham T, Raff R, Sale GE, Schuening F, Appelbaum FR. Prevention of transfusion-induced sensitization to minor histocompatibility antigens on DLA-identical canine marrow grafts by gamma irradiation of marrow donor blood. *Transplantation* 1991; 52: 956-960.
7. Storb R, Deeg HJ, Farewell V, Doney K, Appelbaum F, Beatty P, Bensinger W, Buckner CD, Clift R, Hansen J, Hill R, Longton G, Lum L, Martin P, McGuffin R, Sanders J, Singer J, Stewart P, Sullivan K, Witherspoon R, Thomas ED. Marrow transplantation for severe aplastic anemia: Methotrexate alone compared with a combination of methotrexate and cyclosporine for prevention of acute graft-versus-host disease. *Blood* 1986; 68: 119-125.
8. Deeg HJ, Storb R, Weiden PL, Raff RF, Sale GE, Atkinson K, Graham TC, Thomas ED. Cyclosporin A and methotrexate in canine marrow transplantation: Engraftment, graft-versus-host disease, and induction of tolerance. *Transplantation* 1982; 34: 30-35.

9. Deeg HJ, Storb R, Appelbaum FR, Kennedy MS, Graham TC, Thomas ED. Combined immunosuppression with cyclosporine and methotrexate in dogs given bone marrow grafts from DLA-haploidentical littermates. *Transplantation* 1984; 37: 62-65.
10. Camitta B, Ash R, Menitove J, Murray K, Lawton C, Hunter J, Casper J. Bone marrow transplantation for children with severe aplastic anemia: Use of donors other than HLA-identical siblings. *Blood* 1989; 74: 1852-1857.
11. Bowden RA. Infections in patients with graft-vs.-host disease. In: Burakoff SJ, Deeg HJ, Ferrara J, Atkinson K, eds. *Graft-Vs.-Host Disease: Immunology, Pathophysiology, and Treatment.* New York: Marcel Dekker, Inc., 1990: 525-538.
12. Socié G, Henry-Amar M, Cosset JM, Devergie A, Girinsky T, Gluckman E. Increased incidence of solid malignant tumors after bone marrow transplantation for severe aplastic anemia. *Blood* 1991; 78: 277-279.
13. Witherspoon RP, Storb R, Pepe M, Longton G, Sullivan KM. Cumulative incidence of secondary solid malignant tumors in aplastic anemia patients given marrow grafts after conditioning with chemotherapy alone (Letter). *Blood* 1992; 79: 289-292.
14. Deeg HJ, Socié G, Schoch G, Henry-Amar M, Witherspoon RP, Gluckman E, Storb R. New malignancies in patients with aplastic anemia treated by marrow transplantation: analysis of the Seattle and Paris results (Abstract). *Blood* 1994; 84(Suppl 1): 249a.
15. Doney K, Pepe M, Storb R, Bryant E, Anasetti C, Appelbaum FR, Buckner CD, Sanders J, Singer J, Sullivan K, Weiden P, Hansen JA. Immunosuppressive therapy of aplastic anemia. Results of a prospective, randomized trial of antithymocyte globulin (ATG), methylprednisolone and oxymetholone to ATG, very high-dose methylprednisolone and oxymetholone. *Blood* 1992; 79: 2566-2571.
16. Doney K, Dahlberg SJ, Monroe D, Storb R, Buckner CD, Thomas ED. Therapy of severe aplastic anemia with anti-human thymocyte globulin and androgens: The effect of HLA-haploidentical marrow infusion. *Blood* 1984; 63: 342-348.
17. Doney K, Storb R, Appelbaum FR, Buckner CD, Sanders J, Singer J, Hansen JA. Recombinant granulocyte-macrophage colony stimulating factor followed by immunosuppressive therapy for aplastic anaemia. *Br J Haematol* 1993; 85: 182-184.
18. Tichelli A, Gratwohl A, Wursch A, Nissen C, Speck B. Late haematological complications in severe aplastic anaemia. *Br J Haematol* 1988; 69: 413-418.
19. Appelbaum FR, Fefer A, Cheever MA, Sanders JE, Singer JW, Adamson JW, Mickelson EM, Hansen JA, Greenberg PD, Thomas ED. Treatment of aplastic anemia by bone marrow transplantation in identical twins. *Blood* 1980; 55: 1033-1039.
20. Storb R, Doney KC, Thomas ED, Appelbaum F, Buckner CD, Clift RA, Deeg HJ, Goodell BW, Hackman R, Hansen JA, Sanders J, Sullivan K, Weiden PL, Witherspoon RP. Marrow transplantation with or without donor buffy coat cells for 65 transfused aplastic anemia patients. *Blood* 1982; 59: 236-246.
21. Storb R, Prentice RL, Sullivan KM, Shulman HM, Deeg HJ, Doney KC, Buckner CD, Clift RA, Witherspoon RP, Appelbaum FR, Sanders JE, Stewart PS, Thomas ED. Predictive factors in chronic graft-versus-host disease in patients with aplastic anemia treated by marrow transplantation from HLA-identical siblings. *Ann Intern Med* 1983; 98: 461-466.
22. Storb R, Leisenring W, Deeg HJ, Anasetti C, Appelbaum F, Bensinger W, Buckner CD, Clift R, Doney K, Hansen J, Martin P, Sanders J, Stewart P, Sullivan K, Thomas ED, Witherspoon R. Long-term follow-up of a randomized trial of graft-versus-host disease prevention by methotrexate/cyclosporine versus methotrexate alone in patients given marrow grafts for severe aplastic anemia (Letter). *Blood* 1994; 83: 2749-2756.
23. Beatty PG, Di Bartolomeo P, Storb R, Clift RA, Buckner CD, Sullivan KM, Doney K, Appelbaum FR, Anasetti C, Witherspoon R, Sanders J, Stewart P, Martin PJ, Ciancarelli M, Hansen JA, Thomas ED. Treatment of aplastic anemia with marrow grafts from related donors other than HLA genotypically-matched siblings. *Clin Transplant* 1987; 1: 117-124.
24. Anasetti C, Hansen JA. Bone marrow transplantation from HLA-partially matched related donors and unrelated volunteer donors. In: Forman SJ, Blume KG, Thomas ED, eds. *Bone Marrow Transplantation.* Boston, MA: Blackwell Scientific Publications, 1994: 665-680.
25. Deeg HJ, Anasetti C, Storb R, Doney K, Hansen JA, Petersdorf E, Sanders J, Sullivan KM, Appelbaum FR. Cyclophosphamide plus ATG conditioning is insufficient for sustained hematopoie-

tic reconstitution in patients with severe aplastic anemia transplanted with marrow from HLA-A, B, DRB matched unrelate donors (Letter). *Blood* 1994; 83: 3417-3418.
26. Kernan NA, Bartsch G, Ash RC, Beatty PG, Champlin R, Filipovich A, Gajewski J, Hansen JA, Henslee-Downey J, McCullough J, McGlave P, Perkins HA, Phillips GL, Sanders J, Stroncek D, Thomas ED, Blume KG. Analysis of 462 transplantations from unrelated donors facilitated by The National Marrow Donor Program. *N Engl J Med* 1993; 328: 593-602.

Résumé

Pour tous les malades de moins de 50 ans atteints d'aplasie médullaire grave, la greffe de moelle à partir d'un donneur familial phéno ou géno HLA-identique est le traitement de choix. Avec les conditionnements et les traitements préventifs actuels de la GVH, la survie actuarielle est de plus de 90%. Chez les malades n'ayant pas de donneur identique, les résultats de la transplantation sont moins bons, et le traitement immunosuppresseur par ATG, CsA, corticoïdes, avec ou sans facteurs de croissance hématopoïétiques, est utilisé en première intention. Néammoins, les malades qui ne répondent pas à ce traitement doivent être traités par greffe de moelle provenant d'autres donneurs. Les greffes à partir de donneurs familiaux non HLA identiques pour un antigène donnent une survie de l'ordre de 50%. Si le donneur est non apparenté HLA identique ou avec un antigène différent, la survie est de 30%. La prise est observée chez presque tous les malades, mais l'incidence de la GVH est élevée et ses complications, en particulier infectieuses, sont responsables d'une mortalité élevée.

Bone marrow transplantation for severe aplastic anemia. A report from the International Bone Marrow Transplant Registry

Mary M. Horowitz, Jakob R. Passweg, Kathleen A. Sobocinski, Melodee Nugent and John P. Klein, for the Advisory Committee

International Bone Marrow Transplant Registry, Health Policy Institute, Medical College of Wisconsin, Milwaukee, USA, tel.: (414) 456 8325, fax: (414) 266 8471

Summary

Bone marrow transplantation is an effective treatment for severe aplastic anemia (SAA). SAA accounts for 10-15% of allogeneic transplants worldwide. Three-year survival after an HLA-identical sibling transplant for SAA is about 70% with results influenced by prior transfusions and time to transplant. Survival after transplants from unrelated donors is lower, around 35%.

Since 1972, the International Bone Marrow Transplant Registry (IBMTR) has collected data from over 300 institutions performing allogeneic bone marrow transplants worldwide. The IBMTR database includes information for about 40% of all allogeneic transplants done between 1968 and 1994, with data for over 20,000 transplant recipients. Between 10 and 15% of these transplants were for severe aplastic anemia (SAA) *(Figure 1)*.

Bone marrow transplantation is now the treatment of choice for young patients with aplastic anemia who have an HLA-identical sibling. Characteristics of 525 recipients of HLA-identical sibling transplants for SAA between 1988 and 1994, reported to the IBMTR, are shown in Table I. Median age was 20 years. Over one-half received their transplant within two months of diagnosis. Twenty-one percent received a transplant within one month of diagnosis.

Approaches to bone marrow transplantation for aplastic anemia changed substantially over the past 20 years, with improved methods for preventing graft-versus-host disease (GVHD) and infection. About two-thirds of current transplants use combined methotrexate and cyclosporine for GVHD prophylaxis *(Table I)*. The incidence of grade II-IV acute GVHD decreased from about 40% in 1976-87 to about 20% in 1988-94.

The one-year probability (95% confidence interval) of graft failure for the 525 patients described in Table I was $13 \pm 3\%$. The 100-day probability of grade II-IV acute GVHD was $19 \pm 4\%$ and the three-year probability of chronic GVHD, $30 \pm 5\%$. The three-year probability of survival was $68 \pm 4\%$. Survival rates differ significantly for patients receiving few versus many pre-transplant transfusions *(Figure 2)* and for those transplanted early versus late after diagnosis *(Figure 3)*. Addition of radiation or antithymocyte globulin to cyclophosphamide may decrease graft failure but does not significantly increase survival *(Figure 4)*.

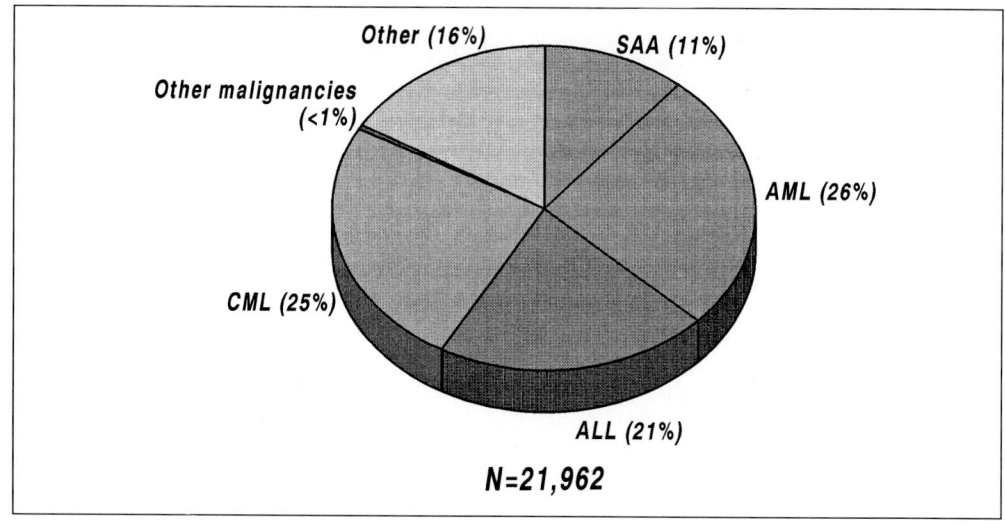

Figure 1. Diseases for which transplants are done as reported to the IBMTR between 1968 and 1994.

Table I. Characteristics of 525 patients receiving HLA-identical sibling transplants for SAA between 1988 and 1994 and reported to the IBMTR.

Age, median (range) yrs	20 (1-51)
Number of pretransplant transfusions, median (range)	25 (0-833)
Prior treatment, N (%)	
Any	276 (53%)
ATG	76 (15%)
Androgens	116 (22%)
Corticosteroids	186 (35%)
Time to transplant, median (range) mos	2 (<1-232)
Conditioning regimen, N (%)	
Cy alone	268 (51%)
Cy + TBI	24 (5%)
Cy + LFR	162 (31%)
Cy + ATG	50 (9%)
Other	21 (4%)
GVHD prophylaxis, N (%)	
MTX ± other	7 (1%)
CSA ± other	143 (27%)
MTX + CSA	353 (68%)
T-depletion	15 (3%)
Other	7 (1%)
Prophylactic acyclovir, N (%)	384 (73%)
Intravenous immune globulin, N (%)	243 (46%)
Prophylactic ganciclovir, N (%)	33 (6%)

ATG = antithymocyte globulin; Cy = cyclophosphamide; TBI = total body irradiation; LFR = limited field radiation; GVHD = graft-versus-host disease; MTX = methotrexate; CSA = cyclosporine

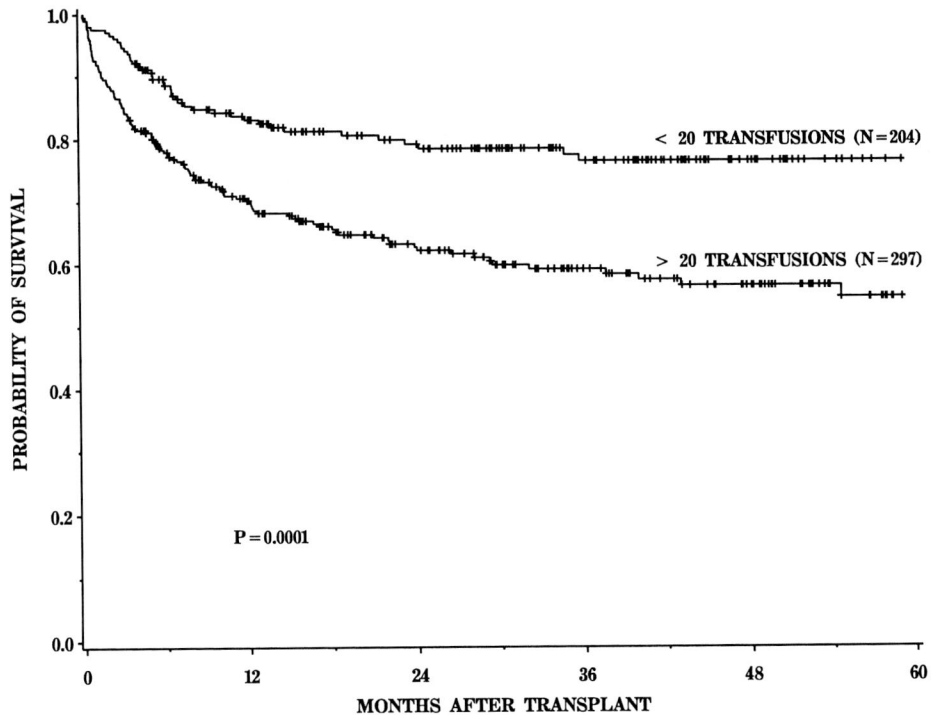

Figure 2. Actuarial probability of survival after HLA-identical sibling transplants for SAA according to number of pretransplant transfusions.

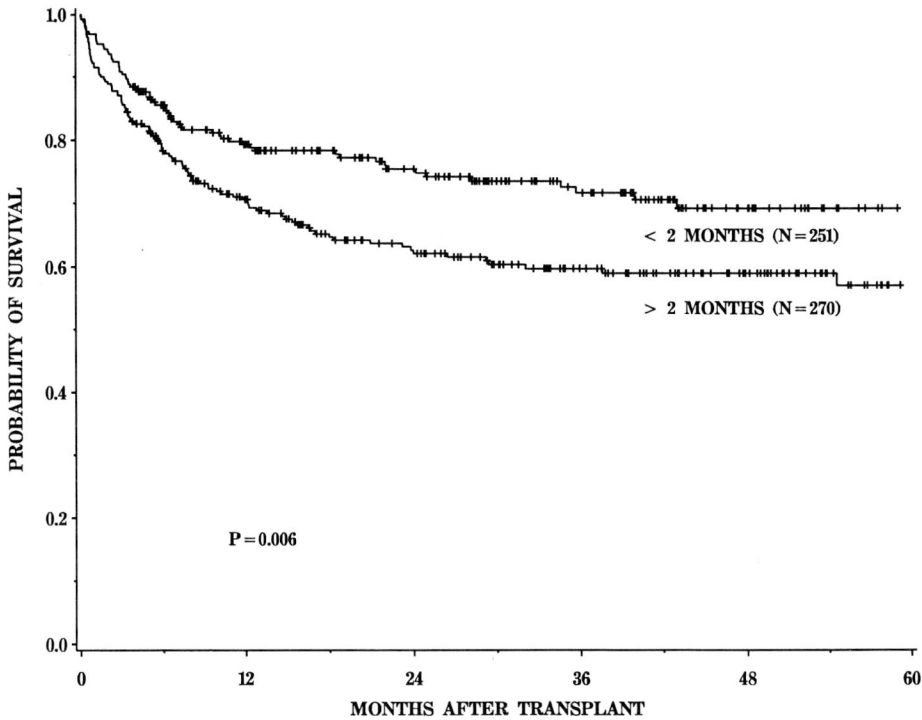

Figure 3. Actuarial probability of survival after HLA-identical sibling transplants for SAA according to interval between diagnosis and transplant.

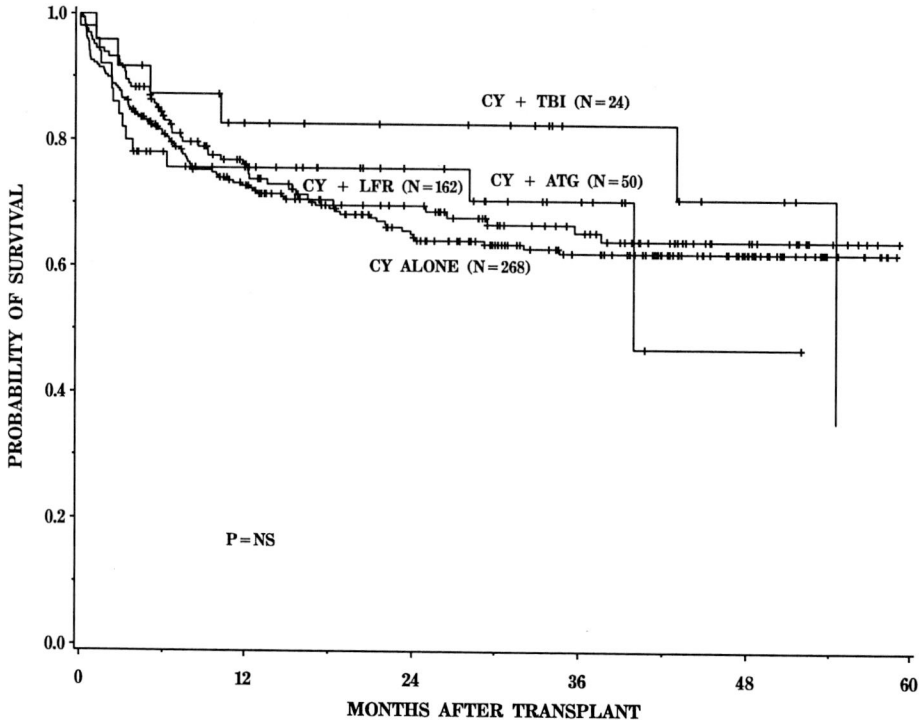

Figure 4. Actuarial probability of survival after HLA-identical sibling transplants for SAA according to conditioning regimen. LFR=limited field radiation; TBI=total body irradiation; ATG=antithymocyte globulin; CY=cyclophosphamide.

Analyses of HLA-identical sibling transplants reported to the IBMTR for transplants done between 1976 and 1992 indicate an improvement in three-year survival from about 50% in 1976-80 to about 70% in 1988 to 1992. Improved outcome does not appear to result from significant changes in patient characteristics but may result primarily from improved GVHD prophylaxis with cyclosporine.

Since only 20-30% of patients with SAA have an HLA-identical sibling, there is growing interest in use of alternative donors. Among 64 recipients of unrelated donor transplants reported to the IBMTR, the three-year probability of survival is 36 ± 14%. Lower survival results primarily from more GVHD- and infection-related deaths. Hopefully, these results will improve with more efficient donor identification, earlier transplants and improved approaches to preventing GVHD in this setting.

Supported by Public Health Service Grant PO1-CA-40053 from the National Cancer Institute, the National Institute of Allergy and Infectious Diseases, and the National Heart, Lung and Blood Institute, and Contract No CP-21161 from the National Cancer Institute of the US Department of Health and Human Services; and grants from Activated Cell Therapy, Inc; Alpha Therapeutic Corporation; Amgen, Inc; Armour Pharmaceutical Company; Applied Immune Science; Astra Pharmaceutical; Baxter Healthcare Corporation; Biogen; Lynde and Harry Bradley Foundation; Bristol-Myers Squibb Company; Frank G Brotz Family Foundation; Burroughs-Wellcome Company; Center for Advanced Studies in Leukemia; Charles E Culpeper

Foundation; Eleanor Naylor Dana Charitable Trust; Deborah J Dearholt Memorial Fund; Eppley Foundation for Research; Hewlett-Packard Company; Immunex Corporation; Kettering Family Foundation; Robert J Kleberg, Jr and Helen C Kleberg Foundation; Herbert H. Kohl Charities; Eli Lilly Company Foundation; Nada and Herbert P Mahler Charities; Marion Merrell Dow Inc; Milstein Family Foundation; Milwaukee Foundation/Elsa Schoeneich Research Fund; Samuel Roberts Noble Foundation; Ortho Biotech Corporation; John Oster Family Foundation; Elsa U Pardee Foundation; Jane and Lloyd Pettit Foundation; Pharmacia; RGK Foundation; Roche Laboratories; Roerig Division of Pfizer Pharmaceuticals; Sandoz Pharmaceuticals; Schering-Plough International; Walter Schroeder Foundation; Stackner Family Foundation; Starr Foundation; Joan and Jack Stein Charities; StemCell Technologies, Inc; Therakos; Upjohn Company; and Wyeth-Ayerst Laboratories.

Résumé

La greffe de moelle est un traitement efficace de l'aplasie médullaire et représente 10% à 15% des greffes de moelle osseuse allogéniques faites dans le monde. La survie à 3 ans après greffe avec un donneur familial HLA identique est de 70%, les résultats sont influencés par l'existence de transfusions antérieures et l'intervalle entre le diagnostic et la greffe. La survie après greffe de moelle à partir d'un donneur non apparenté est de 35%.

Allogeneic bone marrow transplantation in Fanconi anemia

Eliane Gluckman

Service d'Hématologie-Greffe de Moelle, Hôpital Saint-Louis, 1, avenue Claude-Vellefaux, 75475 Paris Cedex 10, France, tel.: (33 1) 42 49 96 44, fax: (33 1) 42 49 96 34

Fanconi's anemia (FA) was originally described as an autosomal recessive disorder, characterized by progressive pancytopenia, diverse congenital abnormalities, and increased predisposition to malignancy [1]. FA cells show a high level of chromosomal breakage, both spontaneously or when induced by cross-linking agents such as mitomycin C, nitrogen mustard, diepoxybutane or photoactivated psoralens [2, 3]. Four genetic complementation groups (A-D) have been described [4]. The cDNA for the group C has been cloned and located on chromosome 9 [5]. The function of the FA group C gene is, however, still unknown [6-8].

FA is an heterogeneous disorder with both genetic and phenotypic variability. Bone marrow failure is the most frequent hematological abnormality occurring typically around 5 years of age, but aplasia can appear later. Clonal abnormalities including a high frequency of monosomy 7 and duplications involving 11q can be observed on marrow cytogenetic analysis as a sign of transformation to myelodysplastic syndrome or acute myeloblastic leukemia [9, 10]. Without curative treatment, spontaneous survival is poor, death occurring during the second decade of life from aplastic anemia, leukemia or cancer.

Bone marrow failure seems to occur early in life, and bone marrow studies including clonogenic assays and long-term marrow cultures show a decrease of hematopoietic stem cell pool without gross microenvironmental defect [11]. It is not known if normal hematopoietic stem cells can persist for a while. Although the molecular expression of the *c-kit* proto-oncogene and *kit* ligand in long term marrow culture is normal [12], there is evidence of a subtle microenvironment defect consisting of dysregulation of cytokines such as interleukin-6(IL-6), tumor necrosis factor (TNF) and GM-CSF, which may contribute to marrow failure [13].

Treatment with androgens, steroids or hematopoietic growth factors can give a transient improvement but cannot cure the patients [14].

HLA identical sibling transplants results

Bone marrow transplantation is the only treatment which restores definitively normal hematopoiesis. Cyclophosphamide (Cy), which is used for the conditioning of patients with idiopathic aplastic anemia at the total dose of 200mg/kg, has been proven to be too toxic for the FA patients, leading to a high rate of transplant-related mortality [15]. This was shown in-vitro as well as in-vivo. Radiosensitivity studies, both *in vitro* and *in vivo*, have shown a delay in skin radio-induced lesions, an increased intensity of skin damage, and an absence of repair after fractionated irradiation [16]. For this reason, the conditioning regimen for bone marrow transplantation was modified by our team in 1980; it includes Cyclophosphamide 20mg/kg given IV over 4 days and a 5 Gy thoraco-abdominal irradiation, followed by Cyclosporin A alone for prevention of GVH [17]. In the study performed by our center, including 45 patients who had received a HLA identical sibling bone marrow or a cord blood transplant, the 5 years actuarial disease-free survival was 75,6%. The causes of death observed in 15 patients were: bone marrow failure (2 pts), infection (1pt), hemolytic and uremic syndrome (1pt), interstitial pneumonitis (1pt), chronic GVH and infection (5 pts), secondary tumor (3 pts) and post hepatitis B cirrhosis (1 pt) [18]. Study of chimerism showed that all engrafted patients were of donor type with no residual host cells. This confirms that the decrease of the dose of immunosuppression was sufficient to induce long-term tolerance and absence of autologous reconstitution [19].

Reports from the international bone marrow transplant registry and from individual centers have confirmed that regimens including low dose Cyclophosphamide(CY) gave a better survival than regimens using > 100mg/kg CY [20-22].

Some centers, however, report that doses of Cy in the order of 100mg to 140mg/kg with or without ATG and without irradiation gave a long term survival of about 50 to 80% [23, 24]. They were small series of patients and the overall toxicity was reported as high, but these results raise the possibility that the sensitivity to alkylating agents might vary according to the type of the genetic defect which is reflected *in vivo* by the heterogeneity of the phenotypic expression and *in vivo* by the variability of the number of chromosomal breaks. Some genetic defects might be more severe than others.

The observation of secondary tumors after transplant is of major concern. The probability of developing malignant tumors is very high in this population because of the addition of several risk factors including the method of conditioning with or without irradiation, environmental exposure and chromosome instability that is characteristic of the disease.

All secondary tumors (ST) were observed in males at an interval of 6 to 11 years after transplant. They were all head and neck squamous carcinoma [24, 25]. A joint analysis between the Seattle group and the Paris group has shown that the relative risk of ST was 42% and that irradiation was not the only risk factor as the Seattle group never used irradiation in the conditioning regimen. In a multivariate analysis, the factors associated with high risk to develop secondary tumors were acute GVH (RR:77) and increasing age (RR:1.3). The fact that only solid tumors and no lympho myeloproliferative malignancies were observed post-transplant is consistent with the fact that transplantation provided patients with a normal hematopoietic system, but did not affect the congenital defect in other tissues.

The good results of allogeneic bone marrow transplantation with an HLA identical sibling raises several questions about the optimal date of BMT and the best conditioning regimen.

Concerning the date of transplant, there is a general agreement to use BMT with an HLA identical sibling, as first line therapy, without trying androgens or steroids which have secondary effects. When blood counts show the criteria of severe aplastic anemia(Hb<8g/100ml, PMN<500/mm3 or platelets<20000/mm3), transfusions are necessary and therefore, this limit seems suitable for indication of BMT. During this waiting period, it is very important to perform regular bone marrow aspiration and cytogenetic analysis for detection of clonal abnormalities or signs of leukemic transformation. Results show that transplant performed late after a long period of aplasia or during leukemic transformation gives poor results.

The problem of the best conditioning regimen is more difficult to solve for several reasons. First, because the number of patients is too small for a prospective randomised multicenter study. Second, there is not, for the moment, any *in vitro* test for predicting the sensitivity of a given patient to the conditioning regimen. There is no information about the sensitivity of cell subsets to alkylating agents. The sensitivity of leukemic cells seems to be increased, as some remissions have been obtained after low dose chemotherapy or after conditioning with low dose Cy without any attempt to induce remission, but these cases are rare and most of the patients treated for acute leukemia do not tolerate standard dose chemotherapy and have a very poor prognosis. It is possible that the genetic diagnosis, which will be performed in the future, will delineate criteria for disease severity. For this reason, it is highly important to report all the new cases in the Registries. In Europe, the EUFAR group has begun to register all the cases of familial aplastic anemias including Fanconi's anemia [26].

Third; because it will be very difficult to prove any further improvement, when most survival curves show more than 75% long-term survival. Furthermore, the absence of irradiation in the conditioning regimen did not seem to diminish the risk of secondary tumors, which are also related to the genetic defect and to the environment, as shown by the observation of different phenotypic expression of the disease in homozygous twins (unpublished observations).

Alternative donor transplants

During recent years, the development of large Registries including more than 2 million donors throughout the world has lead to the possibility to find donors in patients without HLA identical siblings. In Fanconi anemia, the results of mismatched family transplants or transplants performed with HLA identical unrelated donors have been disappointing. In our series of 18 patients, only 2 are surviving. The causes of death have been: multivisceral failure (6 pts), acute GVH (5 pts), rejection (2 pts) and interstitial pneumonitis (2 pts). Of 41 patients with alternative donors reported to the IBMTR, actuarial 2 year survival was 29%; the probability of rejection was 24%; the probability of grade II-IV GVHD: 51%; of chronic GVHD: 46% and of IP 25%. The number of patients was to small to analyse risk factors [28].

Several modifications of the transplant procedure can be used experimentally for overcoming the risks of toxicity, GVH and rejection. To overcome GVH, T cell depletion can be used either by positive selection of $CD34^+$ cells on columns or magnetic beads, or by depletion with elutriation or lyse with monoclonal antibodies. This approach is likely to increase the frequency of rejection. As increasing the conditioning regimen will certainly increase the risk of toxicity, it is possible to use agents not yet tested such as Myleran or Thiothepa in the conditioning, or to increase the number of stem cells infused by adding to the $CD34^+$ cells from the marrow donor G-CSF mobilised peripheral blood $CD34^+$ cells. The add-back of lymphocytes after transplant might also improve the engraftment in patients without GVH.

New strategies for therapy

Recently,after the first successful HLA identical cord blood transplant in a patient with Fanconi anemia [29], unrelated cord blood matched or partially mismatched transplants have shown very interesting results with good engraftment and limited incidence of GVH. This alternative might be particularly valuable for Fanconi anemia patients in whom any modification of the conditioning might lead to severe toxicity or to late complications due to severe GVH.

Autologous transplants have been discussed but seem of very limited value in Fanconi anemia where the few CD34$^+$ cells isolated from G-CSF mobilised HSC from the blood do not grow in long-term culture and are unlikely to give a short or a long-term engraftment.

Gene therapy is currently under investigation but several questions remain unsolved: integration of the gene in primitive hematopoietic stem cells, level of integration necessary for the correction of the disease, long term expression of the transfected gene, selective growth advantage of transfected cells, and function of the FA group C gene protein.

On the other hand, prenatal diagnosis and early recognition of the disease as well as detection of the heterozygous state is very likely to diminish the incidence of the disease.

References

1. Auerbach AD, Rogatko A, Schroeder-Kurth TM. International Fanconi anemia registry: Relation of clinical symptoms to diepoxybutane sensitivity. *Blood* 1989; 73: 391-396.
2. Auerbach AD, Wolman SR. Susceptibility of Fanconi anaemia fibroblasts to chromosome damage by carcinogens. *Nature* 1976; 261: 494-496.
3. Berger R, Bernheim A, Gluckman E. *In vitro* effect of Cyclophosphamide metabolites on chromosomes of Fanconi's anaemia patients. *Br J of Haematol* 1980; 45: 565-568.
4. Strathdee CA, Duncan AMV, Buchwald M. Evidence for at least four Fanconi anaemia genes including FACC on chromosome nine. *Nature Genet* 1992; 1: 196-198.
5. Strathdee CA, Gavish H, Shannon WR, Buchwald M. Cloning of cDNAs for Fanconi's anaemia by functional complementation. Nature. 1992; 356: 763-767.
6. Yamashita T Barber DL, Zhu Y, Wu N, D'andrea AD. The Fanconi anemia polypeptide FACC is localised to the cytoplasm. *Proc Natl acad Sci USA* 1994; 91: 6712-6716.
7. Walsh CE, Nienhuis AW, Samulski RJ, Brown MG, Miller JM, Young NS, Liu JM. Phenotypic correction of Fanconi anemia in human hematopoietic cells with a recombinant adeno-associated virus vector. *J Clin Invest* 1994. 94: 1440-1448.
8. Segal GM, Magenis RE, Brown M, Keeble W, Smith TD, Heinrich MC, Bagby GC. Repression of Fanconi anemia gene(FACC) expression inhibits growth of hematopoietic progenitor cells. *J of Clin Invest* 1994. 94; 846-852.
9. Butturini A, Gale RP, Verlander PC, Adler-Brecher B, Gillio AP, Auerbach AD. Hematological abnormalities in Fanconi anemia: an international Fanconi anemia registry study. *Blood* 1994; 84: 1650-1655.
10. Auerbach AD, Allen RG. Leukemia and preleukemia in Fanconi anemia patients. *Cancer Genet cytogenet* 1991; 51: 1-12.
11. Stark R, Thierry D, Richard P, Gluckman E. Long-term bone marrow culture in Fanconi's anaemia. *Br J of Haematol* 1993; 83: 554-559
12. Stark R, Andre C, Thierry D, Cherel M, Galibert F, Gluckman E. The expression of cytokine and cytokine receptor genes in long-term bone marrow culture in congenital and acquired bone marrow hypoplasias. *British J of Haematol* 1993; 83: 560-566.
13. Rosselli F, Sanceau J, Gluckman E, Wietzerbin J, Moustacchi E. Abnormal lymphokine production a novel feature of the genetic disease Fanconi anemia: II *in vitro* and *in vivo* spontaneous overproduction of tumor necrosis factor alfa. *Blood* 83: 1216-1225.
14. Guinan EC, Lopez KD, Huhn RD, Felser JM, Nathan DG. Evaluation of granulocyte-macrophage colony-stimulating factor for treatment of cytopenia in children with Fanconi anemia. *J Pediatr* 1994; 124: 144-150.
15. Gluckman E, Devergie A, Schaison G et al. Bone marrow transplantation in Fanconi anemia. *Br J of Haematol* 1980; 45: 557-564.
16. Dutreix J, Gluckman E. Skin test of radiosensitivity. Application to Fanconi anemia. *J Europ Radiotherap* 1983; 4:3-8.

17. Gluckman E, Devergie A, Dutreix J. Radiosensitivity in Fanconi anemia: application to the conditioning for bone marrow transplantation. *Br J of Haematol* 1983; 54: 431-440.
18. Gluckman E. Bone marrow transplantation for Fanconi anemia. *Baillière's Clin Haematol* 1989; 2: 153-162.
19. Socie G, Gluckman E, Raynal B *et al.* Bone marrow transplantation for Fanconi anemia using low dose cyclophosphamide/thoraco abdominal irradiation as conditioning regimen: chimerism study by the polymerase chain reaction. *Blood* 1993; 82: 2249-2256.
20. Gluckman E, Auerbach AD, Horowitz M. Bone marrow transplants for Fanconi anemia. International bone marrow transplant registry. *Exp Hematol* 1990; 20:831 abstract.
21. Hows JM, Chapple M, Marsch JCW, Durrant S, Vin JL, Swirsky D. Bone marrow transplantation for Fanconi anaemia: the Hammersmith experience 1977-1989. *Bone Marrow Transplant* 1989; 4: 629-634.
22. Kohli-Kumar M, Morris C, Delaat C, Sambrano J, Masterson M, Mueller R, Shahidi NT, Yanik G, Desantes K, Friedman DJ, Auerbach AD, Harris RE. Bone marrow transplantation in Fanconi anemia using matched sibling donors. *Blood* 1994; 84: 2050-2054.
23. Flowers MED, Doney KC, Storb R, *et al.* Marrow transplantation for Fanconi anemia with or without leukemic transformation: an update of the Seattle experience. *Bone Marrow Transpl* 1992; 9: 167-173.
24. Zanis-Neto J, Ribeiro RC, Meideros C, Andrade RJ, Ogasawara V, Hush M, Magdalena N, Friedrich ML, Bitencourt MA, Bonfim C, Pasquini R. Bone marrow transplantation for patients with Fanconi anemia: a study of 24 cases from a single institution. *Bone Marrow transpl* 1995; 15: 293-298.
25. Socie G, Henry-Amar M, Cosset JM, Devergie A, Girinsky T, Gluckman E. Increased incidence of solid malignant tumors after bone marrow transplantation for severe aplastic anemia. *Blood* 1991; 78-277-279.
26. Deeg HJ, Socie G, Schoch G, Henry-Amar M, Flowers M, Witherspoon RP, Devergie A, Sullivan KM, Gluckman E, Storb R. Malignancies after marrow transplantation for aplastic anemia and Fanconi anemia: a joint Seattle and Paris analysis of results in 700 patients Submitted in Blood. 1995.
27. Gluckman E, Joenje HJ. Fanconi anemia research: current status and prospects. *Europ J cancer* 1995; 31A: 268-272.
28. Gluckman E *et al.* Bone marrow transplantation in Fanconi anemia from the International bone marrow transplant registry. Submitted. 1995.
29. Gluckman E, Broxmeyer HE, Auerbach AD *et al.* Hematopoietic reconstitution in a patient with Fanconi anemia by means of umbilical cord blood from HLA identical sibling. *New Engl J Med* 1989; 321: 1174-1178.
30. Liu JM, Buchwald M, Walsh CE, Young NS. Fanconi anemia and novel strategies for therapy. *Blood* 1994; 84: 3995-4007.

Résumé

La maladie de Fanconi est une maladie héréditaire caractérisée par de multiples malformations et une aplasie médullaire. La maladie se caractérise par une instabilité chromosomique, les cassures sont augmentées par les agents alkylants. Au moins 4 groupes de complémentation ont été décrits et le cDNA du gène du groupe C a été cloné. Bien que l'aplasie soit le plus souvent sensible à une androgénothérapie, ce traitement devient progressivement inefficace et la maladie évolue de façon fatale par aggravation de l'aplasie médullaire ou par transformation en leucémie aiguë. Il a été démontré que le pool de cellules souches hématopoïétiques est anormal dès la naissance et que la diminution du nombre de colonies en culture n'est pas toujours corrélée avec la numération formule sanguine. Le mécanisme de l'aplasie médullaire n'est pas connu, mais il est le plus souvent attribué à un défaut de la cellule souche hématopoïétique plus qu'à une atteinte du microenvironnement. Il a été démontré que ces patients avaient une sensibilité augmentée aux agents alkylants utilisés pour le conditionnement à la greffe. Pour cette raison, les doses de Cyclophosphamide (CY) ont été diminuées de 10 fois. Nous avons traité 45 patients avec un conditionnement comportant CY 20mg/kg et 5 GY d'irradiation thoraco-abdominale. La survie actuarielle à 5 ans est de 75,6%. Les résultats n'ont pas été aussi favorables lorsqu'un donneur non apparenté HLA identique a été utilisé, 2 patients seulement sur 14 ont survécu. Les échecs sont liés à l'augmentation de fréquence et de gravité de la réaction du greffon contre l'hôte (GVH) (55,6%). Les greffes de sang de cordon apparentés ou non apparentés donnent des résultats encourageants en raison de la diminution de la fréquence de la GVH. La comparaison avec les résultats des autres équipes montre que le conditionnement par des petites doses de CY comparé aux fortes doses donne de meilleurs résultats dans les greffes à partir de donneurs de la fratrie HLA identiques. La surveillance à long terme montre une augmentation de fréquence des tumeurs malignes de siège ORL. Le rôle de la maladie, de l'irradiation et de l'immunosuppression est discuté.

Unrelated or mismatched bone marrow transplants for aplastic anemia: experience at four major centers

Bruce Camitta[1], H. Joachim Deeg[2], Hugo Castro-Malaspina[3] and Norma K.C. Ramsay[4]

[1] The Midwest Children's Cancer Center of the Medical College of Wisconsin and Children's Hospital of Wisconsin, Milwaukee, WI, tel.: (414) 266 4170, fax: (414) 266 4623; [2] the Fred Hutchinson Cancer Center, Seattle, WA; [3] the Memorial Sloan-Kettering Cancer Center, New York, NY; [4] the University of Minnesota, Minneapolis, MN, USA

Bone marrow transplantation from a histocompatible sibling donor is the treatment of choice for children and young adults with severe aplastic anemia. However, because of decreasing family size as well as medical and social considerations, only 20% to 35% of patients have an available genotypically matched sibling donor. Alternate donor sources are needed if marrow transplantation is to be extended to the majority of individuals.

Partially matched family members have been utilized as marrow donors. However, early attempts were marked by high rates of graft rejection and graft vs. host disease (GvHD) [1]. Similar problems were reported by the National Marrow Donor Program (NMDP) for the use of unrelated matched or partially matched donors [2].

The above problems have encouraged more rigorous marrow transplant preparative regimens and prophylaxis of GvHD. This report summarizes the results of 83 unrelated donor bone marrow transplants for aplastic anemia at four USA centers with a special interest in that disease.

Patients and methods

Details of patient characteristics, transplant regimens and outcomes were contributed by four centers: the Midwest Children s Cancer Center (MCCC), the University of Minnesota (MINN), the Memorial Sloan-Kettering Cancer Center (MSKI), and the Fred Hutchinson Cancer Center (SEATTLE). The majority of the patients in this report were not included in the previous publication of the NMDP.

Patient characteristics (age and donor-recipient histocompatibility) are summarized in *Table I*. Transplant preparatory regimens and GvHD prophylaxis are summarized in *Table II*. Details of chemotherapy doses can be obtained from previous publications or by writing to the authors.

Table I. Patient age, donor-recipient histocompatibility and transplant outcome.

	MCCC		MINN		MSKI		Seattle		Total	
AGE: < 18 yr	27	(15)	5	(2)	1	(0)	12	(9)	45	(22)
≥ 18 yr	1	(1)	12	(2)	3	(2)	22	(6)	38	(11)
HLA: ABDR=	10	(7)	4	(2)	2	(2)	25	(8)	41	(19)
A or B mm	16	(9)	6	(1)	0		2	(0)	24	(10)
DR or Dw mm	1	(0)	6	(0)	2	(0)	6	(2)	15	(2)
Other	1*	(0)	1**	(1)	0		1#	(1)	3	(2)

Numbers in parentheses indicate numbers of survivors in each category. mm = mismatch; * = BB mm; ** = B + DR mm; # = unknown.

Table II. Transplant regimens and GvHD prophylaxis.

	MCCC	MINN	MSKI	Seattle	Total
PreBMT Regimen					
CTX + ALG	0	0	0	5	5
CTX + ALG + TBI	0	0	0	7#	7
CTX + TBI	0	17**	4***	19##	40
CTX + ARA C + TBI	28*	0	0	0	28
Other	0	0	0	3	3
GvHD Prophylaxis					
MTX	No	Yes	No	Yes	
CSA	Yes	15	No	Yes	
T-Depletion	$T_{10}B_9$	No	SBA/ER	No	
Other	ALG(9)	Xoma(3)			
		Pred (3)			

Abbreviations: CTX = cyclophosphamide; ALG = antilymphocyte globulin; TBI = total body irradiation; MTX = methotrexate; CSA = cyclosporine; $T_{10}B_9$ = anti-T-cell monoclonal antibody; SBA/ER = soybean agglutinin/E-rosetting; Xoma = XomaZyme; Pred = prednisone.
TBI regimens :   * 1400 cGy/9 fractions/3 days or 1332 cGy/6 fractions/3days
          : ** 1320 cGy/8 fractions/4 days
          : *** 1375 cGy (1), 1500 cGy (3)
          : # 400 - 600 cGy/2-3 fractions/2-3 days
          : ## 1200 cGy/6 fractions/6 days or 920 cGy in 1 fraction

Results

Engraftment

Nine patients failed to engraft and seven rejected their transplant after variable periods of engraftment *(Table III)*. Two of these patients survived: one with graft recovery after treatment with ATG and one with persistent marrow hypoplasia. Graft failure was seen with all types of

Table III. Engraftment, graft rejection, graft vs host disease and survival.

	MCCC	MINN	MSKI	Seattle	Total
No Graft	3	3	1	2	9
Rejection	0	0	2 (1)	5	7 (2)
GvHD ≥ II	8/25*	9/14	0/3	19/27	36/68
Survival	16	4	2	11	33

* = number with GvHD/number at risk; ( ) = number survived

donor-recipient histocompatibility patterns [MCCC (A mm, B mm, BB mm), MINN (A mm, DR mm, ABDR=), MSKI (DR mm, DR mm, ABDR=), SEATTLE (all ABDR=)]. There was no relationship of graft failure to conditioning regimens or to the use of T-cell depletion to prevent GvHD.

Graft vs host disease

Acute GvHD ≥ grade II occurred in 36 of 68 patients at risk *(Table III)*. There was no clear relationship of acute GvHD to the degree of histocompatibility. Acute GvHD was less frequent after regimens using T-cell depletion (MCCC and MSKI). Preliminary analysis suggests that this is not explained by differences in patient ages. Detailed information on chronic GvHD was not collected for all centers. At the MCCC, chronic GvHD was seen in one third of patients and was severe in only one individual.

Survival

Raw survival numbers for each center are given in the Tables. The reader is cautioned against making detailed comparisons due to multiple differences in dates of accrual, patient characteristics, preparatory regimens, GvHD prophylaxis, and length of follow-up.
Thirty-three patients survived. Survival was better in children than in adults *(Table I and Figure 1)*. Survival also appeared to be affected by donor-recipient histocompatibility: ABDR= (19/41) better than A or B mm (10/24) better than DR mm (3/16) *(Table I)*. Patients with acute GvHD ≥ grade II had a worse outcome but lack of detailed information on individual patients limited further analyses.

Discussion

Bone marrow transplantation from a matched unrelated donor (MUD) can be used successfully for treatment of aplastic anemia. However, overall results are significantly worse than when matched siblings are used as donors. This may reflect in part later referral of patients for MUD transplants. Prolonged prior treatment may result in organ damage, general debility or sensitization to blood products.

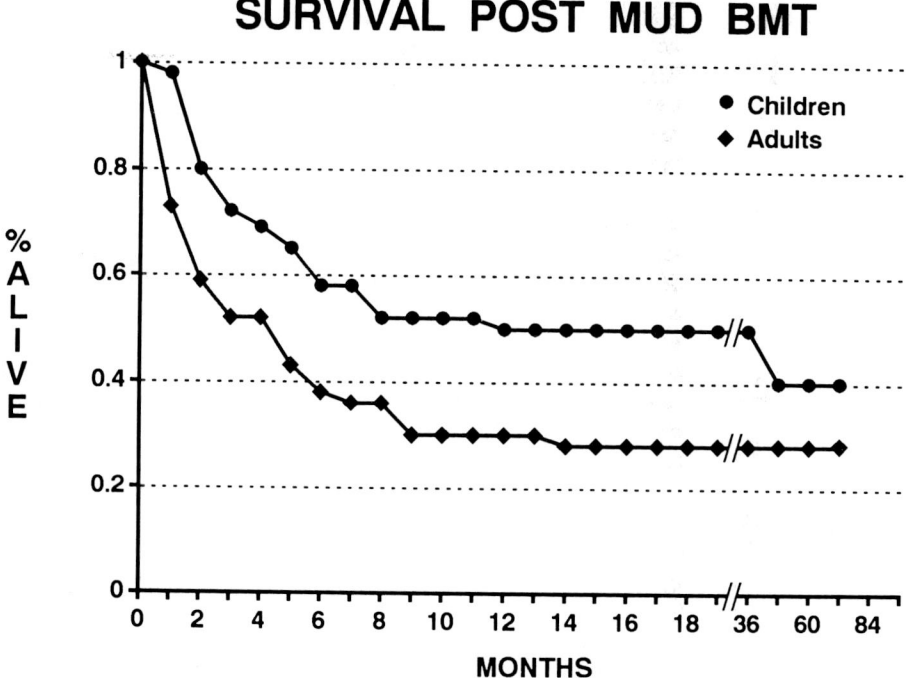

Figure 1. Survival post unrelated donor bone marrow transplantation in relation to patientage. Children = < 18 years at time of transplant.

Other factors contributing to the poor prognosis of MUD bone marrow transplants relate to graft failure, GvHD, and regimen-related toxicities. Histoincompatibility increases the risk of graft failure (nonengraftment or graft failure) in patients with hematologic malignancies who receive marrow transplants from related donors [3]. A similarly increased risk of graft failure was seen with the use of unrelated donors [2]. Patients with aplastic anemia may have a greater risk of graft failure because they are less immunosuppressed both before and during preparation for marrow transplantation. Thus, graft failure rates of up to 23% have been reported (despite the use of additional pretransplant immune suppression) in transfused patients with aplastic anemia who receive a matched sibling bone marrow transplant [4]. The graft failure rate in this series was 18% (22% in ABDR= transplants, 15% in single A, B or DR mismatched transplants). The increased intensity of pretransplant preparatory regimens for MUD transplants may compensate in part for the increased histoincompatibility of MUD grafts.

GvHD is increased with increasing histoincompatibility in related donor marrow transplants [5]. It is uncertain whether this is also true in recipients of grafts from unrelated donors [2]. There were insufficient numbers of non-T-depleted transplants to determine the relationship between histoincompatibility and GvHD in our patients. As in the NMDP report [2], GvHD was less severe in patients who received T-depleted grafts in our series. However, caution is urged in analysis of this data because of the multiple other differences between the centers.

Age is an important factor in the outcome of bone marrow transplantation. The better results in younger patients are apparent in this report as well. A decreased incidence of GvHD and better overall functional status prior to transplantation may contribute to the greater success of marrow transplants in children and young adults.

The increased risk of graft failure in MUD bone marrow transplants for aplastic anemia has led to the use of more intensive preparatory regimens. The increased toxicities from such treatments may contribute to the worse outcome of MUD transplants. A preparatory regimen that allowed reliable engraftment without use of total body irradiation would be a major contribution. Data from Seattle suggest that the antithymocyte globulin plus cyclophosphamide regimen, successful for second marrow transplants between matched siblings, is inadequate to prevent graft failure in MUD transplants [6].

Matched sbling bone marrow transplants are more successful in previously untreated (untransfused) patients [7]. However , if a sibling donor is not available, 2 to 5 months are required to locate an appropriate unrelated donor. While searching for a donor, patients should be treated with an immunosuppressive regimen (± cytokines). If there is no response to immunosuppression after 4 months, consideration should be given to a MUD bone marrow transplant as the secondary treatment of choice. This is certainly true for younger patients where long term results of delayed MUD marrow transplants appear similar to results of primary treatment with immunosuppression. In adults results of MUD marrow transplants for aplastic anemia are suboptimal. Secondary therapy in older patients should be guided by local expertise and patient preference.

Supported in part by the Midwest Athletes Against Childhood Cancer (BC); USPHS grants HL 3644 and CA 18221, and a grant from the National Marrow Donor Program/Baxter Health Care Division (HJD); the Children's Cancer Research Fund, University of Minnesota (NKCR).

References

1. Beatty PG, DiBartolomeo P, Storb R, Clift RA, Buckner CD, Sullivan KM, Doney K, Applebaum FR, Anasetti C, Witherspoon R, Sanders J, Stewart P, Martin PJ, Ciancarelli M, Hansen JA, Thomas ED. Treatment of aplastic anemia with marrow grafts from related donors other than HLA genotypically-matched siblings. *Clin Transplant* 1987; 1: 117-24.
2. Kernan NA, Batrsch G, Ash RC, Beatty PG, Champlin R, Filipovich A, Gajewski J, Hansen JA, Henslee-Downey J, McCullough J, McGlave P, Perkins H, Phillips GL, Sanders J, Stroncek D, Thomas ED, Blume KG. Analysis of 462 transplantations from unrelated donors facilitated by the National Marrow Donor Program. *N Engl J Med* 1993; 328: 593-602.
3. Anasetti C, Amos D, Beatty PG, Applebaum FR, Bensinger W, Buckner CD, Clift R, Doney K, Martin PJ, Mickelson E, Nisperos B, O Quigley J, Ramberg R, Sanders JE, Stewart P, Storb R, Sullivan KM, Witherspoon RP, Thomas ED, Hansen JA. Effect of HLA compatibility on engraftment of bone marrow transplants in patients with leukemia of lymphoma. *N Engl J Med* 1989; 320: 197-204.
4. Storb R, Etzioni R, Anasetti C, Applebaum FR, Buckner CD, Bensinger W, Bryant E, Clift R, Deeg J, Doney K, Flowers M, Hansen J, Martin P, Pepe M, Sale G, Sanders J, Singer J, Sullivan KM, Thomas ED, Witherspoon RP. Cyclophosphamide combined with antithymocyte globulin in preparation for allogeneic marrow transplants in patients with aplastic anemia. *Blood* 1994; 84: 941-9.
5. Beatty PG, Clift RA, Mickelson EM, Nisperos BB, Flournoy N, Martin PJ, Sanders JE, Stewart P, Buckner CD, Strob R, Thomas ED, Hansen JA. Marrow transplantation from related donors other than HLA-identical siblings. *N Engl J Med* 313: 765-71.
6. Deeg HJ, Anasetti C, Petersdorf E, Storb R, Doney K, Hansen JA, Sanders J, Sullivan KM, Applebaum FR. Cyclophosphamide plus ATG conditioning is insufficient for sustained hematopoietic reconstitution in patients with severe aplastic anemia transplanted with marrow from HLA-A, B, DRB matched unrelated donors. *Blood* 1994; 83: 3417-8.
7. Anasetti C, Doney KC, Storb R, Meyers JD, Farewell VT, Buckner CD, Applebaum FR, Sullivan KM, Clift RA, Deeg HJ, Fefer A, Martin PJ, Singer JW, Sanders JE, Stewart PS, Witherspoon RP, Thomas ED. Marrow transplantation for severe aplastic anemia: Long term outcome in fifty untransfused patients. *Ann Intern Med* 1986; 104: 461-6.

Résumé

Quatre-vingt-trois patients provenant du Midwest Children Cancer center (MCCC), de l'Université du Minnesota (MINN), du Memorial Sloan-Kettering Cancer Center (MSKI) et du Fred Hutchinson Cancer Center (Seattle) ont été analysés. Les degrés de compatibilité, les conditionnements et les méthodes de traitement sont différents d'un centre à l'autre, ce qui rend toute comparaison difficile. La survie globale est de 33/83, le rejet 16/83 de GVH>II 36/68. Les enfants ont une meilleure survie que l'adulte. La survie est meilleure lorsque le donneur est HLA-identique. Ces résultats sont clairement inférieurs à ceux des greffes à partir de donneurs HLA identiques, le problème des indications reste posé, cette indication doit être relativement précoce surtout chez l'enfant.

Alternative donor bone marrow transplantation for severe aplastic anaemia: the European experience*

J. Hows[1], A. Bacigalupo, T. Downie[1], R. Brand

[1] *Department of Transplantation Sciences, University of Bristol, Westbury-on-Trym, Bristol BS10 5NB, UK, tel.: (44) 272 50 50 50, fax: (44) 272 59 31 54*

It remains generally accepted that bone marrow transplantation (BMT) is the treatment of choice for severe acquired aplastic anaemia (SAA) in younger patients who have an available HLA identical sibling [1]. In older patients primary therapy with immunosuppression (IS) using antithymocyte globulin (ATG) in combination with cyclosporin is generally recommended because of the increased risk with age of transplant related mortality and persistent chronic graft versus host disease (C-GVHD) [2]. The upper age limit for performing HLA identical sibling BMT varies from centre to centre but in Europe is in the range of 35-55 years. Previously published data from the European Bone Marrow Transplant Group (EBMTG) SAA working party indicate that children and patients with very severe aplastic anaemia (VSAA), defined by $<0.2 \times 10^9/l$ peripheral blood neutrophils have a low probability of survival after IS therapy [2, 3]. Thus patients in this poor risk group have been considered for alternative donor (ALT) BMT, either from a partially matched family member or from a HLA phenotypically matched unrelated donor [4]. Another reason for considering ALT-BMT in young patients with VSAA is the 50% probability of late clonal diseases including paroxysmal nocturnal haemoglobinuria, myelodysplastic syndrome and acute myeloblastic leukaemia after IS treatment [5] but not after successful BMT.

Patients with Fanconi anaemia (FA) and the other rare congenital forms of aplastic anaemia do not respond to IS and treatment with human recombinant growth factors has been disappointing. The majority of patients with FA who develop severe aplasia despite the use of androgenic steroids are considered appropriate candidates for HLA identical sibling BMT. In the absence of a HLA identical sibling ALT-BMT has been attempted but data are sparse because of the rarity of the congenital aplastic anaemias [6].

The preliminary data outlined below are intended to summarize current thinking in Europe on the indications for ALT-BMT in acquired SAA and FA. Data are based on studies in progress in the EBMTG SAA working party and from analyses performed on prospectively collected data

---

* A preliminary report from the European Bone Marrow Transplant Group (EBMTG), working party for severe aplastic anaemia and on behalf of the BMT centres participating in the IMUST study.

from unrelated donor BMT performed in centres participating in the International Marrow Unrelated Search and Transplant (IMUST) Study [7].

Alternative donor BMT from the EBMTG SAA working party

A preliminary retrospective analysis of the EBMTG SAA database has been performed to investigate the success of both HLA partially mismatched family donor (FAM) and phenotypically matched unrelated donor (UD) BMT for FA and acquired SAA. The EBMTG SAA database contains 993 evaluable cases, 883 transplanted from HLA identical siblings or twins, and 110 transplanted from ALT donors, 49 of which were UD and 61 FAM transplants. Fifty five ALT transplants were performed between 1974 and 1988 and 55 between 1989 and 1994. Thirty one of 110 ALT-BMT were for FA, the remainder for SAA. Forty three ALT-BMT recipients were children less than 15 years old and 67 were adults. Fifty nine ALT-BMT were carried out within one year of diagnosis, and 51 at a later stage of the disease. By unifactorial analysis results of ALT BMT were significantly worse than HLA identical sibling BMT with 20% versus 65% actuarial survival at 10 years after BMT. Within the ALT-BMT group, the following factors did not predict survival by unifactorial analysis, a diagnosis of FA compared with SAA, patient age at BMT, or whether the donor was FAM or UD. The length of time between diagnosis and BMT did predict survival, with a probability of 40% for patients transplanted within one year of diagnosis compared with 20% for patients transplanted more than one year after diagnosis (p=0.002). There was a trend towards better survival of patients transplanted after 1989, 40% at one year compared with patients transplanted in the earlier transplant era, 30% at one year (p= 0.16). Multifactorial analysis using proportional hazards regression confirmed that the most important predictors of survival after ALT-BMT were transplant era, relative risk (RR) 0.55 (0.30-1.00), p=0.05, and time from diagnosis to BMT, RR 2.0, (1.20-3.40), p=0.01.

Unrelated donor BMT for SAA: results from the IMUST study

The IMUST Study group prospectively collected and analysed the results of 305 UD-BMT performed between 1989 and 1993. Of these 24 were transplants for SAA. Although this is a small group prospective data collection made causes of failure easier to identify than from the retrospective EBMTG database. The mean age of this group of patients was 16 years, and 11 patients were transplanted within one year of diagnosis and 13 at a later stage in their disease. Seventeen patients were transplanted from HLA-A,B,DR serologically matched donors, and 4 from HLA mismatched donors, in 3 cases HLA typing was incomplete. Twenty one of the 24 patients were transplanted with intensive immunosuppressive protocols, including total body irradiation and cyclophosphamide, (CY), high dose total lymphoid irradiation, and CY or busulfan and CY. Seventeen of the 21 intensively conditioned patients also received Campath-1G or ATG pre-transplant as additional pre-graft immunosuppression. Only 3 patients were conditioned with CY alone. The actuarial survival at one year was 42%. The main cause of death was engraftment failure with 8 patients suffering initial graft failure, and 4 additional patients developing late graft failure. It is notable that none of the 3 patients conditioned with CY alone achieved sustained engraftment, although one is a long-term survivor following autologous marrow reconstitution.

Should alternative donor BMT be considered as first-line therapy for SAA?

The results of ALT-BMT outlined above show some improvement in recent years, but are still significantly inferior to the results of HLA identical sibling BMT. Bacigalupo and Brand on behalf of the EBMTG SAA working party are currently analysing the results of IS treatment over the period 1990-93, in comparison with the results of IS from 1975-89. There has been a marked improvement in survival after IS therapy since 1990 compared with 1975-1989 due both to improvements in IS protocols, and in supportive care. Multifactorial estimates of survival of patients with SAA or VSAA treated with IS have been made. Estimated survival at 5 years for patients treated in 1990-91 are as follows: age 10 years-79%; age 15 years-77%; age 20 years-74%; age 25 years-72%; age 30 years-69%; age 35 years-66%; age 40 years-63%; age 45 years-60%; age 50 years-56%. Although the survivors of IS treatment are still at risk of late clonal evolution of their disease these data are very encouraging. As a result it is suggested that ALT-BMT should not be attempted as first-line treatment for patients with SAA or VSAA. The place of ALT-BMT for salvage treatment of patients who fail to respond to IS requires further study and may be a reasonable option in selected younger patients with well matched unrelated donors.

Should alternative donor BMT be considered in treatment of FA?

Young patients with FA are considered for HLA identical sibling BMT when their disease has become resistant to low dose androgen therapy, and before they become heavily transfusion dependent. In contrast to patients with SAA there is no alternative treatment at this stage of the disease apert from supportive care alone. Provided a well matched unrelated marrow donor can be found ALT-BMT should be considered. Recently human umbilical cord blood cells have been successfully used to transplant children with FA [8]. In the future umbilical cord blood banks may be routinely used to provide suitable donations for FA children who lack a HLA identical sibling.

Conclusion

Current concepts of the use of ALT-BMT in Europe have been presented. The most important implication for treatment planning comes from recently improved results of IS treatment of SAA and VSAA.. At present the risk of transplant related mortality especially from graft failure after ALT-BMT for SAA is too high to consider ALT-BMT as first-line treatment. Therefore it is recommended that IS is given in all cases where there is no availible HLA identical sibling. Young patients with FA do not have an alternative to BMT when their disease is progressive. For these patients ALT-BMT or cord blood transplantation are reasonable options.

References

1. Camitta BM, Storb R, Thomas ED. Aplasic anemia: pathogenesis, diagnosis, treatment and prognosis. *Blood* 1982; 306: 645.

2. Bacigalupo A, Hows J, Gluckman E *et al.* Bone marrow transplantation (BMT) versus immunosuppression (IS) for the treatment of severe aplastic anaemia (SAA): a report of the EBMT SAA working party. *Brit J Haematol* 1988; 70: 177.
3. Bacigalupo A, Broccia G, Corda G *et al.* Antilymphocyte globulin, cyclosporin and granulocyte stimulating factor in patients with acquired severe aplastic anaemia (SAA): a pilot studyof the EBMT SAA working party. *Blood* 1995; (in press).
4. Bacigalupo A, Hows JM, Gordon-Smith E *et al.* Bone marrow transplantation for severe aplastic anaemia from donors other than HLA identical siblings: A report of the EBMT SAA working party. *Bone Marrow Transplant,* 1988; 3: 531-535.
5. Speck B, Tichelli A, Gratwohl A, *et al.* Treatment of severe aplastic anaemia: a 12 year follow up of patients after bone marrow transplantation or therapy with anti-lymphocyte globulin In: Nasrollah T, Shahidi N, eds. Aplastic anemia and other bone marrow failure syndromes. New York: Springer Verlag, 1990: 96-103.
6. Gluckman E and Hows JM. Bone Marrow transplantation in Fanconi Anaemia. (1994), Bone Marrow Transplantation Eds Donnall-Thomas E, Blume K, Foreman S. *Blackwell Scientific Publications* 61:902-911.
7. Bradley B, Gore s, Howard M, Hows J. International Marrow Unrelated Search and Transplant (IMUST) Study. *Bone Marrow Transplant* 1989; 12: (suppl 12): 44
8. Gluckman E, Broxmeyer H, Auerbach A *et al.* Hematopoietic reconstitution in a patient with Fanconi anemia by means of umbilical cord blood from a HLA identical sibling. *N Engl J Med* 1989; 321: 1174-1178.

Résumé

Deux types de données sont présentés: le registre européen de l'EBMT et l'étude IMUST.

La première étude a analysé de façon rétrospective 110 malades greffés, soit avec un donneur non apprenté (49), soit un donneur familial non HLA identique (61). La survie actuarielle est de 20%. La survie est significativement meilleure si la greffe est faite dans l'année du diagnostic. Dans l'étude IMUST 24 patients ont été transplantés pour aplasie médullaire sur 305 entrés dans l'étude. La survie actuarielle à 1 an est de 42%. La cause principale d'échec est l'absence de prise Ces résultats font poser le problème des indications de la greffe dans les aplasies médullaires lorsqu'il n'y a pas de donneur HLA-identique dans la fratrie.

Ontogeny of hematopoiesis. Aplastic anemia. Eds E. Gluckman, L. Coulombel.
Colloque INSERM/John Libbey Eurotext Ltd. © 1995, Vol: 235, pp. 335-343.

Results of European trials of immunosuppression for treatment of aplastic anemia

N. Frickhofen[1], H. Schrezenmeier[1] and A. Bacigalupo[2]

[1] Department of Medicine III, University of Ulm, R Koch Strasse 8, D-89081, Ulm, Germany, tel.: (49 73) 15 02 43 92, fax: (49 73) 15 02 43 93 and [2] Divisione Ematologia 2, Ospedale San Martino, Genova, Italy

Summary

Immunosuppressive treatment of aplastic anemia has traditionally been a focus of clinical research in several European centers. In this review, European strategies as they evolved from the early observations of Mathé et al are summarized. Consecutive trials established antilymphocyte globulin as the gold standard; cyclosporine was characterized as the most promising alternative to ALG, and current trials are trying to facilitate treatment, decrease early mortality and further increase response and survival by testing various combinations of immunosuppressive agents and adjuncts like androgens and hematopoietic growth factors. This trial and error approach improved immunosuppressive therapy of aplastic anemia to a point where the outcome is comparable to allogeneic bone marrow transplantation. Since both immunosuppression and bone marrow transplantation have specific advantages and disadvantages, it will be very important to define parameters that will allow the best possible allocation of patients to the various treatment protocols available today.

Antilymphocyte globulin, the gold standard

Horse antithymocyte globulin and antithoracic duct lymphocyte globulin (ALG) (the term ALG will be used here irrespective of the preparation used) have been used for about 20 years to treat patients with aplastic anemia who are not candidates for immediate bone marrow transplantation (BMT). Mathé was the first to observe autologous hematopoietic recovery in patients treated with ALG before infusion with HLA-nonidentical bone marrow [1]. Following his report, many European centers treated patients with various ALG regimens. In an early collection of data from 3 centers, 4 of 29 patients responded [2]. ALG-induced return of blood counts to normal or near normal levels without repTacement of the patient's bone marrow by an allogeneic transplant implied that a significant pool of hematopoietic stem cells persists in aplastic anemia and that they can be salvaged.

The group in Basel was the most prominent proponent of ALG in Europe. Swiss ALG was regarded the reference ALG preparation at that time. Speck *et al* prospectively compared treatment with ALG and BMT and found a response rate to ALG of 62% [3]. Despite these encouraging results, skepticism prevailed until 1983 when two prospective US trials proved superiority of ALG over supportive care [4] or androgens [5].

ALG has since become the gold standard for treatment of aplastic anemia. Response rates vary between 40 and 70% irrespective of the etiology of the disease (reviewed by Camitta *et al* [6]). Response rates have generally been lower in the US than in Europe. Some authors speculated about the quality of different brands or lots of ALG being responsible for these differences. There are in fact differences in the antibody specificities and biologic activities between major brands of ALG [7, 8], but there is no convincing evidence that any of these differences accounts for the variable response of patients with aplastic anemia to ALG. Patient selection due to different treatment policies is probably a better explanation for the variable results in different countries. The component of ALG which is able to induce remission of aplastic anemia has never been identified. Marginal therapeutic activity of ALG preparations which are very potent agents for treatment of rejection in organ transplantation suggests, that lympholytic activity may not be all that is required to treat aplastic anemia [8].

Are there alternatives to ALG?

Although the "first generation" studies clearly established ALG as an effective treatment for aplastic anemia, there have been many attempts to find alternative treatment modalities in "second generation" phase II-studies *(Figure 1)*.

Androgens are definitely inadequate as sole treatment of patients with severe aplastic anemia [9]. However, there are patients with nonsevere disease and single patients with severe aplastic anemia who respond to androgens and require maintenance treatment with androgens [10, 11]. This led several investigators to use androgens as adjunct to immunosuppressive regimens (see below).

Cyclophosphamide has been tested in aplastic anemia. at about the same time as ALG. Encouraged by a case report [12] and by speculations about cyclophosphamide-mediated auto-

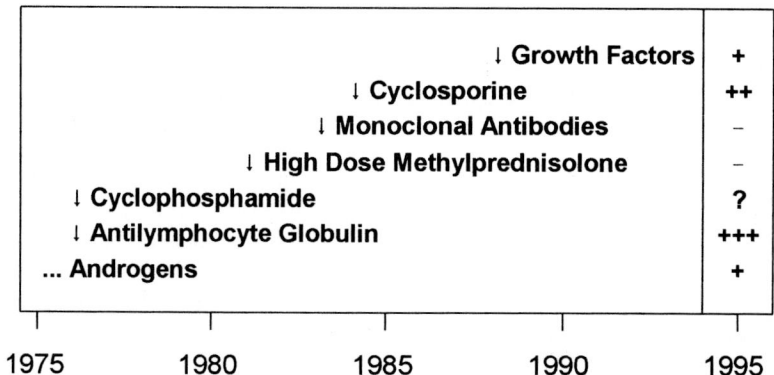

Figure 1. Sequence of testing of various agents for treatment of patients with aplastic anemia. The current place of these agents in the treatment of aplastic anemia is given in the last column.

logous marrow recovery after failed engraftment of allogeneic marrow [13] several patients were treated with cyclophosphamide at conventional doses. This practice was discouraged by a survey among members of the American Society of Hematology which revealed only 3 remissions among 70 patients treated [14]. Since the dose of cyclophosphamide may have made the difference, there is currently renewed interest in this drug. Bacigalupo *et al* were the first to investigate the possibility of megadose immunosuppression followed by autologous transplantation in aplastic anemia, a concept which a first glance seems weird in aplastic anemia. However, data generated so far are encouraging (A Bacigalupo, this volume). Fully exploiting the potent immunosuppressive properties of cyclophosphamide makes perfect sense in a disease that is increasingly viewed as an autoimmune disease related to classical autoimmune diseases like lupus erythematodes (NS Young, this volume p. 191).

Corticosteroids at low doses are ineffective and may even decrease survival of patients with aplastic anemia [15]. Very high doses of methylprednisolone have been described to induce remissions comparable to ALG [16, 17], but significant acute as well as long term adverse effects (like osteonecrosis in 20% of the patients [18]) limit its applicability in aplastic anemia patients. Methylprednisolone is currently mainly used as a short course / low dose regimen parallel to ALG in order to prevent adverse effects of ALG like anaphylaxis and serum sickness.

Monoclonal antibodies directed at T lymphocyte antigens were studied mainly in the US with the idea to replace the poorly standardized, broadly reactive (7) and thereby more toxic ALG. Except for anecdotal case reports (*e.g.* response to treatment with anti-IL2 receptor antibody [19], none of the antibodies tested so far proved to be active in aplastic anemia [20-22].

Cyclosporine A turned out to be the only drug with a therapeutic potential comparable to ALG. Investigators in the US and Europe first reported successful treatment of aplastic anemia with cyclosporine in 1984 [23, 24]. An example of the course of one of these early patients strongly suggesting therapeutic activity of cyclosporine is illustrated in *Figure 2*.

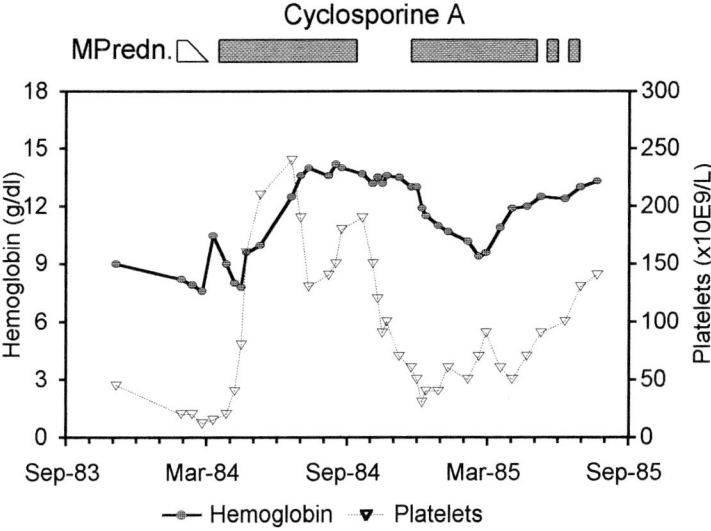

Figure 2. Response, relapse and second response to cyclosporine A in a patient with nonsevere aplastic anemia (cyclosporine was continued until 2/86; N Frickhofen, unpublished). The rapid and complete response of platelets seen in this patient is rarely observed in patients with severe aplastic anemia.

In a retrospective survey on the use of cyclosporine, data from 263 European and 78 American patients treated from 1983 to 1990 could be collected. Three and 6 months after treatment with cyclosporine alone, partial or complete responses were found in 34% and 55% of 109 evaluable patients, respectively. Response kinetics and response rates in patient subgroups were similar to historical data with ALG and there was no significant difference in response or survival whether cyclosporine was given alone or combined with ALG and/or androgens (A Raghavachar and H Schrezenmeier, unpublished). Reporting bias cannot be excluded in this survey and there are single reports which failed to show response to cyclosporine [25]. However, many other studies confirmed the early case reports and helped to establish cyclosporine as the second standard drug next to ALG [26].

The efficacy of cyclosporine is interesting with regard to the pathophysiology of aplastic anemia. Cyclosporine is a potent immunosuppressive drug with much better defined immunosuppressive activity than ALG [27]. However, CsA can also promote rather than suppress immune responses in specific clinical situations [28]. One should thus be cautious to use response to cyclosporine as evidence for a simple model of aplastic anemia as an autoimmune disease caused by autoaggressive T lymphocytes. Complex immunomodulation and interference with negative regulatory cytokine networks is a more likely hypothesis linking ALG and cyclosporine-induced responses in aplastic anemia.

The use of **hematopoietic growth factors** is discussed in detail elsewhere in this volume. All the growth factors increased peripheral blood counts in patients with some residual hematopoiesis, but they did not change the natural history of the disease. Growth factors should thus not be used as sole treatment of aplastic anemia [29], but they may have a significant role in combination with immunosuppressive regrmens (see below).

Phase III studies to replace or supplement ALG

The emergence of cyclosporine as an effective drug for treatment of aplastic anemia had a major impact on the design of "l3rd generation" phase III studies in Europe. *Table I* summarizes strategies and results of recently completed and ongoing European phase III trials.

One set of trials asked the question whether **cyclosporine can replace ALG.** Gluckman *et al* randomized 116 patients with severe aplastic anemia for treatment with ALG and methylprednisolone or cyclosporine [30]. Patients who did not respond at 3 months were crossed over to the alternative regimen. There was no difference in the response rate to ALG and cyclosporine at 3 months (12% vs 16%) and crossover did not change the proportion of responding patients at 12 months (32% vs 30%). Survival at 2 years was similar in patients initially treated with ALG or cyclosporine. However, 13 of 56 patients initially treated with ALG died within 3 months, mostly from infections, whereas only 2 of 60 patients started on CsA died within this period. High early toxicity in the patients treated with ALG was one reason why the response rate to ALG was relatively low in this study. Irrespective of speculations about the low response rate, the study confirmed comparability of ALG and CsA in a multicenter trial.

Encouraged by these results, 2 ongoing European trials are analyzing whether cyclosporine alone (trial of the European Group for Blood and Marrow Transplantation (EBMT) in nonsevere aplastic anemia) or cyclosporine combined with granulocyte-colony-stimulating factor (G-CSF) is similarly effective as cyclosporine combined with ALG (German trial in severe aplastic anemia). Similar efficacy of the regimens without ALG would enable outpatient treatment of aplastic anemia and thereby increase the quality of life of the patients and probably decrease the cost of treatment. ALG combined with cyclosporine is used as the control regimen in both stu-

Table I. All response data refer to patients with severe aplastic anemia[1] evaluated at 3 months, except for the trial of Bacigalupo et al where response was analyzed after 4 months[2].

Strategy of the study		(Investigators)	Response (3/4[2] months)	Survival (2 years)
Can CsA replace ALG?				
→ ALG	vs CsA	(Gluckman, 1992)	16/12%	0.60/0.64
→ ALG + CsA	vs CsA	(EBMT, 1993+)	–	–
→ ALG + CsA	vs CsA + G-CSF	(Germany, 1993+)	–	–
Can other agents improve response to ALG?				
→ ALG	vs ALG + CsA	(Frickhofen, 1991)	58/31%[1]	0.55/0.80[1]
→ ALG	vs ALG + Oxymetholone	(Bacigalupo, 1993)	56/40%[2]	0.71/0.73[2]
→ ALG	vs ALG + GM-CSF	(Gordon-Smith, 1991)	64/18%	(no data)
→ ALG + CsA	vs ALG + CsA + G-CSF	(EBMT, 1994+)	–	–

dies since this combination was considered the most effective treatment modality at the time these trials were designed (see below).

Another set of trials does not intend to replace ALG but rather asks whether adding cyclosporine, androgens or growth factors may further improve response rates and survival. The first trial evaluating a **multiagent immunosuppressive regimen** was a German multicenter trial testing ALG and methylprednisolone versus ALG, methyl-prednisolone and cyclosporine [31]. In contrast to other trials mentioned in *Table I*, this trial included nonsevere (n=24) as well as severe aplastic anemia patients (n=60). Response rate at 3 months was significantly higher in patients treated with cyclosporine (65 vs 39% of all patients) but did not reach the level of significance in patients with severe aplastic anemia (58 vs 31%, p= 0.06). There was a trend towards better survival in patients with severe disease, which however did not hold up in a more recent analysis with longer followup [32]. Many patients who had not responded to ALG where later crossed over to the cyclosporine regimen which precludes reliable evaluation of differences in survival in this trial. Adverse effects of cyclosporine were modest; unexpectedly, cyclosporine even decreased typical adverse effects of ALG like fever and serum sickness.

Favorable results of the addition of cyclosporine to ALG have been confirmed in a small trial in children [33] and in a larger study including mostly adult patients [34]. Based on these results, most recent trials use the combination of ALG and cyclosporlne as the reference treatment of aplastic anemia.

Androgens, although inferior to ALG as single agents, have been found to significantly increase the response rate when added to ALG in an early German study [35]. These results were recently confirmed in a large EBMT trial [36]: 134 patients with severe aplastic anemia were randomized to receive or not to receive oxymetholone for 4 months after ALG. The response rate at 4 months was significantly greater in patients treated with androgen (56% vs 40%; p = 0.04). The difference was most significant in female patients with neutrophils less than 0.5 x 109/1. Long term survival was not different in the two patient groups, but there was a trend towards bctter survival in female patients with low neutrophil counts.

The observation that females respond better to a regimen including androgens may not be surprising. However, a similar trend towards improved response of female patients was also found in the German trial evaluating cyclosporine (N Frickhofen, unpublished analysis [31]). Since the Basel group also observed different results of immunosuppressive therapy in male versus female patients (in their experience, older females did best [37], gender should be evaluated as a variable of immunosuppressive regimens in aplastic anemia.

Growth factors were disappointing when used alone for treatment of aplastic anemia. However they were still thought to be valuable as adjunct to immunosuppression for 2 reasons: (1) Early death from infection is a major cause of mortality in all studies reported to date. One could thus argue that a strategy of giving growth factors during the time the patient waits for a response to immunosuppression may decrease early mortality. (2) Maximizing neutrophil production by the addition of growth factors may also accelerate the usually slow kinetics of recovery of hematopoiesis induced by immunosuppression.

Along these lines of reasoning, several centers performed small pilot studies. The study of Gordon Smith et al is the only randomized study published to date [38]. This trial included 22 patients with severe aplastic anemia who were treated with ALG. Two weeks after ALG, patients were randomized to receive either GM-CSF or placebo for 28 days. GM-CSF significantly increased granulocyte counts and there were significantly fewer days of fever in the treatment group compared with placebo. However, the effect was limited to the time of treatment with the growth factor and there was no difference in the response rate and survival. There were significant adverse effects in the patients treated with GM-CSF.

Since emphasis of growth factor trials is on granulocyte counts, G-CSF was considered more effective and less toxic. Therefore, the EBMT is currently running a large randomized study evaluation G-CSF added to ALG and cyclosporine. This trial followed a pilot study of Bacigalupo et al which tested feasibility and safety of the 3 drug-combination [39]. Among 40 patients treated with ALG, cyclosporine and G-CSF, 82% responded at 4 months with an unusually high proportion of 40% complete responses. Actuarial survival at 3 years is 92% which is comparable to the results reported for the most effective BMT regimen of the Seattle group [40].

Lessons from immunosuppressive protocols

From the studies reviewed here and from unpublished analyses of the EBMT database, several lessons can be drawn:
1. A low granulocyte count at diagnosis is the best predictor of response and survival. This criterium should be used to allocate patients to treatment strategies until reliable *in vitro* parameters predicting response to immunosuppression become available (NS Young, this volume).
2. About 50% of the patients who fail a single course to immunosuppression can be rescued by repeated immunosuppression which may or may not include novel agents (H Schrezenmeier, unpublished EBMT data). Considering still unfavorable results of unrelated donor transplants in aplastic anemia (J Hows, this volume), a patient who does not have a sibling donor should thus undergo at least a second course of immunosuppression.
3. Relapse occurs in about 1 out of 3 patients responding to immunosuppression. Fortunately, most of these patients respond to repeated immunosuppressive therapy [41].
4. ncomplete response, relapse and clonal diseases after successful immunosuppressive treatment are of concern (G Socie, this volume). These observations illustrate that ALG and cyclosporine modulate rather than cure the disease in many patients.

If the ongoing randomized EBMT study on the use of G-CSF in addition to immunosuppression confirms the high response rate and good long term survival of the pilot study, it will be very important to metaanalyze in detail current BMT and immunosuppression trials. It will be important, since long term survival is probably the most important treatment result for a patients with aplastic anemia. However, survival is by no means all that is required to qualify for a successful treatment strategy. Quality of life and long term adverse effects will be crucial parameters to assess the role of the different treatment strategies in the future.

Acknowledgements

We would like to thank our colleagues from all over Europe who contributed data to the national and EBMT databases.

References

1. Mathé G, Amiel JL, Schwarzenberg L, Choay J, Trolard P, Schneider M, et al. Bone marrow graft in man after conditioning by antilymphocytic serum. *Br Med J* 1970; 2: 131-136.
2. Speck B, Gluckman E, Haak HL, van Rood JJ. Treatment of aplastic anemia by antilymphocyte globulin with and without allogeneic bone marrow infusions. *Lancet* 1977; 2: 1145-1148.
3. Speck B, Gratwohl A, Nissen C, Leibundgut U, Ruggero D, Osterwalder B, et al. Treatment of severe aplastic anaemia with antilymphocyte globulin or bone marrow transplantation. *Br Med J [Clin Res]* 1981; 282: 860-863.
4. Champlin R, Ho W, Gale RP. Antithymocyte globulin treatment in patients with aplastic anemia: a prospective randomized trial. *N Engl J Med* 1983; 308: 113-118.
5. Camitta B, O'Reilly RJ, Sensenbrenner L, Rappeport J, Champlin R, Doney K, et al. Antithoracic duct lymphocyte globulin therapy of severe aplastic anemia. *Blood* 1983; 62: 883-888.
6. Camitta BM, Doney K. Immunosuppressive therapy for aplastic anemia: indications, agents, mechanisms, and results. *Am J Pediatr Hematol Oncol* 1990; 12: 411-424.
7. Raefsky EL, Gascon P, Gratwohl A, Speck B, Young NS. Biological and immunological characterization of ATG and ALG. *Blood* 1986; 68: 712-719.
8. Taniguchi Y, Frickhofen N, Raghavachar A, Digel W, Heimpel H. Antilymphocyte immunoglobulins stimulate peripheral blood lymphocytes to proliferate and release lymphokines. *Eur J Haematol* 1990; 44: 244-251.
9. Camitta BM, Thomas ED, Nathan DG, Gale RP, Kopecky KJ, Rappeport JM, et al. A prospective study of androgens and bone marrow transplantation for treatment of severe aplastic anemia. *Blood* 1979; 53: 504-514.
10. Najean Y, Haguenauer O. Long-term (5 to 20 Years) evolution of nongrafted aplastic anemia. *Blood* 1990; 76: 2222-2228.
11. Stebler C, Tichelli A, Gratwohl A, Hoffmann T, Nissen C, Speck B. Androgen dependence in patients with severe aplastic anemia after antilymphocyte globuline therapy. *Bone Marrow Transplant* 1991; 7 Suppl 2:101
12. Baran DT, Griner PF, Klemperer MR. Recovery from aplastic anemia after treatment with cyclophosphamide. *N Engl J Med* 1976; 295: 1522-1523.
13. Speck B, Cornu P, Jeannet M, et al. Autologous marrow recovery following allogeneic marrowtransplantation in a patientwith severe aplastic anemia. *Exp Hematol* 1976; 4: 131-137.
14. Griner PF. A survey of the effectiveness of cyclophosphamide in patients with severe aplastic anemia. *Am J Hematol* 1980; 8: 55-60.
15. Najean Y, Pecking A, LeDanvic M. Androgen therapy of aplastic anemia - a prospective study of 352 cases. *Scand J Haematol* 1979; 22: 343-356.
16. Bacigalupo A, Podesta M, van Lint MT, Vimercati R, Cerri R, Rossi E, et al. Severe aplastic anaemia: correlation of *in vitro* tests with clinical response to immunosuppression in 20 patients. *Br J Haematol* 1981; 47: 423-432.

17. Gluckman E, Devergie A, Poros A, Degoulet P. Results of immunosuppression in 170 cases of severe aplastic anaemia. Report of the European Group of Bone Marrow Transplant (EGBMT). *Br J Haematol* 1982; 51: 541-550.
18. Marsh JC, Zomas A, Hows JM, Chapple M, Gordon Smith EC. Avascular necrosis after treatment of aplastic anaemia with antilymphocyte globulin and high-dose methylprednisolone. *Br J Haematol* 1993; 84: 731-735.
19. Schwinger W, Urban C, Lackner H, Mache C. Treatment of aplastic anemia with a monoclonal antibody directed against the interleukin-2 receptor. *Ann Hematol* 1993; 66: 181-184.
20. Jansen J, Gratama JW, Zwaan FE, *et al*. Therapy with monoclonal antibody OKT3 in severe aplastic anemia. *Exp Hematol* 1984; 12, Suppl 15: 46-47.
21. Champlin R, Ho W, Feig SA, *et al*. Lack of efficacy for intravenous monoclonal antibody (T101) for aplastic anemia: a randomized controlled trial. *Blood* 1984; 64, Suppl 1: 132a Abstract.
22. Doney K, Martin P, Hansen J, Storb R, Thomas ED. A randomized trial of antihuman thymocyte globulin versus murine monoclonal antihuman T-cell antibodies as immunosuppressive therapy for aplastic anemia. *Exp Hematol* 1985; 13: 520-524.
23. Finlay JL, Toretsky J, Hoffman R, Bruno E, Shahidi NT. Cyclosporine A (CyA) in refractory severe aplastic anemia *(M)*. *Blood* 1984; 64, Suppl 1: 104a Abstract.
24. Stryckmans PA, Dumont JP, Velu T, Debusscher L. Cyclosporine in refractory severe aplastic anemia [letter]. *N Engl J Med* 1984; 310: 655-656.
25. Jacobs P, Wood L, Martell RW. Cyclosporin A in the treatment of severe acute aplastic anaemia. *Br J Haematol* 1985; 61: 267-272.
26. Schrezenmeier H, Schlander M, Raghavachar A. Cyclosporin A in aplastic anemia – report of a workshop. *Ann Hematol* 1992; 65: 33-36.
27. Briggs JD. A critical review of immunosuppressive therapy. *Immunol Lett* 1991; 29: 89-94.
28. Prud'homme GJ, Parfrey NA, Vanier LE. Cyclosporine-induced autoimmunity and immune hyperreactivity. *Autoimmunity* 1991; 9: 345-356.
29. Marsh JC, Socie G, Schrezenmeier H, Tichelli A, Gluckman E, Ljungman P, *et al*. Haemopoietic growth factors in aplastic anaemia: a cautionary note. European Bone Marrow Transplant Working Party for Severe Aplastic Anaemia. *Lancet* 1994; 344: 172-173.
30. Gluckman E, Esperou-Bourdeau H, Baruchel A, Boogaerts M, Briere J, Donadio D, *et al*. Multicenter randomized study comparing cyclosporine-A alone and antithymocyte globulin with prednisone for treatment of severe aplastic anemia. *Blood* 1992; 79: 2540-2546.
31. Frickhofen N, Kaltwasser JP, Schrezenmeier H, Raghavachar A, Vogt HG, Herrmann F, *et al*. Treatment of aplastic anemia with antilymphocyte globulin and methylprednisolone with or without cyclosporine. *N Engl J Med* 1991; 324: 1297-1304.
32. Frickhofen N. Antilymphocyte globulin and methylprednisolone with or without cyclosporine A for treatment of aplastic anemia. Updated results of a German randomized trial. In: Raghavachar A, Schrezenmeier H, Frickhofen N, editors. *Aplastic anemia. Current perspectives on the pathogenesis and treatment*. Vienna: Blackwell-MZV, 1993 :118-125.
33. Matloub YH, Bostrom B, Golembe B, Priest J, Ramsay NK. Antithymocyte globulin, cyclosporine, and prednisone for the treatment of severe aplastic anemia in children. A pilot study. *Am J Pediatr Hematol Oncol* 1994; 16: 104-106.
34. Rosenfeld SJ, Kimball J, Vining D, Young NS. Intensive immunosuppression with antithymocyte globulin and cyclosporine as treatment for severe aplastic anemia. *Blood* 1995; 85: 3058-3065.
35. Kaltwasser JP, Dix U, Schalk KP, Vogt H. Effect of androgens on the response to antithymocyte globulin in patients with aplastic anaemia. *Eur.J.Haematol.* 1988; 40: 111-118.
36. Bacigalupo A, Chaple M, Hows J, van Lint MT, McCann S, Milligan D, *et al*. Treatment of aplastic anaemia (M) with antilymphocyte globulin (ALG) and methylprednisolone (MPred) with or without androgens: a randomized trial from the EBMT SAA working party. *Br J Haematol* 1993; 83: 145-151.
37. Nissen C, Gratwohl A, Tichelli A, Stebler C, Wursch A, Moser Y, *et al*. Gender and response to antilymphocyte globulin (ALG) for severe aplastic anemia. *Br J Haematol* 1993; 83: 319-325.
38. Gordon Smith EC, Yandle A, Milne A, Speck B, Marmont A, Willemze R, *et al*. Randomised placebo controlled study of RH-GM-CSF following ALG in the treatment of aplastic anaemia. *Bone Marrow Transplant* 1991; 7 Suppl 2: 78-80.

39. Bacigalupo A, Broccia G, Corda G, Arcese W, Carotenuto M, Gallamini A, *et al.* Antilymphocyte globulin, cyclosporin, and granulocyte colony-stimulating factor in patients with acquired severe aplastic anemia (SAA): a pilot study of the EBMT SAA Working Party. *Blood* 1995; 85: 1348-1 353.
40. Storb R, Etzioni R, Anasetti C, Appelbaum FR, Buckner CD, Bensinger W, *et al.* Cyclophosphamide combined with antithymocyte globulin in preparation for allogeneic marrow transplants in patients with aplastic anemia. *Blood* 1994; 84: 941-949.
41. Schrezenmeier H, Marin P, Raghavachar A, McCann S, Hows J, Gluckman E, *et al.* Relapse of aplastic anaemia after immunosuppressive treatment: a report from the European Bone Marrow Transplantation Group SAA Working Party. *Br J Haematol* 1993; 85: 371-377.

Résumé

Les traitements immunosuppresseurs de l'aplasie médullaire ont été l'objet de plusieurs études européennes. Ces études consécutives ont été faites à la suite de l'observation par G. Mathé du rôle du sérum anti-lymphocytaire dans le traitement des aplasies médullaires. Les études consécutives ont confirmé cette efficacité. Dans un second temps, il a été démontré que la ciclosporine était active. Les études actuelles esssaient d'optimiser les traitements, de diminuer la mortalité et d'augmenter la réponse et la survie en testant des associations d'agents immunosuppresseurs et l'addition d'androgènes ou de facteurs de croissance hématopoïétiques. Cela a permis d'améliorer les résultats qui deviennent comparables à ceux de la greffe de moelle à partir d'un donneur familial HLA-identique. Chaque traitement a ses avantages et ses inconvénients, il devient alors très important de définir des paramètres permettant de choisir entre les divers traitements

ns* Ontogeny of hematopoiesis. Aplastic anemia. Eds E. Gluckman, L. Coulombel.
Colloque INSERM/John Libbey Eurotext Ltd. © 1995, Vol. 235, pp. 345-352.

Hematopoietic growth factors in the treatment of aplastic anemia. Emphasis on European studies

A. Gratwohl

Division of Hematology, Department of Internal Medicine, Kantonsspital, CH-4031 Basel, Switzerland, tel.: (4161) 26 54 254, fax: (4161) 26 54 450

Summary

Hemorrhagic and infectious complications are the main cause of death for patients with severe aplastic anemia (SAA). Several recombinant human hematopoietic growth factors are available today for clinical use: Erythropoietin (Epo), granulocyte-colony stimulating factor (G-CSF), granulocyte-macrophage-colony stimulating factor (GM-CSF), Interleukin -1, -3 and -6 (IL-1, IL-3, IL-6) and most recently, stem cell factor (SCF) and thrombopoietin. They are used in aplastic anemia in an attempt to increase peripheral blood values, reduce the risks of complications caused by pancytopenia and eventually, to induce a sustained multilineage response. Despite many reports, results are not yet conclusive. G-CSF and GM-CSF have been very widely tested. Both induce a dose dependent transient response in patients with residual bone marrow function but fail in patients with most severe aplastic anemia. G-CSF is postulated to induce multilineage response after prolonged treatment, its role is currently being investigated in a prospective randomized European study. IL-3 can induce a transient increase of neutrophils, no multilineage response has been described when given as a single agent. IL-6 has no effect but can aggravate thrombopenia and anemia. Erythropoietin can reduce the need for red cell transfusions in a small subgroup of patients with late clonal complications and low erythropoietin levels. No data are yet available concerning SCF and thrombopoietin. Combinations of growth factors are now being evaluated, mainly G-CSF and Epo. No prospective randomized controlled study has yet been published in detail. Despite a multitude of case reports, the role of hematopoietic grwoth factors in the treatment of SAA still needs to be defined. Application of growth factors outside clinical studies cannot be recommended.

Bone marrow transplantation (BMT) is the treatment of choice for young patients with severe aplastic anemia (SAA) and an HLA-identical sibling donor. 60-80% of these patients are likely to be alive and free of disease at ten years post transplant [1-3]. This is illustrated by the constant and steadily increasing number of allogeneic BMT for patients with SAA in Europe. Since 1990 the European Group for Blood and Marrow Transplantation (EBMT) has been collecting transplant data on an annual basis according to indication and donor source from

European transplant teams. in 1990 164 transplants were performed for SAA, 227 in 1994 [4]. These patients recover donor type hemopoiesis post transplant and do not need hematopoietic growth factors. The treatment of choice for those patients without a suitable donor or beyond the age of 50 years remains therapy with antilymphocyte or antithymocyte globulin (ALG/ATG) associated with or without cyclosporin, androgens or prednison. Cyclosporin as single immunosuppression has also been advocated. Results with immunosuppression at ten years are comparable to BMT as regards survival. There are, however, marked discrepancies. Patients with very severe disease or young patients have a considerably better chance of survival with BMT. Patients with milder disease or older patients fare better with immunospuppression [5]. Moreover, patients treated with immunosuppression retain stigmata of their disease and a significant percentage can develop late clonal complications such as myelodysplastic syndromes, leukemia or paroxysmal nocturnal hemoglobinuria [6]. Response after immunosuppressive therapy with ALG/ATG takes time. Patients remain at risk for infectious or hemorrhagic complications during a prolonged period of time. The advent of hematopoietic growth factors capable of stimulating precursor cells into proliferation raises hopes for a new therapeutic tool in the treatment of SAA as an adjuvant therapy to reduce complications of pancytopenia or, eventually, as an alternative treatment to BMT or immunosuppression. The present report summarises data from published studies and some past and ongoing trials in Europe.

Methods

Study design

For the present analysis we summarized our own clinical studies with hematopoietic growth factors in the treatment of SAA. We reviewed published material, obtained data from selected concluded studies and some ongoing or planned clinical trials. The report concentrates on studies conducted with G-CSF, GM-CSF, IL-3, IL-6, Epo, combinations thereof and to a limited extent on SCF.

Results

Publications

In a medline search more than a hundred publications have appeared concerning the use of any of the above growth factors in patients with SAA. Most reports are case reports or pilot studies. Only one prospective randomized placebo controlled study has been concluded. It is published so far only as proceedings [7].

Erythropoietin

Serum erythropoietin levels are elevated in most patients with SAA at diagnosis. In some patients this increase might be to a lower extent than expected for the respective hemoglobin level. Epo levels decline with improvement of the disease [1, 3, 8]. Few studies describe the use of EPO in SAA. We treated two patients with PNH as a late clonal complication secondary to SAA and ALG therapy. One patient responded to a dose of 500 U/kg Epo 3 times a week [9].

Single cases of response to Epo in SAA have been published. No clear study with Epo has been perfomed in SAA. Yoshida *et al* treated 7 patients with doses up to 24000 U t.i.w. A response was observed in 3 patients, but only as long as Epo was given [8]. Epo has been combined with G-CSF or GM-CSF. Several case reports with sustained multilineage response following this therapy have been published. All these patients were pretreated with ALG or received cyclosporin additionally. No conclusive data are available.

In a phase II study Epo is currently tested in combination with cyclosporin and G-CSF for patients with refractory or relapsed SAA at a dose of 150 U/kg. The study is single armed. (Contact: Dr A Raghavachar, Ulm.)

GM-CSF

GM-CSF has been the first hematopoietic growth factor to be tested prospectively in patients with SAA. Initially, Champlin *et al* [10] reported good responses in 4 patients. We tested GM-CSF in poor risk patients. Four patients with very severe refractory SAA or who relapsed after ALG were treated with increasing courses of GM-CSF from 4 to 32 (g/kg *i.v.* for 14 days. One patient with minimal residual myelopoiesis responded transiently to two separate courses of GM-CSF. Septicemia and bilateral pneumonia that had been resistant to conventional therapy were resolved. Three patients with no bone marrow reserve showed no response. The apparent clinical response of one patient was the basis for the following study [11].

In a prospective randomized placebo controlled trial at five institutions (London, Paris, Munich, Leyden, Basel) 27 patients with newly diagnosed SAA were treated with ALG, followed immediately by a course of GM-CSF 300 g (13 patients) or placebo (14 patients) for 28 days s.c. or as a continuous infusion. When data were analysed, a significant difference in neutrophil, eosinophil and monocyte counts was observed between the two groups. Counts were constantly higher in the GM-CSF group. Following withdrawal leukocyte counts declined rapidly in the GM-CSF group, counts were no longer different in the two groups at 7 days post treatment. Initial neutrophil count was the most important response factor in the GM-CSF group. Only patients with some residual marrow function showed an increase. There was a significant reduction in days with fever in the GM-CSF group ($p < 0.05$) and a trend for fewer days on antibiotics. There was no difference in platelet and red cell transfusion requirements and no difference in overall treatment response and survival [7].

Several other groups have investigated the role of GM-CSF. The Seattle group were able to show that pretreatment with GM-CSF does not interfere with subsequent ALG treatment. The role of GM-CSF remains unclear [12]. The Huston group advocated the use of very low dose GM-CSF in combination with Epo. Again, the role remains unclear and no subsequent studies confirmed these results [13]. No subsequent trials with prolonged GM-CSF application have been established. Recently, Khan *et al* reported on nine children with SAA treated solely with GM-CSF for up to 42 days [14]. None of these patients showed inprovement in the disease nor clearance of infections. Thus, GM-CSF without immunosuppression should not be given to SAA patients.

G-CSF

G-CSF is a potent stimulating agent of myelopoiesis. Single cases of successful treatment of patients with SAA have been reported. A first larger series of children with SAA was published by Kojima [15]. Ten children with SAA were given 400-2000 mg/m2 for 4 weeks. Six out of 10 showed an increase in neutrophils, their infections cleared and they are alive.

The EBMT working party for SAA piloted the use of long term G-CSF, 5 ug/kg/d, s.c. for 90 days, in 40 patients with newly diagnosed SAA [16]. All were uniformly treated with horse ALG, 15 mg/kg/d for 5 days, combined with cyclosporin, 5 mg/kg/d for 180 days, and methylprednisolone, 2 mg/kg/d for 5 days, then at a tapered dose. The median age was 16 years, from 2 to 72 years and the median time from diagnosis to trreatment was 24 days with a range from 12 to 71 days. 21 patients had very severe SAA with neutrophils $< 0.2 \times 10^9/l$. Treatment was well tolerated with minimal side effects. There were 3 early deaths due to infection (8%), 4 patients (10%) showed no recovery. 33 of the 40 patients (82%) had trilineage reconstitution and became transfusion independent within a median of 115 days post treatment. All patients with a granulocyte count $> 0.2 \times 10^9/l$ are alive.

The results from this pilot trial are in line with a recent report of the Japanese pediatric group. Imashuku et al [17] treated 45 children with G-CSF, 200 to 400 ug/kg/d for 4-24 weeks (15 median). 43 of the 45 patients showed an increase in neutrophils and 7 of the 45 patients (16%) experienced a trilineage response, two of which without any other therapy. These data are encouraging and form the basis for a prospective randomized trial of the EBMT currently in progress: Patients with newly diagnosed SAA are treated with the same regimen of ATG, cyclosporin and prednisone and randomized to receive additional treatment with G-CSF, 5 ug/kg/d for 90 days or no other treatment. About xx patients have been entered so far into this study. No data are yet available. The trial is ongoing and teams are invited to participate. (Coordinators: E Gluckman, Paris and A Bacigalupo, Genova). Concomitantly the German multicenter study for SAA is also investigating the role of G-CSF for patients with SAA. Newly diagnosed patients are randomized to be treated with ALG, cyclosporin and methylprednisolone or with cyclosporin alone combined with G-CSF. No results are yet available. (Coordinator: Dr A Raghavachar, Ulm).

Several isolated case reports have been described about recovery of trilineage response following long term (> 3 months) application of G-CSF alone or combined with Epo [18-21]. Interpretation is difficult, most patients were pretreated with ALG and or cyclosporin. Results of ongoing trials are eagerly awaited.

IL-3

IL-3 acts as an early regulator of hemopoiesis and induces a trilineage response in normal individuals. Ganser [22] reported a platelet response in one and reticulocyte response in 4 patients with SAA. In a collaborative two center prospective open labelled phase I/II trial we tested efficacy and tolerability of IL-3. 15 patients, *i.e.* 7 male, 8 female, 13-40 years old with idiopathic (12 patients) or secondary (3 patients) refractory or relapsed SAA were included. IL-3 was given at 5 escalating dose levels of 1, 2, 4, 8 and 16 (g/kg/d as a continuous infusion for 21 days. IL- 3 was prematurely withdrawn in 2 patients for adverse events. Nine of 15 patients showed an increase in leukocytes; 2/6 at the 1-2 (g/kg level, 7/9 at the 4-16 (g/kg level. Increase in leukocytes was dose dependent and transient in all patients. No patient showed a response in platelet or reticulocyte counts or a change in transfusion requirements. We failed to repeat the previously described erythroid or megakaryocytic response. Occurence of side effects was dose dependent and dose limiting at 8 (g/kg. Anti IL-3 antibodies were detected in 5/9 patients given 4-16 µg/kg [23]. This study indicates that IL-3 as single growth factor is of minimal benefit in patients with refractory SAA and is in line with the report of Nimer *et al*, showing also a dose dependent neutrophil response [24].

Few case reports have appeared with combined treatment of IL-3 and GM-CSF or G-CSF. Most patients were pretreated with ALG and or combined with cyclosporin, rendering interpretation difficult. It remains open whether IL-3 might sensitize response to G-CSF as has been postulated in a case report [25].

IL-3 is integrated in the German multicenter protocol for patients with refractory or relapsed SAA. Previous non responders to G-CSF will be treated with cyclosporin and IL-3 at a dose of 5 (g/kg/d. No data are yet available. (Coordinator: Dr A Raghavachar, Ulm)

IL-6

IL-6 is a maturational stimulator of megakaryocytopoiesis and increases platelet counts in normal individuals. IL-6 was assessed in a two center open labelled phase I/II trial for its efficacy and safety in SAA. 11 patients with refractory or relapsed SAA either acquired (10 patients) or Fanconi's SAA were treated with 0.5, 1, 2.5 and 5 (g/kg/d s.c. for 28 days for 1 or 2 cycles. One of the 11 patients showed a sustained increase in platelet counts from 18 to 72 x 10 9/l. Bleeding occured in 4 patients and caused premature discontinuation of IL-6 therapy in 3 patients. 9/11 patients showed a deterioration of their preexisting anemia. No changes were observed in leukocyte counts during the first cycle. Peripheral blood monocyte counts dropped significantly during th second cycle. Lack of response and side effects caused premature closure of this study [26]. There are few other reports of the use of IL-6 in patients with SAA. To our knowledge no current clinical protocol investigates the role of IL-6 alone or in combination in patients with SAA.

SCF

SCF acts on a very early level of the human hematopoietic precursor cells. It has been shown that some patients with SAA have low serum levels of SCF.Potentially , treatment with SCF could be of benefit to a subgroup of patients with SAA. A current phase I/II trial investigates the role of SCF in patients with refractory or relapsed SAA. Increasing doses of SCF of 5, 10, 15, 20, 25, 35 (g/kg /d s.c. for 28 days x 2 are given. SCF is well tolerated at dose levels up to 20 (g/kg. No information is yet available concerning therapeutic efficacy. (Contact in Europe. A Gratwohl, Basel).

Toxicities

All hematopoietic growth factors are potent drugs with substantial side effects. Toxicities observed in SAA patients are not different from those seen in other patient categories with some exceptions. Particular problems relating to SAA patients can be summarized as follows. Local reactions at the injection site of s.c. injections such as bleeding, infections or cytokine release associated pustular eruptions can lead to severe systemic disease in SAA patients. Careful observation and stringent techniques are required.

The potential hypertension following Epo administration could be an excessive risk in thrombopenic SAA patients. no intracerebral bleeding in such a patient has yet been reported. Splenic infarction following Epo administration to a patient with SAA has been described [28]. It might be an isolated event.

GM-CSF, IL-3 and IL-6 induce secondary cytokine release. Vascular damage with thromboembolic complications, vascular endothelial leakeage with diffuse hemorrhages into the tissue have been reported at higher doses. This fits with observations of hemophagocytosis in bone marrow specimens in patients treated with IL-3 [29, 30]. Sweet's syndrome, as reported in one patient with SAA might also be the consequence of cytokine release [31].

Paradoxically, given to reduce complications of pancytopenia, some growth factors mainly IL-3 and IL-6 can reduce circulating platelet counts, increase the risk of bleeding and aggravate anemia [26]. One major late event of SAA treated with immunosuppression is developement of late clonal complications. Emergence of acute leukemia follwoing trreatment with G-CSF has been reported [32, 33]. It remains to be evaluated in prospective trials whether the incidence of such clonal evolutions is increased by the use of growth factors.

The greatest risk is induced if patients are treated with growth factors alone and specific treatment is withheld or delayed because of a transient response to growth factors [3]. There is no evidence that they can correct the underlying defect of the hemopoietic precursor cells or of the autoimmune component of the disease.

Discussion

SAA is not due to a deficiency of any known hematopoietic growth factor. Most patients have high circulating concentrations of factors such as G-CSF, GM-CSF and Epo. Aplastic marrow stromal cells release normal or increased amounts of G-CSF, GM-CSF and IL-6 and mRNA expression of these factors including IL-1 and SCF are normal, increased or in few patients only decreased [1-3]. No distinct pattern of growth factor deficiency is recognized in SAA. In principle, from a pathophysiological point of view, no basic change could be expected from exogenously administered growth factors.

Nevertheless, growth factors have been tried and continue to be given in an attempt to increase peripheral blood values, reduce the risk of pancytopenia and eventually alter the course of the disease. So far, in most patients with SAA treated with G-, GM-CSF or IL-3 a transient increase in neutrophil counts is observed the extent of the rise being proportional to the amount of residual myelopoiesis. Side effects in addition and of IL-6 can be serious. There is no clear evidence yet, despite the claims of several case reports, that hematopoietic growth factors have changed the course of the disease. The promising results of some pilot studies, however, justify the ongoing and planned randomized studies.

In summary, the currently available recombinant human hematopoietic growth factors are fascinating tools to investigate regulation of hematopoiesis and promising agents to improve outcome of patient with SAA. Despite almost a decade of investigations, clear answers are lacking. The recommendations of the Working Party SAA of the EBMT can only be reiterated. Patients with newly diagnosed SAA should not be treated with growth factors outside of a clinical protocol. Such protocols designed to assess the role of hematopoietic growth factors are still urgently needed. Inappropriate use of growth factors could reduce the excellent chance of long term cure after transplantation or delay the administsration of effective immunosuppressive therapy. In contrast, well designed clinical trials will allow us to establish the role of hematopoietic growth factors and their combination and further improve the current results.

References

1. Young NS, Alter BP. Aplastic anemia: Acquired and inherited. WB Saunders, Philadelphia, 1994
2. Young NS, Barrett AJ. The treatment of severe acquired aplastic anemia. *Blood* 1995 (in press)
3. Marsh JC, Socie G, Schrezenmeier H, Tichelli A, Gluckman E, Ljungman P, McCann SR, Raghavachar A, Marin P, Hows JM, *et al*. Haemopoietic growth factors in aplastic anaemia: a cautionary note. European Bone Marrow Transplant Working Party for Severe Aplastic Anaemia. *Lancet* 1994; 344: 172-173
4. Gratwohl A, Hermans J. Bone marrow transplant activity in 1993. *Clinical transplants* 1995 (in press)
5. Bacigalupo A, Chaple M, Hows J, McCann S, Milligan D, Chessels J, Goldstone AH. Treatment of aplastic anemia with antilymphocyte globulin and methylprednisolone with or without androgens. *Blood* 1992; 80337-80345

6. Tichelli A, Gratwohl A, Nissen C, Signer E, Stebler Gysi Ch, Speck B. Morphology in patients with severe aplastic anemia with antilymphocyte globulin and methylprednisolone with or without androgens. A randomised EBMT study. *Br J Haematol* 1993; 83: 145
7. Gordon-Smith EC, Yandle A, Milne A, Speck B, Marmont A, Willemze R, Kolb H. Randomised placebo controlled study of Rh-GM-CSF following ALG in the treatment of aplastic anaemia. *Bone Marrow Transplant* 1991; 7 (Suppl 2): 78-80
8. Yoshida Y, Anzai N, Kawabata H, Kohsaka Y, Okuma M. Serial changes in endogenous erythropoietin levels in patients with myelodysplastic syndromes and aplastic anemia undergoing erythrpoietin treatment. *Ann Hematol* 1993; 66: 175-180
9. Stebler C, Tichelli A, Dazzi H, Gratwohl A, Nissen C, Speck B. High dose recombinant human erythropoietin for treatment of anemia in myelodysplastic syndromes and paroxysmal nocturnal hemoglobinuria: a pilot study. *Exp Hematol* 1990; 18: 1204-1208
10. Champlin RE, Nimer SD, Ireland P Oette DH, Golde DW. Treatment of refractory aplastic anemia with recombinant human granulocyte macrophage colony stimulating factor. *Blood* 1989; 73: 694-99
11. Nissen C, Tichelli A, Gratwohl A, Speck B, Milne A, Gordon-Smith EC, Schädelin J. Failure of recombinant human Granulocyte macrophage colony-stimulating factor therapy in aplastic anemia patients with very severe neutropenia. *Blood* 1988; 72: 2045-2047
12. Doney K, Storb R, Appelbaum FR, Buckner CD, Sanders J, Singer J, Hansen JA. Recombinant granulocyte-macrophage colony stimulating factor followed by immunosuppressive therapy for aplastic anaemia. *Br J Haematol* 1993; 85: 182-184
13. Kurzrock R, Talpaz M, Gutterman JU. Very low doses of GM-CSF administered alone or with erythropoietin in aplastic anemia. *Am J Med* 1992; 93: 41-48
14. Khan MA, Hameed A, Tahir M, Gandapur AJ, Rehman HU, Durrani FM, Ahmad A. Haemopoietic growth factor GM-CSF for aplastic anaemia in children (letter). *Lancet* 1995; 345: 199
15. Kojima S, Fukuda M, Miyajima Y, Matsuyama T, Horibe K. Treatment of aplastic anemia in children with recombinant human granulocyte colony-stimulating factor. *Blood* 1991; 77: 937-941
16. Bacigalupo A, Broccia G, Corda G, Arcese W, Carotenuto M, Gallamini A, Locatelli F, ori PG, Saracco P, Todeschini A, Coser P, Iacopino P, van Lint MT, Gluckman E. Antilymphocyte globulin, cyclosporin and granulocyte colony stimulating factor in patients with acquired severe aplastic anemia: A pilot study of the EBMT SAA working party. *Blood* 1995 (in press)
17. Imashuku S, Akiyama Y, Nakajiama F, Hibi S, Oguni T, Koike M. Multilineage response to G-CSF in pediatric aplastic anemia. *Lancet* 1994; 344: 1236-1237
18. Bessho M, Toyoda A, Itoh Y, Sakata T, Kawai N, Jinnai I, Saito M, Hirashima K. Trilineage recovery by combination therapy with recombinant human granulocyte colony-stimulating factor (rhG-CSF) and erythropoietin (rhEpo) in severe aplastic anaemia. *Br J Haematol* 1992; 80: 409-411
19. Takahashi M, Aoki A, Mito M, Nikkuni K, Ohtsuka T, Saitoh H, Moriyama Y, Shibata A. Combination therapy with rhGM-CSF and rhEpo for two patients with refractory anemia and aplastic anemia. *Hematol Pathol* 1993; 153-158.
20. Weide R, Lyttelton M, Samson D, Gorg C, Koppler H, Pfluger KH, Havemann K. Sustained trilineage response in a patient with ALG-resistant severe aplastic anaemia after treatment with G-CSF, erythropoietin and cyclosporin A: Association of recovery with marked elevation of serum alkaline phosphatase. *Br J Haematol* 1993; 85: 608-610
21. Nawata J, Toyoda Y, Nisihira H, Honda K, Kigasawa H, Nagao T. Hacmatological improvement by long-term administration of recombinant human granulocyte-colony stimulating factor and recombinant human erythropoietin in a patient with severe aplastic anaemia. *Eur J Pediatr* 1994; 153: 325-327
22. Ganser A, Lindemann A, Seipelt G, Ottmann OG, Eder M, Falk S, Herrmann F, Kaltwasser JP, Meusers P, Klausmann M, Frisch J, Schulz G, Mertelsmann R, Hoelzer D. Effects of recombinant human interleukin-3 in aplastic anemia. *Blood* 1990; 76: 1287-1292
23. Bargetzi M, Gluckman E, Tichelli A, Devergie A, Esüperou H, Kabata J, Nissen C, Speck B, Gratwohl A. Recombinant human interleukin-3 in refractory severe aplastic anemia: A phase I/II trial. *Bone Marrow Transplant* 1995 (in press)
24. Nimer SD, Paquette RL, Ireland P, Resta D, Young D, Golde DW. A phase I/II study of interleukin-3 in patients with aplastic anemia and myelodysplasia. *Exp Hematol* 1994; 22: 875-880

25. Schleuning M, Thomssen C, Kolb HJ, Sauer HJ, Wilmanns W. Treatment of refractory severe aplastic anemia with granulocyte colony stimulating factor and interleukin 3 (letter). *Am J Hematol* 1994; 46: 250-251
26. Schrezenmeier H, Marsh J, Stromeyer P, Heimpel H, Gordon-Smith EC, Raghavachar A. A phase I/II trial of recombinant human interleukin-6 in patients with aplastic anemia. *Blood* 1995 (in press)
27. Wodnar-Filipowicz A, Tichelli A, Zsebo KM, Speck B, Nissen C. Stem cell factor stimulates the *in vitro* growth of bone marrow cells from aplastic anemia patients. *Blood* 1992; 79: 3196-3202
28. Imashuku S, Nakagawa Y, Hibi S. Splenic infarction after erythropoietin therapy (letter). *Lancet* 1993; 342: 182-183
29. Herrmann F, Lindemann A, Lange W, Kochling G, Raghavachar A, Schrezenmeier H, Frickhofen N, Mertelsmann RH. Medullary histiocytosis following treatment of severe aplastic anemia with recombinant human interleukin-3 in combination with methylprednisolone. *Ann Hematol* 1991; 63: 229-231
30. Nachbaur D, Gratwohl A, Herold M, Tichelli A, Slanicka M, Nissen C, Niederwieser D, Speck B. Cytokine serum levels during treatment with high-dose recombinant human IL-3 in a patient with severe aplastic anemia. *Ann Hematol* 1993; 66: 71-75
31. Fukutoku M, Shimizu S, Ogawa Y, Takeshita S, Masaki Y, Arai T, Hirose Y, Sugai S, Konda S, Takiguchi T. Sweet's syndrome during therapy with granulocyte colony-stimulating factor in a patient with aplastic anaemia. *Br J Haematol* 1994; 86: 645-648
32. Kojima S, Tsuchida M, Matsuyama T. Myelodysplasia and leukemia after treatment of aplastic anemia with G-CSF (letter). *N Engl J Med* 1992; 326: 1294-1295
33. Izumi T, Muroi K, Takatoku M, Imagawa S, Hatake K, Miura Y. Development of acute myeloblastic leukaemia in a case of aplastic anaemia treated with granulocyte colony-stimulating factor. *Br J Haematol* 1994; 87: 666-668

Résumé

Les complications infectieuses et hémorragiques sont les principales causes de mort chez les malades atteints d'aplasie médullaire. Plusieurs facteurs de croissance hématopoïétiques sont actuellement disponibles pour la clinique: l'érythropoïétine, (Epo), le facteur stimulant les colonies de granulocytes et de macrophages (GM-CSF), le facteur stimulant les colonies de granuleux (G-CSF), les interleukines-1,-3,et -6 (IL-1, IL-3, IL-6) et, plus récemment, le *stem cell factor* (SCF) et la thrombopoïétine (MPL). Ils sont utilisés dans les aplasies médullaires dans le but d'améliorer la numération, de diminuer les complications cliniques de la pancytopénie et, éventuellement, de stimuler les cellules souches hématopoïétiques. Malgré de nombreux articles, les résultats sont loin d'être concluants. Le G-CSF et le GM-CSF ont été les plus utilisés. Tous les deux induisent une réponse transitoire dépendante de la dose chez les malades les moins graves chez lesquels une hématopoïèse résiduelle persiste, mais ils ne produisent qu'une réponse limitée chez les malades les plus graves. Le G-CSF pourrait induire une réponse sur les 3 lignées après un traitement prolongé, son rôle est actuellement à l'étude dans une étude européene prospective randomisée. L'IL-3 peut entraîner une augmentation transitoire des neutrophiles , mais aucune réponse des autres lignées n'a été observée; l'IL-6 n'a pas d'effet et aggrave l'anémie et la thrombopénie. L'érythropoïétine peut réduire les besoins transfusionnels dans un petit groupe de patients atteints de complications clonales tardives, avec des taux bas d'érythropoïétine. Aucun résultat n'est actuellement disponible sur le SCF et la thrombopoïétine.

Des associations de facteurs de croissance, surtout Epo et G-CSF, sont actuellement à l'étude mais aucune étude prospective randomisée n'a été publiée. Devant cette absence de preuve d'efficacité de ces traitements, il n'est pas recommandé de les utiliser en dehors d'études cliniques contrôlées.

The role of cytokines in the pathogenesis and treatment of aplastic anemia and myelodysplastic syndromes

Stephen D. Nimer

Memorial Sloan-Kettering Cancer Center, 1275 York Avenue, Box 575, New York, NY 10021, USA, tel.: (212) 639 7871, fax: (212) 794 5849

Summary

Cytokine production has been studied more extensively in patients with aplastic anemia than in patients with MDS. Abnormalities in lymphocyte populations and cytokine generation are seen in AA, consistent with the idea that immunologic suppression of hematopoiesis plays a critical role in the pathogenesis of this disease. In contrast, MDS generally presents as a stem cell disorder, often times with identifiable clonal population(s) of hematopoietic progenitor cells. Our current laboratory investigations of cytokine abnormalities in AA do not permit us to rationally choose initial therapy (immunosuppressive therapy vs. BMT), but perhaps someday this will be possible.

The defects in both AA and MDS are complex, and thus far are not corrected by cytokine administration. Many patients do have populations of cytokine responsive progenitors that can be stimulated, at least transiently, to produce mature effector cells such as neutrophils, and occasionally erythrocytes or platelets. Although cytokine therapy has not been very effective in patients who have failed immunosuppressive therapy, cytokines may have greater activity if used earlier in the course of the disease. The judicious use of cytokines in AA or MDS may be helpful in certain circumstances; in general their use should be restricted to well designed clinical trials.

Aplastic anemia and myelodysplastic syndromes

The most common causes of primary bone marrow failure are aplastic anemia and myelodysplastic syndromes. Both result in peripheral blood cytopenias although the bone marrow morphologies in these two conditions are usually distinct. A variety of therapeutic advances have significantly changed the prognosis for patients with aplastic anemia [1, 2] whereas most patients with myelodysplasia continue to receive predominantly supportive rather than definitive or potentially curative therapies. The role of cytokine abnormalities in the pathogenesis of these diseases and the results of cytokine trials in the treatment of these disorders will be discussed.

Aplastic anemia

Aplastic anemia (AA) can be stratified into moderately severe, severe or very severe based upon the peripheral blood counts, which has both prognostic and therapeutic significance [3]. The diagnosis of aplastic anemia is usually straightforward, but other disorders such as myelodysplasia, paroxysmal nocturnal hemoglobinuria or acute leukemia must also be thoughtfully considered. The underlying etiology of most cases of aplastic anemia is unknown but even in situations where an offending or triggering agent can be implicated, such as post-hepatitis virus infection or following drug exposure, only a subset of the individuals at risk develop aplastic anemia.

The immune mediated suppression of hematopoiesis, that can be implicated in the majority of aplastic anemia patients, may have a genetic basis. Several studies, from Switzerland, Japan, England, and the U.S., have suggested an association of aplastic anemia with the HLA DR2 phenotype [4-7]. We examined the incidence of HLA-DR2 positivity in 75 patients with aplastic anemia and observed a ~1.9 fold greater than expected incidence (P<0.0005) [6]. The presence of HLA DR2 (which is now serologically split into DR15 and DR16) has been suggested to predict for a response to immunosuppressive therapy, such as ATG or cyclosporin A, although this correlation was not seen in our study, which examined a more ethnically heterogeneous group of patients. 33 of the 37 patients who received immunotherapy (usually ATG alone) were evaluable for a response and response rates were equivalent in the DR2+ and DR2- patients (50% vs. 36.8%, p = .50). In contrast to these results, the response rate to cyclosporin A (CsA) in a group of 15 Japanese patients with AA was strongly dependent on the DR2 status of the patient [5]. This data suggests that ATG and CsA may work via different mechanisms, as does the increased response rate to ATG and CsA compared to either agent alone [8]. A specific HLA haplotype (DRB1*1501-DQA1*0102-DQB1*0602) is consistently seen in Japanese patients whose hematopoiesis is dependent on continuous cyclosporin A administration [9]. The genetic component to the hematopoietic responses seen in aplastic anemia could relate to differences in the etiology or the pathogenesis of this disease. A better understanding of the genetic component of this disease may lead to a more informed choice of therapy.

The efficacy of immunosuppressive or immunomodulatory agents in treating aplastic anemia, and several decades of *in vitro* studies of hematopoiesis in AA patients, have identified the presence of cells and/or cytokines that inhibit hematopoiesis in AA. A variety of lymphocyte populations capable of *in vitro* suppression of hematopoiesis have been identified in the peripheral blood of patients with aplastic anemia. The phenotype of these cells is often that of activated suppressor cells (*i.e.* they are CD8+,HLA-DR+,Tac+) [10], although other phenotypes have also been reported. Numerous studies have examined the production of stimulatory or inhibitory lymphokines by lymphocytes from aplastic anemia patients. Production of positive acting hematopoietic growth factors by peripheral blood lymphocytes or mononuclear cells has generally been normal or elevated [11-15], except for deficient production of IL-1 [16-17]. We examined granulocyte-macrophage colony-stimulating factor (GM-CSF) production in 29 patients with AA; GM-CSF was secreted by PHA-stimulated lymphocytes in 28 of 29 AA patients [13]. The amount of GM-CSF produced was similar in the AA patients and the normal controls. GM-CSF was not detected in the serum of six AA patients, using a sensitive radio immunoassay, but GM-CSF is not normally detectable in serum.

Enhanced production of inhibitory molecules such as interferon-γ, (IFN-γ) or tumor necrosis factor (TNFα), by lectin activated lymphocytes from AA patients has been demonstrated *in vitro* and elevated circulating levels of γ-IFN has also been reported [18-21]. Despite some controversy about whether γ-IFN is a marker of immune activation or is the suppressor of hematopoietic interferon-γ is being increasingly implicated in the pathogenesis of the cytopenias seen in this disease [20].

Serum levels of cytokines produced by "stromal" cells in the bone marrow microenvironment have also been examined. Although bone marrow levels of stem cell factor (SCF, kit ligand, mast cell growth factor), an early acting HGF produced by a variety of mesenchymal cells including bone marrow stromal cells has not been examined, serum levels of SCF have been found to be slightly but significantly lower than normal in patients with AA [22, 23]. Serum SCF levels did not correlate with the duration or severity of the aplastic anemia, and SCF serum levels are similarly decreased in patients with MDS. Clinical trials of SCF in patients with AA are ongoing.

ATG

Anti-thymocyte globulin (ATG) has been used to treat aplastic anemia for greater than 10 years and numerous clinical trials have demonstrated a response rate of approximately 50% [24, 25]. This response rate can be improved upon by the addition of cyclosporin but overall survival may not be improved, except in patients with very severe AA, who tend not to respond to ATG alone [8]. A randomized study from France compared the use of cyclosporine and prednisone to ATG therapy and found them to be equivalent [26]. Although commonly referred to as immunosuppressive therapy, it is not clear that the effectiveness of these agents relates solely to their immunosuppressive properties. Corticosteroids and monoclonal antibodies directed against human T cells, though immunosuppressive, are ineffective treatments in aplastic anemia.

In the French randomized trial, some patients who failed to respond to ATG responded to CsA, and vice versa, suggesting that at least in some patients these agents may restore hematopoiesis by different mechanisms [26]. Although both are referred to as immunosuppressive therapy, ATG has been shown to have immunostimulatory effects, stimulating thymidine uptakes, IL-2 secretion and the production of GM-CSF and IL-3 by T cells. In contrast, CsA inhibits the expression of these cytokines, at least in part by interfering with the formation of the NF-AT (nuclear factor-activated T cells) transcription factor [27]. A variety of factors have been examined for their ability to predict for a clinical response to ATG therapy including the duration of aplastic anemia, disease severity, the presence of bone marrow inflammatory cells, or the *in vitro* production of γ-interferon [18]. None of these factors have consistently correlated with a response to ATG at multiple institutions, except for the severity of neutropenia, which also correlates with long term survival [28].

A response to ATG typically takes 8-12 weeks, during which time significant morbidity or mortality may occur, primarily related to infectious complications. The use of G-CSF during this period, to decrease the risk of serious infections, has recently been reported by the European BMT SAA working group [29]. Forty patients with SAA received G-CSF, ATG and cyclosporin A in this very encouraging study. These patients had a high response rate (82%), low early mortality (8%) and excellent survival thus far. Many centers are exploring the addition of G-CSF to ATG alone, CsA alone or ATG and CsA, to reduce early mortality due to infection.

Clinical trials of CSFs

Recombinant hematopoietic growth factors have been used in aplastic anemia patients 1) who fail to respond to immunosuppressive therapy, 2) as an adjunct to immunosuppressive therapy to hasten blood count recovery, 3) for patients with frequent or severe recurrent bacterial infections, and 4) in the management of patients with sepsis, in addition to antibiotics and other supportive measures. Numerous trials have examined the ability of GM-CSF, granulocyte-CSF (G-CSF) or interleukin-3 (IL-3) to stimulate hematopoiesis in patients with aplastic anemia [30-34]. Although most patients will have an increase in the number of circulating neutrophils while on G-CSF or GM-CSF therapy, neither of these cytokines, consistently increases platelet counts or hemoglobin levels.

We recently reported a phase I/II trial of the multilineage colony-stimulating factor rhIL-3, given for 21 days as a subcutaneous injection at a dose of 0.5, 1.25, 2.5, 5.0 or 10 µg/kg/d to 21 patients with severe aplastic anemia or myelodysplastic syndrome (MDS) [34]. Patients with aplastic anemia were required to have failed ATG and be ineligible for, or refuse bone marrow transplantation, and have an absolute neutrophil count < 1,000/mL, or a platelet count < 50,000/mL, or a hemoglobin < 10 gm/dL. Patients with MDS were required to have < 20% blasts in the bone marrow and an absolute neutrophil count < 1500/mL, or a platelet count < 50,000/mL, or a hemoglobin < 10 gm/dL. A single dose escalation was possible for non-responding patients receiving less than 10 µg/kg/d, and responding patients could receive multiple cycles of IL-3, each cycle consisting of 21 days of therapy and 10-14 days of washout.

IL-3 was administered according to this schedule for up to nine months in some patients and 19 patients completed at least one 21 day cycle of IL-3. Frequent toxicities of IL-3 included headache, low grade fever, and erythema at the injection site; at higher doses weight gain and peripheral edema was seen. Of the twenty evaluable patients, eight had increases in absolute neutrophil counts (seven patients with MDS, one with AA) including six of the nine patients receiving ≥ 5.0 µg/kg/day. One AA patient became transfusion independent for eight months, while another AA patient had decreased transfusion requirements. Three patients with MDS had at least a doubling of their platelet count and one patient with AA experienced a 1.9-fold increase in platelet count (24,000 to 42,000/ml). Eleven patients developed eosinophilia. One patient with RAEB progressed to aleukemic AML by the end of one treatment cycle. Interleukin-3 was reasonably well-tolerated but multilineage effects were seen in only 25% of patients with primary bone marrow failure states (5 of 20 evaluable), more commonly in patients with MDS. The optimal use IL-3 may be as part of combination hematopoietic growth factor therapy.

Of these three cytokines (GM-CSF, G-CSF and IL-3) G-CSF administration may be associated with a higher incidence of multilineage response. Although multilineage effects have been seen with G-CSF administration, many additional patients must be studied to confirm this effect. The effects of growth factor therapy are transient, and blood counts rapidly return to baseline once the cytokine therapy is stopped. Thus, unlike ATG or cyclosporine, the CSFs do not alter the underlying pathogenesis of this disease. There are also several reports of patients who received IL-3, who later acquired responsiveness to GM-CSF [35]; the basis of this effect is not known. Few patients have had a multilineage response to the CSFs and patients with very severe AA tend not to respond to growth factor therapy. The role of newer cytokines, such as recombinant human stem cell factor (SCF), a growth factor with potentially trilineage hematopoietic stimulatory capability, or the recently cloned thrombopoietin, a glycoprotein that stimulates platelet production in mice and non-human primates, remains to be determined. Combinations of cytokines are being evaluated in clinical trials.

Myelodysplastic syndromes (MDS)

The number of patients with MDS appears to be increasing. Although most cases are idiopathic, exposure to toxins such as benzene, or to chemotherapy and radiation can lead to MDS, usually referred to as secondary or treatment-related MDS (t-MDS). The clinical course of MDS is highly variable, but is typically characterized by progressive refractory anemia, thrombocytopenia, and/or granulocytopenia lasting for several years. Some patients will present without symptoms and will require no therapy. Other patients will present with signs or symptoms related to their cytopenias and will have a rapidly progressing disease. For these patients, frequent RBC and platelet transfusions may be required to ameliorate symptoms of anemia and avoid bleeding.

Therapy for MDS has been generally unsatisfactory. Transfusions of RBCs and platelets are palliative at best and alloimmunization can greatly reduce the efficacy of platelet transfusions. Based upon *in vitro* culture data, a variety of potential myeloid differentiating agents have been tried in MDS patients, however they have not shown much efficacy. More recent trials of differentiating agents, such as hexamethylene bisacetamide (HMBA) or 5-Azacytidine have shown some activity in MDS although further studies are needed. Combination differentiation therapy trials (with or without CSFs) are being initiated at several centers.

Hematopoietic growth factors have been used in clinical trials to ameliorate cytopenias in patients with MDS. Both G-CSF and GM-CSF can raise total leukocyte counts (particularly neutrophils), but they have little effect on platelet counts or red blood cell production. IL-3 has more modest effects on neutrophil numbers, but increases in platelet counts and red blood cell production have been seen in some patients. There is little evidence that these agents can stimulate differentiation of immature hematopoietic cells. Several patients with >15% blasts have progressed to acute leukemia while on CSF therapy, which may or may not simply reflect the natural progression of this disease.

We administered interleukin-6 (IL-6), a pleiotropic cytokine involved in numerous physiological processes related to host defense, to patients with MDS in a phase I/II trial, with variable hematologic responses [36]. Twenty-two patients with MDS, a platelet count < 100,000/ml, and <5% bone marrow (BM) blasts received one of four doses of IL-6 (1.0, 2.5, 3.75, and 5.0 µg/kg/day) as a subcutaneous injection on day 1, followed by a seven day wash-out period, and then received 28 days of IL-6 therapy. Dose-limiting toxicities of fatigue, fever, and elevated alkaline phosphatase were seen at 5.0 µg/kg/day; the maximum tolerated dose was 3.75 µg/kg/day, much lower than the dose tolerated by patients with solid tumors. All patients experienced at least grade II fever and all had an increase in acute phase proteins. Other side effects included cutaneous erythema and/or rash, edema and weight gain, and alterations in serum proteins and cholesterol.

Eight patients experienced at least a transient improvement in platelet counts; three (14%) fulfilled the criteria for response, while five others had clinically significant rises which failed to meet response criteria. Various IL-6-related toxicities prevented more than three patients from receiving maintenance. Two of the three patients who received maintenance IL-6 therapy had a persistent increase in platelet counts during 3 and 12 months of IL-6 therapy, respectively. Laboratory studies indicated that IL-6 increased the frequency of higher ploidy megakaryocytes but did not significantly increase the number of assayable megakaryocytic progenitor cells, suggesting that IL-6 acts as a maturational agent rather than a megakaryocyte CSF. Patient characteristics that could predict a response to IL-6 were not identified, although patients who had more than a transient response to IL-6 had relatively normal levels of CFU-MK. Although IL-6 therapy can promote thrombopoiesis in some MDS patients, its limited activity and significant therapy-related toxicity preclude its use as a single agent in this patient population. We have not used IL-6 in patients with AA because of its effects as an immune activator, which could potentially worsen the disease. IL-1 has been given to AA patients, but it was very poorly tolerated [37].

References

1. Bacigalupo A, Hows J, Gluckman *et al*. Bone marrow transplantation versus immunosuppression for the treatment of severe aplastic anemia; a report of the EBMT SAA working party. *Br J Haematol* 1988; 70: 177-82.
2. Paquette RL, Tebyani N, Frane M, *et al*. Long-term outcome of aplastic anemia in adults treated with antithymocyte globulin: comparison with bone marrow transplantation. *Blood* 1995; 85: 283-290.
3. Camitta BM, Thomas ED, Nathan DG, *et al*. Severe aplastic anemia: a prospective study of the effect of early marrow transplantation on acute mortality. *Blood* 1976; 48: 63-9.
4. Chapuis B, Von Fliedner VE, Jeannet M *et al*. Increased frequency of DR2 in patients with aplastic anemia and increased DR sharing in their parents. *Br J Haematol* 1986; 63: 51-57.
5. Nakao S, Yamaguchi M, Yasue S *et al*. HLA-DR2 predicts a favorable response to cyclosporine therapy in patients with bone marrow failure. *Am J of Hematology* 1992; 40: 239.
6. Nimer SD, Ireland P, Meshkinpour A, and Frane M. An increased HLA DR2 frequency is seen in aplastic anemia patients. *Blood* 1994; 84: 923-927.
7. Rigman FP, Ashby D, Davies JM. Does HLA-DR predict response to specific immunosuppressive therapy in aplastic anemia? *Br J of Haematol* 1990; 74: 545-546.
8. Frickhofen N, Kaltwasser JP, Schrezenmeier *et al*. Treatment of aplastic anemia with antilymphocyte globulin and methylprednisolone with or without cyclosporin. *N Engl J Med* 1991; 324: 1297-130.
9. Nakao S, Takamatsu H, Chuhjo T, *et al*. Identification of a specific HLA class II haplotype strongly associated with susceptibility to cyclosporine-dependent aplastic anemia. *Blood* 1994; 84: 4257-4261.
10. Zoumbos NC, Gascon P, Djeu JY, Trost SR, Young NS. Circulating activated suppressor T-lymphocyte in aplastic anemia. *N Engl J Med* 1985; 312: 257-265.
11. Gascon P, Zoumbos NC, Scala G *et al*. Lymphokine abnormalities in aplastic anemia: implications for the mechanism of action of anti-thymocyte globulin. *Blood* 1985; 65: 407-413.
12. Hinterberger W, Adolf G, Aichinger G, *et al*. Further evidence for lymphokine overproduction in severe aplastic anemia. *Blood* 1988; 72: 266-272.
13. Nimer SD, Golde DW, Kwan K, *et al*. In vitro production of granulocyte-macrophage colony-stimulating factor in aplastic anemia: possible mechanisms of action of antithymocyte globulin. *Blood* 1991; 78: 163-168.
14. Taniguchi Y, Frickhofen N, Raghavachar A, Digel W, Heimpel H. Antilymphocyte immunoglobulins stimulate peripheral blood lymphocytes to proliferate and release lymphokines. *Eur J Haematol* 1990; 44: 244-251.
15. Tong J, Bacigalupo A, Piaggio G, *et al*. In vitro response of T cells from aplastic anemia patients to antilymphocyte globulin and phytohemagglutinin: colony-stimulating activity and lymphokine production. *Exp Hematology* 1991; 19: 312-316.
16. Gascon P and Scala G. Decreased interleukin-1 production in aplastic anemia. *Am J of Med* 1988; 85: 668-700.
17. Nakao S, Matsushima K, Young N. Decreased interleukin-1 in aplastic anaemia. *Br Journal of Haematol* 1989; 71: 431-436.
18. Laver J, Castro-Malaspina H, Kernan N, *et al*. In-vitro interferon-gamma production by cultured T-cells in severe aplastic anemia: correlation with granulomonopoietic inhibition in patients who respond to anti-thymocyte globulin. *Br J Haematol* 1988; 69: 545-550.
19. Nakao S, Yamaguchi M, Shiobara S, *et al*. Interferon-γ gene expression in unstimulated bone marrow mononuclear cells predicts a good response to cyclosporine therapy in aplastic anemia. *Blood* 1992; 79: 2532-2535.
20. Nistico A, and Young NS. Gamma-interferon gene expression in the bone marrow of patients with aplastic anemia. *Ann Intern Med* 1994; 120;463-469.
21. Shinohara K, Ayame H, Tanaka M, *et al*. Increased production of tumor necrosis factor-a by peripheral blood mononuclear cells in the patients with aplastic anemia. *American Journal of Hematology* 1991; 37: 75-79.
22. Nimer SD, Leung DHY, Wolin MJ, and Golde DW. Serum stem cell factor levels in patients with aplastic anemia. *Int Journal of Hematology* 1994; 60: 185-189.
23. Wodnar-Filipowicz A, Yancik S, Moser Y, *et al*. Levels of soluble stem cell factor in serum of patients with aplastic anemia. *Blood* 1993; 81: 3259-3264.

24. Champlin R, Winston H, Gale RP. Antithymocyte globulin treatment in patients with aplastic anemia: a prospective randomized trial. *The New England Journal Of Medicine* 1983; 308: 113-118.
25. Young N, Griffith P, Brittain E, *et al*. A multicenter trial of antithymocyte globulin in aplastic anemia and related diseases. *Blood* 1988; 72: 1861-1869.
26. Gluckman E, Esperou-Bourdeau H, Baruchel A, *et al*, and the Cooperative Group on the Treatment of Aplastic Anemia. Multicenter randomized study comparing cyclosporine-A alone and antithymocyte globulin with prednisone for treatment of severe aplastic anemia. *Blood* 1992; 79: 2540-2546.
27. Emmel EA, Cornelis LV, Durand DB, *et al*. Cyclosporin A specifically inhibits function of nuclear proteins involved in T cell activation. *Science* 1989; 246: 1617-1620.
28. Marsh JCW, Hows JM, Bryett KA, *et al*. Survival after antilymphocyte globulin therapy for aplastic anemia depends on disease severity. *Blood* 1987; 70: 1046-1052.
29. Bacigalupo A, Broccia G, Corda G, *et al*. Antilymphocyte globulin, cyclosporin, and granulocyte colony-stimulating factor in patients with acquired severe aplastic anemia (SAA): a pilot study of the EBMT SAA working party. *Blood* 1995; 85: 1348-1353.
30. Champlin RE, Nimer SD, Ireland P, Oette D, Golde DW. Treatment of refractory aplastic anemia with recombinant human granulocyte-macrophage colony stimulating factor. *Blood* 1989; 73: 694-699.
31. Ganser A, Lindemann A, Seipelt G, *et al.* Effects of recombinant human interleukin-3 in aplastic anemia. *Blood* 1990; 76: 1287-1292.
32. Kojima S, Matsuyama T. Stimulation of granulopoiesis by high-dose recombinant human granulocyte colony-stimulating factor in children with aplastic anemia and very severe neutropenia. *Blood* 1994; 83: 1474-1478.
33. Kurzrock R, Talpaz M, Estrov Z, Rosenblum MG, and Gutterman JU. Phase I study of recombinant human interleukin-3 in patients with bone marrow failure. *J Clin Oncol* 1991; 9: 1241-1250.
34. Nimer SD, Paquette RL, Ireland P, *et al*. A phase I/II study of interleukin-3 in patients with aplastic anemia and myelodysplasia. *Exp Hematology* 1994; 22: 875-880.
35. Herrmann F, Lindemann A, Raghavachar A, Heimpel H, and Mertelsmann R. *In vivo* recruitment of GM-CSF-response myelopoietic progenitor cells by interleukin-3 in aplastic anemia. *Leukemia* 1990; 4: 671-672.
36. Gordon MS, Nemunaitis J, Hoffman R, *et al*. A phase I trial of recombinant human interleukin-6 in patients with myelodysplastic syndromes and thrombocytopenia. *Blood* (in press) 1995.
37. Walsh CE, Liu JM, Anderson SM, *et al*. A trial of recombinant human interleukin-1 in patients with severe refractory aplastic anaemia. *Br Journal of Haematol* 1992; 80: 106-110.

Résumé

La production de cytokines a été plus étudiée dans les aplasies que dans les myélodysplasies. Dans les aplasies, des anomalies des populations lymphocytaires et de la production de lymphokines sont un argument en faveur de l'origine autoimmune de la maladie. A l'inverse, la myélodysplasie est une maladie de la cellule souche, associée souvent à une ou des populations clonales de cellules souches hématopoïétiques. Les résultats actuels des explorations des anomalies des cytokines dans les aplasies médullaires ne permettent pas aujourd'hui de choisir de façon rationnelle entre un traitement par immunosuppresseurs et une greffe de moelle. Les anomalies observées à la fois dans les aplasies et les myélodysplasies sont très complexes et ne sont pas corrigées par l'administration de cytokines. Un grand nombre de patients ont des populations cellulaires comme les granuleux ou occasionnellement les globules rouges ou les plaquettes capables de répondre aux cytokines. Bien que le traitement par facteur de croissance n'ait pas été très efficace chez les patients n'ayant pas répondu aux traitements immunosuppresseurs, leur efficacité serait peut-être meilleure s'ils étaient utilisés plus tôt. On peut conclure que la place des facteurs de croissance hématopoïétiques dans le traitement des aplasies médullaires et des myélodysplasies n'est pas définie et que des études cliniques contrôlées sont encore nécessaires.

Molecular approaches to the treatment of Fanconi anemia

J.M. Liu

National Institutes of Health, Building 10 Acrf, Room 7C103, MD 20205 Bethesda, USA, tel.: (301) 496 5093, fax: (301) 496 8396

Summary

Fanconi anemia (FA) is a genetic syndrome manifested by bone marrow failure, physical anomalies, and cancer susceptibility. Marked by genotypic and phenotypic heterogeneity, FA consists of four distinct complementation groups: A, B, C, D. The defective gene responsible for the C group of FA, FACC, was identified by cDNA complementation cloning. The hallmark of the FA cell phenotype is extreme sensitivity to cross-linking agents such as mitomycin C (MMC), suggesting an inability to tolerate specific DNA damage. We have used two approaches to deduce the molecular function of the FACC polypeptide. First, we have over-expressed FACC in transgenic mice and in baculovirus-infected insect cells. Second, we have used recombinant viral vectors to transduce normal copies of the FACC cDNA to cell lines bearing FACC mutations. Phenotypic correction was demonstrated following viral transduction by resistance to MMC-induced cell death and insusceptibility to induced chromosomal aberrations. In conjunction with cell cycle analyses, our findings suggest that FACC is responsible for diminishing DNA damage prior to the G2 phase of the cell cycle. We next demonstrated that CD34-enriched hematopoietic progenitors isolated from FA patients exhibit the same hypersensitivity to MMC characteristic of cultured FA cells. Gene transduction of FA(C) progenitor cells using a viral vector containing the FACC cDNA significantly improved colony formation in clonogenic assays in the absence, as well as in the presence, of low dose MMC. Improved colony growth may reflect the genetic rescue of progenitor cells following transduction with the normal FACC cDNA. The two types of vectors we have used to transduce FACC are the Moloney retrovirus and the human adeno-associated virus (AAV). We demonstrated that an AAV vector carrying the FACC cDNA can mark human cord blood hematopoietic cells engrafted in SCID/hu mice. In addition, we documented retroviral-mediated transfer of the normal human FACC cDNA to long-term reconstituting stem cells of mice. Based on these preclinical studies, we have proposed a clinical trial of gene therapy for FA(C) patients. FA stem cells rescued by gene transduction should have a selective growth advantage within the hypoplastic FA marrow environment in vivo, suggesting a novel therapeutic approach to marrow reconstitution.

Bone marrow failure can result from genetic defects which arise from congenital or acquired etiologies [1]. The paradigm for constitutional bone marrow failure is Fanconi anemia (FA) [2]. FA is a heterogeneous genetic disorder characterized clinically by progressive bone marrow failure, congenital physical abnormalities, and a predisposition to malignancy. At the cellular level, the hallmark of the FA phenotype is hypersensitivity to DNA cross-linking agents resulting in chromosomal instability and cell death. Complementation of this cellular hypersensitivity was achieved by somatic cell fusion, studies which established that FA cell lines could be divided into four groups, termed A, B, C, and D [3]. Transfection of cDNAs from an expression library into a cell line from complementation group C led to the identification of the gene defect in group C cells [4]. This novel gene, termed FACC for Fanconi anemia C complementing, has a coding region of 1,677 basepairs. The 558 amino acid FACC protein has a molecular mass of 63kD and contains abundant hydrophobic amino acids. Sequence analysis has revealed no consensus motifs that would be informative of the protein's function. FACC maps to chromosome 9q and encodes a set of RNAs that share the same coding region but differ at both 5' and 3' untranslated regions. Mutational analysis of FACC has thus far identified six different disease-associated mutations constituting 10-15% of the patients and families tested [2].

Results

Development of a clinical protocol for gene therapy of FA

Although FA is known to be a heterogeneous disorder, the majority of patients will develop life-threatening hematologic disease [1]. Allogeneic bone marrow transplantation is limited to patients with an unaffected matched sibling donor. Consequently, rational therapies based on the molecular and cellular pathophysiology of FA are needed. We have approached the problem of FA therapy by direct gene complementation [5, 6]. Our studies have also shed light on the nature of the FA genetic defect.

Phenotypic correction of FA(C) hematopoietic cells. The hallmark of the FA cell phenotype is extreme sensitivity to cross-linking agents such as mitomycin C (MMC). FA cell lines were transduced by our FACC viral vectors and were distinguished by their ability to grow at concentrations of MMC several orders of magnitude higher than those concentrations inhibitory of parental controls [5, 6]. The genetically corrected cell lines were analyzed for susceptibility to MMC-induced chromosomal breakage and were found to have been normalized. These two different assays confirmed that our vectors were capable of transferring a functional FACC gene to lymphoid cell lines established from FA(C) patients.

Transduction and expression of FACC in FA(C) lymphoblasts. Transformed lymphoblast cell lines have been established from FA patients bearing mutant FACC alleles. Cell lines representing three different types of mutations were tested by functional complementation with the FACC retrovirus. The HSC 536 line carries a T-to-C transition at base 1,661 of the FACC open reading frame, resulting in an amino acid substitution of leucine$_{554}$ to proline (designated L554P) [4]. The PD-4L line carries a G deletion at nucleotide position 322 (designated ΔG322), causing a frameshift and a truncated message. We independently established the GM12794 line from the same FA(C) patient from whom PD-4L was derived. The BD0215 line contains a C-to-T nonsense mutation causing premature termination of translation at amino acid residue 185. We used these lines to test our retroviral vector [5]. Supernatant infections were performed with each FA(C) line, and neomycin-resistant pools of cells were derived. These transduced cells were then cultured in varying concentrations of MMC to determine sensitivity. As shown in Fig. 1A, all parental FA(C) lines were markedly sensitive to MMC with an EC_{50} of 0.5nM MMC. In contrast, gene-corrected cells were completely altered so that MMC sensitivity was equivalent to lymphoid cells established from a normal individual *(Figure 1B)*. Controls included a FA(C) cell line, GM 12794, which was transduced with a retroviral vector not including the FACC gene: these cells remained markedly sensitive to MMC. In addition, a transformed lymphoid line derived from a normal individual was not altered by transduction with the FACC retroviral vector.

Transduction of FA(C) $CD34^+$ hematopoietic progenitors. We next tested the FACC retroviral vector for the ability to transduce hematopoietic progenitors [5] from a patient bearing a splice mutation (IVS+4A→T) in the FACC gene. This patient had been maintained on G-CSF prior to leukapheresis. A total of 3×10^9 mononuclear cells were obtained by leukapheresis. Following immunoaffinity selection with an anti-CD34 antibody and column purification, 1.5×10^6 $CD34^-$ enriched cells were obtained. These were infected at a concentration of 1×10^5/ml with FACC viral supernatant, in a mixture with recombinant human interleukin-3, interleukin-6, stem cell factor, and protamine. Each day the cells were pelleted and resuspended in fresh supernatant and cytokines. Following infection, hematopoietic cells were plated in methylcellulose and varying concentrations of MMC to assay progenitor growth in the absence and presence of MMC. *Figure 2* shows the macroscopic appearance of progenitor colony growth in MMC. No colony growth was observed in the absence or presence of MMC. In contrast, progenitor cells transduced by the FACC retroviral vector led to markedly enhanced colony growth in the absence and presence of up to 5 nM MMC. The microscopic appearances of these colonies were suggestive of CFU-G or CFU-GM colonies.

FACC over-expression in mice and preclinical studies

Experiments with W/W^V mice. No animal model exists for FA. We have sought to study the effects of constitutive expression of FACC in a murine transplantation model [7]. Bone marrow cells from C57/BL6 mice were infected with the FACC vector by standard methods. $1-2 \times 10^6$ infected mononuclear cells were injected intravenously into eight female W/W^V recipient mice. We analyzed hemoglobin electrophoresis patterns from these transplanted mice 8 weeks after transplantation. All mice analyzed showed the donor pattern of hemoglobin electrophoresis, indicating successful engraftment. These animals remained healthy, with no evidence of deleterious effect, until sacrifice at 6 months. Blood counts were evaluated and found to be normal. We performed DNA analyses on peripheral blood of all animals at approximately 3.5 months following transplantation. Using primer pairs specific for the neomycin resistance gene, we detected proviral DNA by PCR in the peripheral blood cells of all seven animals tested. By using dilutions of peripheral blood DNA from marked animals with mouse DNA and comparing PCR signals to that generated from a transduced cell line, we estimated that most animals had between 10-30% of peripheral blood cells marked with the FACC retrovirus.

Experiments with non-ablated mice: repetitive infusions. Recent experiments have claimed high rates of engraftment of BALB/c marrow infused repetitively into BALB/c hosts. Based in part on these studies, we tested transduction of FACC into seven unprepared host BALB/c animals [7]. A total of $2-5 \times 10^6$ transduced donor bone marrow cells were infused via tail vein injection once every two weeks, for four total injections, into recipient male BALB/c mice. All animals remained healthy until sacrifice at approximately three months following infusion. On two occasions, peripheral blood DNAs were negative for proviral DNA at 30 and 35 cycles of PCR. However, following sacrifice, the bone marrow and spleen of the test and two control animals were dissected and analyzed by DNA PCR: the majority of the test marrow and spleen samples were marked by our FACC vector.

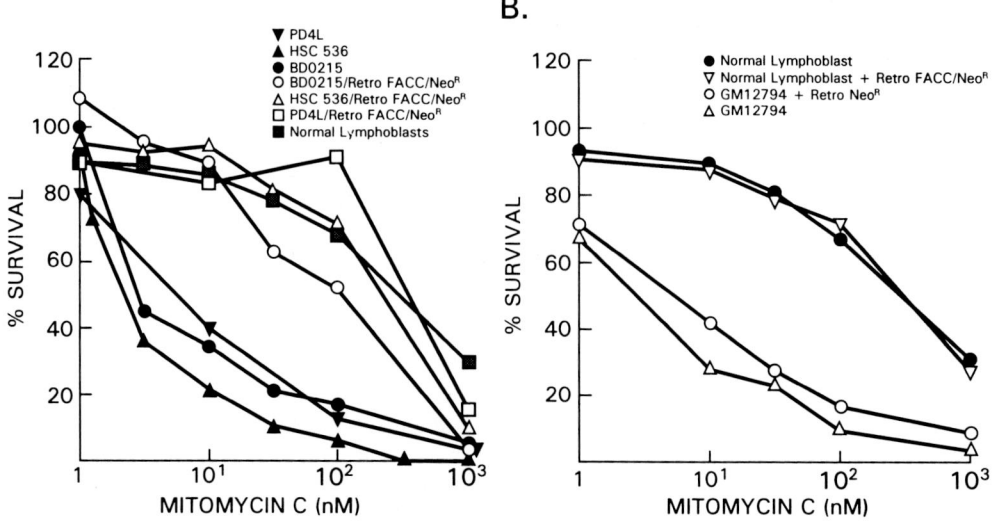

Figure 1

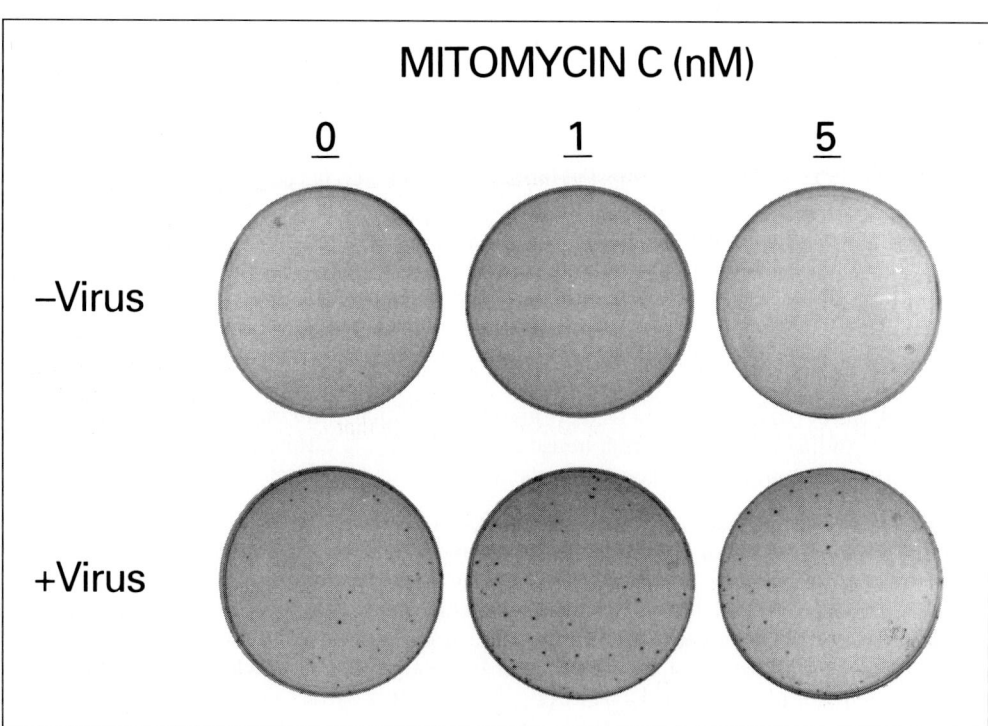

Figure 2

Selective pressure of FACC gene correction. Our studies with gene transfer into non-myeloablated mice suggest that transduction of genes without selective pressure is inefficient. This has also generally been the experience of gene marking studies in humans [8]. Despite the inefficiency of retroviral vectors in targeting human pluripotent stem cells, we would expect that even low-level FACC transduction of FA(C) progenitors might lead to amplification of gene-corrected stem cells through expression of the normal FACC gene. Gene transduction of FA(C) hematopoietic progenitor cells using a viral vector containing the FACC cDNA significantly improved colony formation in methylcellulose culture in the absence as well as the presence of low dose MMC. Increased colony growth may reflect the genetic rescue of progenitor cells following transduction with a copy of the normal FACC gene. This self-selecting growth advantage is apparently conferred by FACC.

Biological role of FACC

The precise biochemical function of the FACC polypeptide is currently unknown. The susceptibility of FA cells to DNA cross-linking agents such as MMC strongly suggests that the FA phenotype involves defective recognition or repair of DNA [2]. However, direct evidence of a defect in cross-link repair has been difficult to establish. Localization of the FACC polypeptide to primarily the cytoplasm has suggested that mechanisms other than direct repair of DNA may be operative. In addition, the cellular pathophysiology of FA suggests other disturbances, such as sensitivity to oxygen and oxygen metabolites [2]. We have recently reported findings from our gene transfer studies which shed light on the biological role of FACC.

Cell kinetics of gene-corrected FA(C) cells. The effect of caffeine, a compound known to inhibit postreplication repair, has been instructive in defining the FA defect. Caffeine potentiates the lethal effects of a variety of DNA damaging agents such as irradiation. Caffeine has also been shown to affect the duration of G2 phase and DNA repair. FA lymphocyte cultures exhibit marked prolongation of G2 phase after irradiation or treatment with MMC. The addition of caffeine during the last 7 hours of culture shortened the duration of G2 phase in both nonirradiated and irradiated FA cells. Chromosome damage was dramatically increased, consistent with loss of the G2 checkpoint and entry of unrepaired DNA into mitosis. We have demonstrated that transfer of the normal FACC cDNA to FA(C) lymphoblasts also shortens the G2 phase prolongation induced by MMC treatment [2, 6]. However, in contrast to the effect of caffeine, the FACC cDNA normalized induced chromosomal aberrations [5, 6]. We believe these experiments demonstrate that FACC can decrease the amount of DNA damage accumulating prior to G2, consequently shortening the duration of G2 phase since fewer unrepaired DNA lesions accumulate *(Figure 3)* [2]. These data constitute evidence that FACC is at least indirectly involved in the repair of DNA.

Transformation susceptibility of FA(C) fibroblasts. FA patients are known to be highly susceptible to cancers, both hematologic and solid organ [1, 2]. *In vitro*, FA primary fibroblasts are 3 to 50 times more sensitive than are normal fibroblasts to transformation in culture by the SV40 virus. We recently confirmed this marked susceptibility to transformation by a FA(C) primary fibroblast cell line, GM449 (again with the IVS+4A→T FACC mutation). We then analyzed what effect FACC gene transduction had on the transformation pattern of GM449. GM449 cells transduced with a copy of the normal FACC cDNA by a FACC-AAV vector were at least tenfold less prone to form transformed foci. This data suggests that the FACC gene may have a tumor suppressor function.

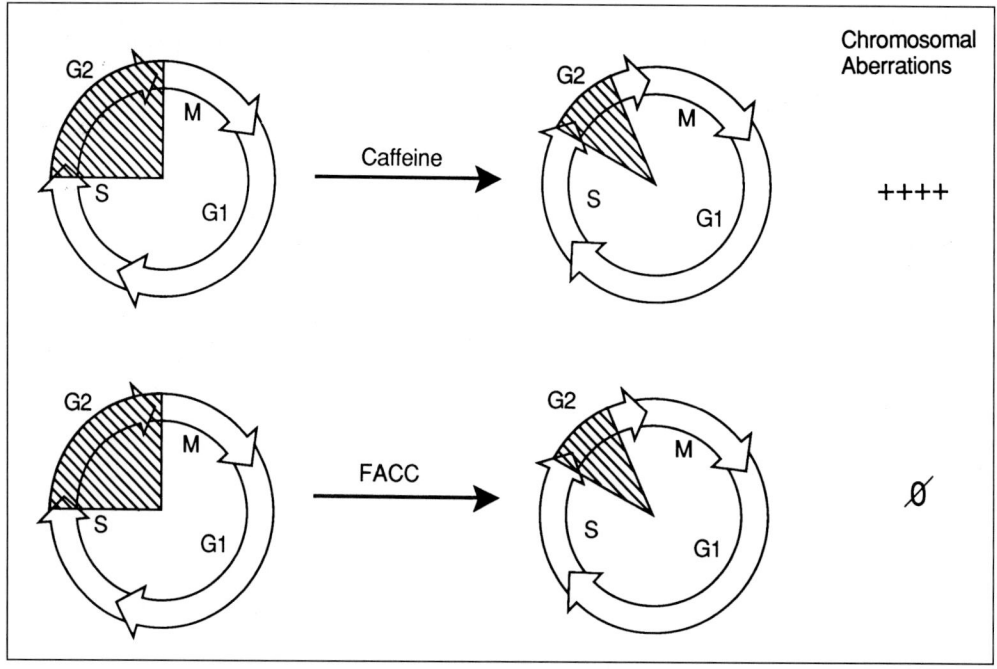

Figure 3

Biochemical purification of FACC polypeptide. The FACC polypeptide is 558 amino acids long with a predicted molecular mass of approximately 63 kD. In an effort to understand the function of FACC, we have overexpressed the polypeptide using both a baculovirus and a yeast expression system. We intend to purify the polypeptide and analyze its function in DNA repair.

Gene therapy for FA and vector targets

Based upon our preclinical data as well as safety studies in mice, we have proposed a protocol for gene therapy of FA. This protocol was recently approved by the Recombinant DNA Advisory Committee and is under review by the U. S. Food and Drug Administration.

Genetic correction of hematopoietic progenitor cells from patients bearing FACC mutant genes may soon become feasible for the treatment of the hematologic manifestations of this disorder. Gene replacement therapy consists of the insertion of a normal functioning gene into an appropriate target cell to correct for the defective gene [8]. Viral vectors are the primary vehicles for gene transfer due to their inherent efficiency in entering cells and transmitting foreign genetic material. Only recombinant retroviruses and adeno-associated virus (AAV) vectors have been demonstrated to stably transduce hematopoietic progenitor cells. These vectors are both capable of genomic integration into the host cell chromosomal DNA, an important feature if the intended outcome is the permanent restoration of hematopoietic lineages. Hematopoiesis in FA patients is defective, presumably due to a failure in maturation and differentiation of the hematopoietic progenitor pool secondary to DNA damage and cell growth disturbances. Transduction of FA progenitor and stem cells might lead to a sustained production of genetically corrected hematopoietic cells of all lineages. However, transduction of stem cells has been difficult due to the need for purification and enrichment of a small number of stem cells as well as cell cycling requirements for retroviral transduction. For FA, gene transduction of hematopoietic cells may circumvent some of these difficulties because of a self-selecting advantage for growth and expansion of gene-corrected hematopoietic cells within the hypoplastic FA bone marrow microenvironment.

AAV vectors may prove to be useful alternatives to standard retroviral vectors [8, 9]. Wild-type AAV, a defective parvovirus [9], has several attractive features including lack of pathogenicity in humans and site-specific integration into a locus on chromosome 19q. These characteristics may be favorable because tumorigenesis via insertional mutagenesis is a well-described phenomenon with wild-type retroviruses, and the potential for replication-competent retrovirus to cause disease has been established in a nonhuman primate model. In addition, AAV may transduce non-dividing cells such as hematopoietic stem cells. For these reasons, we have concurrently used recombinant AAV vectors for transfer of the FACC gene and phenotypic correction of lymphoid and hematopoietic progenitor cells from FA(C) patients.

Umbilical cord blood is enriched for hematopoietic stem and progenitor cells, and placental/umbilical cord blood from HLA-matched siblings was first used for hematopoietic reconstitution of several children with FA [10]. $CD34^+$ and purified $CD34^+$ $CD38^-$ hematopoietic cells from cord blood may be efficiently transduced by our vectors [11]. We anticipate that cord blood gene therapy may overcome some of the potential problems intrinsic to FA, such as a limited stem cell pool.

SCID/hu mouse model for AAV gene transfer. We have further defined the engraftment potential of human umbilical cord blood progenitor cells through the use of severe combined immunodeficient (SCID) mice [12]. The CB17 scid/scid mouse has been shown to support xenografts from human umbilical cord blood cells without the need for hematopoietic growth factor support. We tested the ability of our FACC-AAV vector to transduce human hematopoietic cells in this *in vivo* model. Cord blood progenitor cells enriched for the CD34 antigen were incubated with isopycnic gradient-purified FACC-AAV. Following transduction, 4×10^5 cells were injected into each sublethally-irradiated SCID mouse. Control animals received mock-infected progenitor cells or virus alone. At 11 weeks post-transplantation, mice were sacrificed and analyzed for engraftment by in situ hybridization for human-specific Alu genomic sequences: approximately 5% of the bone marrow cells were determined to be of human origin. PCR analysis of genomic DNA isolated from organs using Neo^R-specific primers revealed viral marking in three of four AAV-infected animals, whereas tissues from the control animals lacked a detectable Neo^R signal. These data suggest that the AAV vectors can transduce human hematopoietic progenitor cells maintained *in vivo* in SCID-hu mice. This is the first demonstration of AAV-mediated gene transfer to human fetal hematopoietic progenitors in a long-term animal model.

Conclusions

We have sought to develop molecular strategies for the treatment of genetic bone marrow failure disorders such as FA. Our gene transfer studies have led to insights regarding the function of the FA gene FACC, including a possible role in tumor suppression.

References

1. Young NS, Alter BP. *Aplastic Anemia, Acquired and Inherited.* Philadelphia: Saunders, 1993.
2. Liu JM, Buchwald M, Walsh CE, Young NS. Fanconi anemia and novel strategies for therapy. *Blood* 1994; 84:3995-4007.
3. Strathdee CA, Duncan AMV, Buchwald M. Evidence for at least four Fanconi anaemia genes including FACC on chromosome 9. *Nature Genet* 1992; 1:196-198.
4. Strathdee CA, Gavish H, Shannon WR, Buchwald M. Cloning of cDNAs for Fanconi's anaemia by functional complementation. *Nature* 1992; 356:763-767.
5. Walsh CE, Grompe M, Vanin E, Buchwald M, Young NS, Nienhuis AW, Liu JM. A functionally active retrovirus vector for gene therapy in Fanconi anemia group C. *Blood* 1994; 84:453-459.
6. Walsh CE, Nienhuis AW, Samulski RJ, Brown MG, Miller JL, Young NS, Liu JM. Phenotypic correction of Fanconi anemia in human hematopoietic cells with a recombinant adeno-associated virus vector. *J Clin Invest* 1994; 94:1440-1448.
7. Liu JM, Kim S, Walsh CE. Retroviral-mediated transduction of the Fanconi anemia C complementing (FACC) gene in two murine transplantation models, submitted 1995.
8. Liu JM, Walsh CE, Nienhuis AW. Gene therapy for hematologic disorders. In: Hoffman R, Benz EJ, Shattil SJ, Furie B, Cohen HJ, Silberstein LE, eds. *Hematology: basic principles and practice.* New York: Churchill Livingstone, 1995:427-435.
9. Walsh CE, Liu JM, Xiao X, Young NS, Nienhuis AW, Samulski RJ. Regulated, high level expression of a human gamma globin gene introduced into erythroid cells by a adeno-associated virus vector. *Proc Natl Acad Sci USA* 1992; 89: 7257-7261.
10. Gluckman E, Broxmeyer HE, Auerbach AD, Friedman HS, Douglas GW, Devergie A, Esperou H, Thierry D, Socié G, Lehn P, Cooper S, English D, Kurtzberg J, Bard J, Boyse EA. Hematopoietic reconstitution in a patient with Fanconi's anemia by means of umbilical-cord blood from an HLA-identical sibling. *N Engl J Med* 1989; 321:1174-1178.
11. Walsh CE, Mann MM, Emmons RVB, Wang S, Liu JM. Transduction of CD34-enriched human peripheral and umbilical cord blood progenitors using a retroviral vector with the Fanconi anemia group C gene, submitted 1994.
12. Walsh CE, Liu JM, Wang S, Xiao X, Hashmi NI, Zwerdling T, Agarwal R. *In vivo* gene transfer with a novel adeno-associated virus vector to human hematopoietic cells engrafted in SCID-hu mice. *Blood* 1994; 84(suppl):256a.

Résumé

La maladie de Fanconi est une maladie génétique caractérisée par une insuffisance médullaire, des anomalies physiques et une augmentation du risque de cancer. Marquée par une hétérogénéité génotypique et phénotypique, la maladie de Fanconi présente 4 groupes de complémentation distincts: A, B, C, D. Le gène défectif responsable du groupe C *(FA-C)* a été identifié par clonage complémentaire du cDNA. La caractéristique des cellules de FA est leur extrême sensibilité aux agents pontants comme la mitomycine C entraînant une incapacité de tolérer des lésions du DNA. Nous avons utilisé deux méthodes pour étudier la fonction moléculaire du polypeptide *FA-C*. Tout d'abord, nous avons hyper-exprimé *FA-C* dans des souris transgéniques et dans des cellules d'insectes infectées par le baculovirus. Puis, nous avons utilisé des vecteurs viraux recombinants pour transduire des copies normales de FAC cDNA dans des lignées cellulaires porteuses de la mutation FAC. Une correction phénotypique a été observée après transduction démontrée par la résistance à la mort cellulaire et la diminution des aberrations chromosomiques induites par la MMC.

Nous avons observé également que *FA-C* diminue les lésions du DNA avant la phase G2 du cycle cellulaire. Ensuite, nous avons démontré que les cellules souches hématopoïétiques enrichies en CD34 isolées des malades FA ont la même sensibilité à la MMC que les cellules en lignées. La transduction du gène *FA-C* avec un vecteur rétroviral contenant le cDNA de *FA-C* dans les cellules souches hématopoïétiques a significativement augmenté la formation de colonies dans des essais clonogéniques en présence ou en absence de MMC. Cette amélioration pourrait démontrer une correction du défaut du gène après transduction avec le gène *FA-C* normal. Les deux types de vecteurs utilisés sont le rétrovirus de Moloney et l'adeno associé virus (AAV). Nous avons démontré que le vecteur AAV transportant le cDNA de *FA-C* peut marquer les cellules souches hématopoïétiques de sang de cordon humaines transplantées chez la souris SCID/hu. De plus, nous avons démontré le transfert rétroviral du cDNA *FA-C* humain normal dans les cellules souches murines capables de repeupler à long terme. Devant ces résultats, nous proposons des essais cliniques de thérapie génique pour les patients atteints de la mutation de *FA-C*. Les cellules transduites par FAC devraient avoir un avantage de croissance sélectif par rapport aux cellules déficientes.

Author index
Index des auteurs

Almeida-Porada G., 89
Alter B.P., 241
Anasetti C., 307
Anderson S., 191
Auerbach A.D., 257
Auerbach R., 33

Bacigalupo A., 203, 331, 335
Barone L., 17
Baumelou E., 291
Bensussan A., 149
Berthier R., 27
Bonnet D., 97
Boumsell L., 149
Brand R., 331
Braun S., 109
Brown K.E., 191
Brownlie A., 17
Broxmeyer H.E., 109, 115
Brubakk A.M., 163
Buchwald M., 249
Bui T.H., 163

Camitta B., 325
Carosella E., 143, 149
Castro-Malaspina H., 325
Chan F.Y., 17
Chaouat G., 71
Charbord P., 37
Charron D., 123
Chen M., 249
Choqueux-Séébold C., 123
Cooper S., 109
Coulombel L., 37, 43, 103
Cumano A., 5, 81
Cumming R., 249

Daly B., 13
Deeg H.J., 209, 307, 325
Dejana E., 27
Dick J.E., 97
Dieterlen-Lièvre F., 5, 37, 81
Detrich III H.W., 17
Di Santo J.P., 63

Dommergues M., 43
Doney K., 307
Downie T., 331
Dragowska W., 49
Dzierzak E., 13

Eaves C.J., 49, 55
Eik-Nes S., 163
Ek S., 163
El Marsafy S., 149
Etienne-Julan M., 109

Figari O., 203
Filippi M.D., 23
Flake A.W., 89
Frickhofen N., 335

Garban F., 123
Garcia-Porrero J., 5
Gaspar M.L., 5
Ge Y., 115
Giambona A., 163
Gillett N., 13
Gluckman E., 149, 183, 319
Godin I., 5, 81
Grassia L., 203
Gratwohl A., 223, 345
Green S.W., 191
Guiguet M., 291

Helgason C.D., 55
Horowitz M.M., 313
Hows J., 331
Hoy C.A., 209
Humeau L., 37
Humphries R.K., 49, 55
Huss R., 209
Huyhn A., 43

Issaragrisil S., 281
Izac B., 43, 103

Jakil C., 163
Joenje H., 265

Katz A., 4, 103
Kieran M., 17
Kirszenbaum M., 143
Kiserud T., 163
Kjaeldgaard A., 163
Klein J.P., 313
Krasnoshtein F., 249
Krieger M.S., 223

Lansdorp P.M., 49, 55
Lapidot T., 97
Laquerbe A., 271
Larochelle A., 97
Le Bouteiller P., 131
Lemieux M.E., 55
Le Pesteur F., 23
Lercari G., 203
Li Z.H., 115
Lightfoot J., 249
Little M.T.E., 49
Liu J.M., 361
Lu L., 109, 115
Lu L.S., 33
Luton D., 37
Lyman S.D., 109

Maciejewski J.P., 191
Maggio A., 163
Mansur I.G., 149
Manz C.Y., 223
Marcos M., 5
Markling L., 163
Marmont A.M., 203
Martin-Sisteron H., 27
Mary J.Y., 291
Mayani H., 49
McClennan H., 17
Medvinsky A., 13
Miles C., 13
Miller C.L., 55
Mitjavila M.T., 23
Mooney N., 123
Moustacchi E., 271
Müller A., 13

Nimer S.D., 353
Nissen C., 223
Nistico A., 191
Nugent M., 313

Olerup O., 163
Orlandi F., 163

Paige C.J., 81
Papadopoulo D., 271
Parker L., 249
Pardanaud L., 5
Passweg J.R., 313
Paw B., 17
Péault B., 37
Pflumio F., 103
Piaggio G., 203
Podesta M., 203
Porada C., 89
Prandini M.H., 27
Pratt S., 17

Raffo M.R., 203
Raghavachar A., 233
Ramsay N.K.C., 325
Ransom D., 17
Rebel V.T., 49, 55

Ringdén O., 163
Rodriguez A.M., 131
Roucard C., 123
Ruthven J., 89

Sainteny F., 23
Sanchez M.F., 13
Sato T., 19
Savoia A., 249
Schiabon V., 149
Schklovskaya E., 223
Schrezenmeier H., 233, 335
Schweitzer A., 27
Serelli C., 191
Sinclair A., 13
Sobocinski K.A., 313
Socié G., 217
Sogno G., 203
Speck B., 223
Srivastava A., 109
Storb R., 307
Svahn B.M., 163

Tavian M., 37
Tedone E., 203
Thomas T.E., 49
Thompson M., 17

Tichelli A., 223
Touraine J.L., 169
Truman J.P., 123

Uzan G., 27

Vainchenker W., 23, 43, 103
Valbonesi M., 203
Van Lint M.T., 203
Verlander P.C., 257
Vittet D., 27
Vormoor J., 97

Wagner J.E., 177
Wang J., 97
Wang S.J., 33
Westgren M., 163
Wodnar-Filipowicz A., 223
Wong S., 191

Young N.S., 191

Zanjani E.D., 89
Ziegler S., 17
Zon L.I., 17

Colloques **INSERM**
ISSN 0768-3154

Other *Colloques* published as co-editions by John Libbey Eurotext and INSERM

133 Cardiovascular and Respiratory Physiology in the
Fetus and Neonate. *Physiologie Cardiovasculaire et Respiratoire du Fœtus et du Nouveau-né.*
Scientific Committee : P. Karlberg,
A. Minkowski, W. Oh and L. Stern;
Managing Editor : M. Monset-Couchard.
ISBN : John Libbey Eurotext 0 86196 086 6
 INSERM 2 85598 282 0

134 Porphyrins and Porphyrias. *Porphyrines et Porphyries.*
Edited by Y. Nordmann.
ISBN : John Libbey Eurotext 0 86196 087 4
 INSERM 2 85598 281 2

137 Neo-Adjuvant Chemotherapy. *Chimiothérapie Néo-Adjuvante.*
Edited by C. Jacquillat, M. Weil and D. Khayat.
ISBN : John Libbey Eurotext 0 86196 077 7
 INSERM 2 85598 283 7

139 Hormones and Cell Regulation (10th European Symposium). *Hormones et Régulation Cellulaire (10ᵉ Symposium Européen).*
Edited by J. Nunez, J.E. Dumont and R.J.B. King.
ISBN : John Libbey Eurotext 0 86196 084 X
 INSERM 2 85598 284 7

147 Modern Trends in Aging Research. *Nouvelles Perspectives de la Recherche sur le Vieillissement.*
Edited by Y. Courtois, B. Faucheux, B. Forette,
D.L. Knook and J.A. Tréton.
ISBN : John Libbey Eurotext 0 86196 103 X
 INSERM 2 85598 309 6

149 Binding Proteins of Steroid Hormones. *Protéines de liaison des Hormones Stéroïdes.*
Edited by M.G. Forest and M. Pugeat.
ISBN : John Libbey Eurotext 0 86196 125 0
 INSERM 2 85598 310 X

151 Control and Management of Parturition. *La Maîtrise de la Parturition.*
Edited by C. Sureau, P. Blot, D. Cabrol, F. Cavaillé and G. Germain.
ISBN : John Libbey Eurotext 0 86196 096 3
 INSERM 2 85598 311 8

Colloques **INSERM**
ISSN 0768-3154

153 Hormones and Cell Regulation (11th European Symposium). *Hormones et Régulation Cellulaire (11ᵉ Symposium Européen).*
Edited by J. Nunez and J.E. Dumont.
ISBN : John Libbey Eurotext 0 86196 104 8
INSERM 2 85598 324 X

158 Biochemistry and Physiopathology of Platelet Membrane. *Biochimie et Physiopathologie de la Membrane Plaquettaire.*
Edited by G. Marguerie and R.F.A. Zwaal.
ISBN : John Libbey Eurotext 0 86196 114 5
INSERM 2 85598 345 2

162 The Inhibitors of Hematopoiesis. *Les Inhibiteurs de l'Hématopoïèse.*
Edited by A. Najman, M. Guignon, N.C. Gorin and J.Y. Mary.
ISBN : John Libbey Eurotext 0 86196 125 0
INSERM 2 85598 340 1

164 Liver Cells and Drugs. *Cellules Hépatiques et Médicaments.*
Edited by A. Guillouzo.
ISBN : John Libbey Eurotext 0 86196 128 5
INSERM 2 85598 341 X

165 Hormones and Cell Regulation (12th European Symposium). *Hormones et Régulation Cellulaire (12ᵉ Symposium Européen).*
Edited by J. Nunez, J.E. Dumont and E. Carafoli.
ISBN : John Libbey Eurotext 0 86196 133 1
INSERM 2 85598 347 9

167 Sleep Disorders and Respiration. *Les Evénements Respiratoires du Sommeil.*
Edited by P. Lévi-Valensi and D. Duron.
ISBN : John Libbey Eurotext 0 86196 127 7
INSERM 2 85598 344 4

169 Neo-Adjuvant Chemotherapy. *Chimiothérapie Néo-Adjuvante.*
Edited by C. Jacquillat, M. Weil, D. Khayat.
ISBN : John Libbey Eurotext 0 86196 150 1
INSERM 2 85598 349 5

171 Structure and Functions of the Cytoskeleton. *La Structure et les Fonctions du Cytosquelette.*
Edited by B.A.F. Rousset.
ISBN : John Libbey Eurotext 0 86196 149 8
INSERM 2 85598 351 7

Colloques INSERM
ISSN 0768-3154

172 The Langerhans Cell. *La Cellule de Langerhans.*
Edited by J. Thivolet, D. Schmitt.
ISBN : John Libbey Eurotext 0 86196 181 1
INSERM 2 85598 352 5

173 Cellular and Molecular Aspects of Glucuronidation. *Aspects Cellulaires et Moléculaires de la Glucuronoconjugaison.*
Edited by G. Siest, J. Magdalou, B. Burchell
ISBN : John Libbey Eurotext 0 86196 182 X
INSERM 2 85598 353 3

174 Second Forum on Peptides. *Deuxième Forum Peptides.*
Edited by A. Aubry, M. Marraud, B. Vitoux
ISBN : John Libbey Eurotext 0 86196 151 X
INSERM 2 85598 354 1

176 Hormones and Cell Regulation (13th European Symposium). *Hormones et Régulation Cellulaire (13ᵉ Symposium Européen).*
Edited by J. Nunez, J.E. Dumont, R. Denton
ISBN : John Libbey Eurotext 0 86196 183 8
INSERM 2 85598 356 8

179 Lymphokine Receptors Interactions. *Interactions Lymphokines-récepteurs.*
Edited by D. Fradelizi, J. Bertoglio
ISBN : John Libbey Eurotext 0 86196 148 X
INSERM 2 85598 359 2

191 Anticancer Drugs (1st International Interface of Clinical and Laboratory responses to anticancer drugs). *Médicaments anticancéreux (1ʳᵉ Confrontation internationale des réponses cliniques et expérimentales aux médicaments anticancéreux).*
Edited by H. Tapiero, J. Robert, T.J. Lampidis
ISBN : John Libbey Eurotext 0 86196 223 0
INSERM 2 85598 393 2

193 Living in the Cold (2nd International Symposium). *La Vie au Froid (2ᵉ Symposium International).*
Edited by A. Malan, B. Canguilhem
ISBN : John Libbey Eurotext 0 86196 234 9
INSERM 2 85598 395 9

Colloques INSERM
ISSN 0768-3154

194 Progress in Hepatitis B Immunization. *La Vaccination contre l'épatite B.*
Edited by P. Coursaget, M.J. Tong
ISBN : John Libbey Eurotext 0 86196 249 4
INSERM 2 85598 396 7

196 Treatment Strategy in Hodgkin's Disease. *Stratégie dans la maladie de Hodgkin.*
Edited by P. Sommers, M. Henry-Amar,
J.H. Meezwaldt, P. Carde
ISBN : John Libbey Eurotext 0 86196 226 5
INSERM 2 85598 398 3

198 Hormones and Cell Regulation (14th European Symposium). *Hormones et Régulation Cellulaire (14e Symposium Européen).*
Edited by J. Nunez, J.E. Dumont
ISBN : John Libbey Eurotext 0 86196 229 X
INSERM 2 85598 400 9

199 Placental Communications : Biochemical, Morphological and Cellular Aspects. *Communications placentaires : aspects biochimique, morphologique et cellulaire.*
Edited by L. Cedard, E. Alsat, J.C. Challier,
G. Chaouat, A. Malassiné
ISBN : John Libbey Eurotext 0 86196 227 3
INSERM 2 85598 401 7

204 Pharmacologie Clinique : Actualités et Perspectives. (6e Rencontres Nationales de Pharmacologie clinique).
Edited by J.P. Boissel, C. Caulin, M. Teule
ISBN : John Libbey Eurotext 0 86196 225 7
INSERM 2 85598 454 8

205 Recent Trends in Clinical Pharmacology (6th National Meeting of Clinical Pharmacology).
Edited by J.P. Boissel, C. Caulin, M. Teule
ISBN : John Libbey Eurotext 0 86196 256 7
INSERM 2 85598 455 6

206 Platelet Immunology : Fundamental and Clinical Aspects. *Immunologie plaquettaire : aspects fondamentaux et cliniques.*
Edited by C. Kaplan-Gouet, N. Schlegel,
Ch. Salmon, J. McGregor
ISBN : John Libbey Eurotext 0 86196 285 0
INSERM 2 85598 439 4

Colloques INSERM
ISSN 0768-3154

207 Thyroperoxidase and Thyroid Autoimmunity.
Thyroperoxydase et auto-immunité thyroïdienne.
Edited by P. Carayon, T. Ruf
ISBN : John Libbey Eurotext 0 86196 277 X
INSERM 2 85598 440 8

208 Vasopressin. *Vasopressine.*
Edited by S. Jard, R. Jamison
ISBN : John Libbey Eurotext 0 86196 288 5
INSERM 2 85598 441 6

210 Hormones and Cell Regulation (15th European Symposium). *Hormones et Régulation Cellulaire (15e Symposium Européen).*
Edited by J.E. Dumont, J. Nunez, R.J.B. King
ISBN : John Libbey Eurotext 0 86196 279 6
INSERM 2 85598 443 2

211 Medullary Thyroid Carcinoma. *Cancer Médullaire de la Thyroïde.*
Edited by C. Calmettes, J.M. Guliana
ISBN : John Libbey Eurotext 0 86196 287 7
INSERM 2 85598 440 0

212 Cellular and Molecular Biology of the Materno-Fetal Relationship. *Biologie cellulaire et moléculaire de la relation materno-fœtale.*
Edited by G. Chaouat, J. Mowbray
ISBN : John Libbey Eurotext 0 86196 909 1
INSERM 2 85598 445 9

215 Aldosterone. Fundamental Aspects. *Aspects fondamentaux.*
Edited by J.P. Bonvalet, N. Farman, M. Lombes, M.E. Rafestin-Oblin
ISBN : John Libbey Eurotext 0 86196 302 4
INSERM 2 85598 482 3

216 Cellular and Molecular Aspects of Cirrhosis. *Aspects cellulaires et moléculaires de la cirrhose.*
Edited by B. Clément, A. Guillouzo
ISBN : John Libbey Eurotext 0 86196 342 3
INSERM 2 85598 483 1

217 Sleep and Cardiorespiratory Control. *Sommeil et contrôle cardio-respiratoire.*
Edited by C. Gaultier, P. Escourrou, L. Curzi-Dascalora
ISBN : John Libbey Eurotext 0 86196 307 5
INSERM 2 85598 484 X

Colloques INSERM
ISSN 0768-3154

218 Genetic Hypertension. *Hypertension génétique.*
Edited by J. Sassard
ISBN : John Libbey Eurotext 0 86196 313 X
INSERM 2 85598 485 8

219 Human Gene Transfer. *Transfert de gènes chez l'homme.*
Edited by O. Cohen-Haguenauer, M. Boiron
ISBN : John Libbey Eurotext 0 86196 301 6
INSERM 2 85598 497 1

220 Medicine and Change: Historical and Sociological Studies of Medical Innovation. *L'innovation en médecine : études historiques et sociologiques.*
Edited by Ilana Löwy
ISBN : John Libbey Eurotext 2 7420 0010 0
INSERM 5 85598 508 0

221 Structures and Functions of Retinal Proteins. *Structures et fonctions des rétino-protéines.*
Edited by J.L. Rigaud
ISBN : John Libbey Eurotext 0 86196 355 5
INSERM 2 85598 509 9

222 Cellular and Molecular Biology of the Adrenal Cortex. *Biologie cellulaire et moléculaire du cortex surrénal.*
Edited by J.M. Saez, A.C. Brownie, A. Capponi, E.M. Chambaz, F. Mantero
ISBN : John Libbey Eurotext 0 86196 362 8
INSERM 2 85598 510 2

223 Mechanisms and Control of Emesis. *Mécanismes et contrôle du vomissement.*
Edited by A.L. Bianchi, L. Grélot, A.D. Miller, G.L. King
ISBN : John Libbey Eurotext 0 86196 363 6
INSERM 2 85598 511 0

224 High Pressure and Biotechnology. *Haute pression et biotechnologie.*
Edited by C. Balny, R. Hayashi, K. Heremans, P. Masson
ISBN : John Libbey Eurotext 0 86196 363 6
INSERM 2 85598 512 9

Colloques INSERM
ISSN 0768-3154

228 Non-Visual Human-Computer Interactions. *Communication non visuelle homme-ordinateur.*
Edited by D. Burger, J.C. Sperandio
ISBN : John Libbey Eurotext 2 7420 0014 3
   INSERM 2 85598 540 4

229 The negative regulation of hematopoiesis, from fundamental aspects to clinical applications. *Régulation négative de l'hématopoïèse, des aspects fondamentaux à l'application clinique.*
Edited by Y. Beuzard
ISBN : John Libbey Eurotext 2 7420 0015 1
   INSERM 2 85598 541 2

230 From Research in Oncology to Therapeutic Innovations. *De la recherche oncologique à l'innovation thérapeutique.*
Edited by P. Tambourin, M. Boiron
ISBN : John Libbey Eurotext 2 7420 0016 X
   INSERM 2 85598 542 0

231 Human Ochratoxicosis and its pathologies. *Ochratoxicose humaine et ses pathologies.*
Edited by E.E. Creppy, M. Castegnaro, G. Dirheimer
ISBN : John Libbey Eurotext 2 7420 0017 8
   INSERM 2 85598 543 9

232 Anxiety : Neurobiology, Clinic and Therapeutic Perspectives. *Anxiété : Neurobiologie, Clinique et Perspectives Thérapeutiques.*
Edited by M. Hamon, H. Ollat, M.-H. Thiébot
ISBN : John Libbey Eurotext 2 7420 0018 6
   INSERM 2 85598 544 7

234 Sickle cell disease and thalassaemias: new trends in therapy. *Dépranocytose et thalassémies : nouvelles tendances thérapeutiques.*
Edited by Y. Beuzard, B. Lubin, J. Rosa
ISBN : John Libbey Eurotext 2 7420 0063 1
   INSERM 2 85598 578 1

236 Human sperm acrosome reaction.
Réaction acrosomique du spermatozoïde humain.
Edited by P. Fénichel, J. Parinaud
ISBN : John Libbey Eurotext 2 7420 0094 1
   INSERM 2 85598 627 3

LOUIS-JEAN
avenue d'Embrun, 05003 GAP cedex
Tél. : 92.53.17.00
Dépôt légal : 704 — Septembre 1995
Imprimé en France